Health Systems and the Challenge of Communicable Diseases

Experiences from Europe and Latin America

Edited by

Richard Coker, Rifat Atun & Martin McKee

Open University Press

Open University Press
McGraw-Hill Education
McGraw-Hill House
Shoppenhangers Road
Maidenhead
Berkshire
England
SL6 2QL
email: enquiries@openup.co.uk
world wide web: www.openup.co.uk
and Two Penn Plaza, New York, NY 10121–2289, USA

First published 2008

A catalogue record of this book is available from the British Library

ISBN-13 978 0 335 23366 3 (pb)   978 0 335 23365 6 (hb)
ISBN-10 0 335 23366 X (pb)   0 335 23365 1 (hb)

Library of Congress Cataloging-in-Publication Data
CIP data applied for

Typeset by RefineCatch Limited, Bungay, Suffolk
Printed in the UK by Bell and Bain Ltd., Glasgow

The *McGraw·Hill* Companies

European Observatory on Health Systems and Policies Series

The European Observatory on Health Systems and Policies is a unique project that builds on the commitment of all its partners to improving health care systems:

- World Health Organization Regional Office for Europe
- Government of Belgium
- Government of Finland
- Government of Greece
- Government of Norway
- Government of Slovenia
- Government of Spain
- Government of Sweden
- Veneto Region
- European Investment Bank
- Open Society Institute
- World Bank
- London School of Economics and Political Science
- London School of Hygiene and Tropical Medicine

The series

The volumes in this series focus on key issues for health policy-making in Europe. Each study explores the conceptual background, outcomes and lessons learned about the development of more equitable, more efficient and more effective health systems in Europe. With this focus, the series seeks to contribute to the evolution of a more evidence-based approach to policy formulation in the health sector.

These studies will be important to all those involved in formulating or evaluating national health care policies and, in particular, will be of use to health policy-makers and advisers, who are under increasing pressure to rationalize the structure and funding of their health system. Academics and students in the field of health policy will also find this series valuable in seeking to understand better the complex choices that confront the health systems of Europe.

The Observatory supports and promotes evidence-based health policy-making through comprehensive and rigorous analysis of the dynamics of health care systems in Europe.

Series Editors

Josep Figueras is Head of the Secretariat and Research Director of the European Observatory on Health Systems and Policies, and Head of the European Centre for Health Policy, World Health Organization Regional Office for Europe.

Martin McKee is Research Director of the European Observatory on Health Systems and Policies and Professor of European Public Health at the London School of Hygiene and Tropical Medicine as well as a co-director of the School's European Centre on Health of Societies in Transition.

Elias Mossialos is Research Director of the European Observatory on Health Systems and Policies, and Brian Abel-Smith Reader in Health Policy, Department of Social Policy, London School of Economics and Political Science and co-director of LSE Health and Social Care.

Richard B. Saltman is Research Director of the European Observatory on Health Systems and Policies, and Professor of Health Policy and Management at the Rollins School of Public Health, Emory University in Atlanta, Georgia.

European Observatory on Health Systems and Policies Series
Series Editors: Josep Figueras, Martin McKee, Elias Mossialos and Richard B. Saltman

Published titles

Primary care in the driver's seat
Richard B. Saltman, Ana Rico and Wienke Boerma (eds)

Human resources for health in Europe
Carl-Ardy Dubois, Martin McKee and Ellen Nolte (eds)

Health policy and European Union enlargement
Martin McKee, Laura MacLehose and Ellen Nolte (eds)

Regulating entrepreneurial behaviour in European health care systems
Richard B. Saltman, Reinhard Busse and Elias Mossialos (eds)

Social health insurance systems in western Europe
Richard B. Saltman, Reinhard Busse and Josep Figueras (eds)

Health care in Central Asia
Martin McKee, Judith Healy and Jane Falkingham (eds)

Hospitals in a changing Europe
Martin McKee and Judith Healy (eds)

Funding health care: options for Europe
Elias Mossialos, Anna Dixon, Josep Figueras and Joe Kutzin (eds)

Regulating Pharmaceuticals in Europe: striving for efficiency, equity and quality
Elias Mossialos, Monique Mrazek and Tom Walley (eds)

Purchasing to improve health systems performance
Joseph Figueras, Ray Robinson and Elke Jakubowski (eds)

Decentralization in Health Care
Richard B. Saltman, Vaida Bankauskaite and Karsten Vrangbæk (eds)

Contents

List of tables

List of figures

List of boxes

List of abbreviations

AIS	*Acoes Integradas de Saúde* (Integrated Health System)
ARV	antiretroviral
BBP	basic benefits package
CDC	Center for Disease Control (United States)
CRS	Congenital Rubella Syndrome
CSG	Clinical Statistical Group
DALY	disability-adjusted life year
DFID	Department for International Development (United Kingdom)
DOT	directly-observed treatment
DOTS	Directly-Observed Treatment, Short-course
DRG	diagnosis-related group
EC	European Commission
ECDC	European Centre for Disease Prevention and Control
EEA	European Economic Area
EEC	European Economic Community
EFTA	European Free Trade Association
Enter-NET	International Surveillance Network for the Enteric Infections Salmonella and verocytotoxin-producing Escherichia coli (VTEC)
EPI	Expanded Program on Immunization (Pan American Health Organization)
EPIET	European Programme for Intervention Epidemiology Training
EU	European Union
EuroHIV	European Centre for the Epidemiological Monitoring of AIDS
EuroTB	European Centre for the Epidemiological Monitoring of

	Tuberculosis
EWGLI	European Working Group for Legionella Infections
EWRS	Early Warning and Response System
FFS	fee-for-service
GDP	gross domestic product
GFATM	Global Fund to Fight AIDS, Tuberculosis and Malaria
GMP	good manufacturing practice
GNP	gross national product
GOARN	Global Outbreak Alert and Response Network
GPHIN	Global Public Health Intelligence Network
HAART	highly active anti-retroviral therapy
HDI	Human Development Index
HIV/AIDS	human immunodeficiency virus/acquired immunodeficiency syndrome
HLWG	High-Level Working Group
HPA	Health Protection Agency (United Kingdom)
ICRC	International Committee of the Red Cross
MDG(s)	Millennium Development Goal(s)
MDR-TB	multidrug-resistant tuberculosis
MRSA	methicillin-resistant *Staphylococcus aureus*
MSF	*Médecins Sans Frontières* ("Doctors without borders")
MSM	men having sex with men
NAFTA	North American Free Trade Agreement
NATO	North Atlantic Treaty Organization
NIHD	National Institute of Health Department
NTP	National Tuberculosis Programme
OBF	"Officially Brucellosis Free"
OECD	Organisation for Economic Co-operation and Development
PAF	Performance Assessment Framework (World Health Organization)
PAHO	Pan American Health Organization
PHRI	Public Health Research Institute
PLWHA	people living with HIV/AIDS
PLWHIV	people living with HIV
PNDST/AIDS	*Programa Nacional de Doencas Sexualmente Transmissíveis*/AIDS National Program on Sexually Transmitted Infections/AIDS
PPP	purchasing power parity
SARS	severe acute respiratory syndrome
SGH	State Guarantees for Health
STI	sexually transmitted infection
SUDS	*Sistema Unificado e Descentralizado de Saúde* (Unified Decentralized Health System (Brazil))
SUS	*Sestima Único de Saúde* (Unified Health System (Brazil))
SYSRA	Systemic Rapid Assessment (toolkit)
TB	tuberculosis
TBE	tick-borne encephalitis
UNAIDS	Joint United Nations Programme on HIV/AIDS
UNGASS	United Nations General Assembly Special Session on AIDS

UNICEF	United Nations Children's Fund
USSR	Union of Soviet Socialist Republics
WHA	World Health Assembly
WHO	World Health Organization
WTO	World Trade Organization
XDR-TB	extremely drug-resistant tuberculosis

List of contributors

Olusoji Adeyi is the Coordinator of Public Health Programs in the Human Development Network of the World Bank.

Andrew J. Amato-Gauci is the deputy head of the Surveillance Unit of the European Centre for Disease Prevention and Control (ECDC).

Andrea Ammon is Head of the Surveillance Unit of the European Centre for Disease Prevention and Control (ECDC).

Rifat Atun is Professor of International Health Management and Director of the Centre for Health Management at Tanaka Business School, Imperial College London.

Enis Baris is a Senior Public Health Specialist in the Middle East and North Africa Region (MNSHD) at the World Bank, Washington, D.C.

Richard Coker is Reader in Public Health in the Department of Public Health and Policy, London School of Hygiene and Tropical Medicine.

Oscar Echeverri worked for 16 years at the World Bank as Senior Public Health Specialist, Unit Chief of the Population Health and Nutrition Unit at the Technical Department for Latin America, and then as Portfolio Manager for the South East Asia region of the Bank.

Jane Falkingham is Professor of Demography and International Social Policy at the University of Southampton.

Eduardo J. Gómez is a PhD Candidate in the Department of Political Science at

Brown University and a Visiting Scientist and Instructor in the Politics and Governance Group of the Harvard School of Public Health.

Ipek Gurol-Urganci is a Research Associate at the Centre for Health Management, Tanaka Business School, Imperial College London.

Wieslaw Jakubowiak, is a Coordinator for the WHO TB Control Programme in the Russian Federation Office of the Special Representative of the WHO Director-General in Russia.

Shazia Karmali is working on Population and Public Health Project Management for the Provincial Health Services Authority of British Columbia, Canada.

Joseph Kutzin is Regional Advisor, Health Systems Financing, for WHO/Europe. He is also Head of the Organization's Barcelona Office and Visiting Fellow, Imperial College Centre for Health Management.

Jeffrey Lazarus works at the STI/HIV/AIDS programme at WHO/Europe and is on the faculty of Copenhagen University, Denmark.

Kelley Lee is Reader in Global Health and Co-Director of the Centre on Global Change and Health at the London School of Hygiene & Tropical Medicine.

Patricio V. Marquez is a Lead Health Specialist in the Europe and Central Asia Region (ECA) of the World Bank.

Martin McKee is Professor of European Public Health at the London School of Hygiene & Tropical Medicine, and Research Director, European Observatory on Health Systems and Policies.

Anthony McMichael is a medical graduate and epidemiologist, currently based at the National Centre for Epidemiology and Population Health, Australian National University, Canberra.

Nata Menabde is Deputy Regional Director of the WHO Regional Office for Europe.

Ana Mensua is a pharmacist specializing in primary care and community pharmacy, with a Masters in Public Health from the London School of Hygiene & Tropical Medicine.

Andrei Mosneaga is a team Leader, on the Regional Tuberculosis Control Programme in the South Caucasus, GOPA Worldwide Consultants/EPOS Health Consultants.

Claudio Politti is a health systems policy analyst at the WHO Regional Office for Europe.

Ralf Reintjes is Professor for Epidemiology and Public Health Surveillance in the Department of Public Health, Life Sciences Faculty at Hamburg University of Applied Sciences.

Nina Schwalbe is Director of Policy at the TB Alliance in New York.

Until his retirement *John Wyn Owen CB* held the post of Secretary of the Nuffield Trust, London from 1st March 1997 to June 2005 having previously been

Director-General of NSW Health and Chairman of the Australian Health Ministers Advisory Council and, until 1994, Director of NHS Wales.

Elena Yurasova is Medical Officer for TB control with WHO, working in the Russian Federation.

Richard Zaleskis, is the Regional Adviser on Tuberculosis Control at the WHO Regional Office for Europe in Copenhagen, Denmark.

Foreword

Any politician or health official who thinks infectious diseases are not a problem for their country would benefit greatly from reading this book.

While the experiences described mainly come from countries in transition, the lessons it contains are just as relevant to the world's richer countries. Put briefly, these are that: 1) microbes excel in their ability to adapt to changing circumstances, and will exploit these to create outbreaks of "new" diseases. 2) where disease control and research efforts are scaled back or axed, "old" infectious diseases rapidly re-emerge;

The countries of the former Soviet Union provide the most dramatic example of what happens when public health systems start to break down: infectious diseases that had been near elimination can rapidly reappear. The epidemic of diphtheria in these countries in the 1990s is a "text book example" of this. The emergency of a significant HIV epidemic in the former Soviet Union over the past decade, and the alarming rise of tuberculosis and multi drug resistant tuberculosis (MDR-TB) there also illustrate this point. All these epidemics (including diphtheria) had other drivers as well, such as socio-economic upheaval, population movements and changing patterns of human behaviour. But it is clear that weaknesses in disease prevention and control systems played a significant role.

Looking to the other side of the world, the authors of this book find similar lessons in Latin America. Efforts to eradicate the *Aedes aegypti* mosquito dwindled in Latin America in the 1970s and early 1980s. By the late 1990s the mosquito was back in large numbers across the region along with outbreaks of dengue fever, a disease that had been nearly eradicated in the Americas.

Of course, public health systems in Latin America did not experience the same dramatic weakening as those in the former Soviet Union. Indeed, in the past two decades they have had some successes: for example, eradicating polio and measles in the Americas and curtailing the re-emergence of cholera. But even with strong public health systems in place, countries face major challenges from infectious disease. As several contributors to this book remark, the evolutionary struggle between microbes and humans is a never ending one requiring constant vigilance and innovation on the part of the human race. Rapid urbanisation, persistent socio-economic inequalities, changes in the environment and the climate – all present opportunities to humankind's microscopic foes. This book is full of examples of how microbes have taken advantage of these opportunities.

Policy makers in middle income countries should take heed of these examples, and of the analysis of what needs to be done. However, there are also lessons to be learned by policy makers in richer countries. "Old" diseases can re-emerge in the rich countries just as easily as in countries in transition. Nor are they immune from the arrival of "new" diseases, as the outbreak of the tropical disease Chikungunya Fever in Italy last summer illustrates[1].

As the 21st century proceeds, and the world becomes ever more interconnected, the mutual interest of all countries – rich, poor or middle income – in fighting infectious diseases has never been more apparent.

Zsuzsana Jakab
Director, European Centre for Disease Prevention and
Control (ECDC)

---

[1] *Mission Report: Chikungunya in italy*, Ecdc and WHO, Stockholm, September 2007.

chapter one

Contemporary emerging and re-emerging communicable diseases: challenges to control

Richard Coker, Rifat Atun, Martin McKee

Introduction

This book is about countries undergoing rapid political, economic and social transition. It focuses on those situated in two regions where the scale of transition has been especially rapid, central and eastern Europe and Latin America. These are regions that, while far from one another in terms of distance, have much in common.

The effects of transition on these societies are apparent in many ways. People and goods are moving in ever greater numbers, and over ever greater distances. Social mores are changing, with implications for many aspects of how people live and behave. Health and social care systems, tasked with responding to these changing circumstances, are themselves undergoing rapid change. As a consequence, there are simultaneous changes impacting on people, health systems and the broader context within which the people and health systems are situated. These changes are not occurring in isolation but interacting with each other to create a highly dynamic and complex ecosystem, whose behaviour is difficult to predict.

The consequences of these changes are especially visible in relation to infectious diseases. Humans are engaged in a constant evolutionary struggle with microorganisms, with the latter poised to exploit changing circumstances. This can be seen in the increases in diseases such as HIV/AIDS, the emergence of new diseases such as severe acute respiratory syndrome (SARS), the re-emergence of ancient diseases such as tuberculosis (TB) and diphtheria, and, looking ahead, the threat of novel strains of infectious agents such as the H5N1 strain of influenza. All of these developments highlight the dynamic consequences of social, medical, cultural, institutional and political change to public health. It is no accident that the two regions that are the focus of this book have experienced especially rapid increases in diseases such as HIV (in eastern Europe), dengue fever (in Latin America) and multidrug-resistant tuberculosis (MDR-TB) in both.

A renewed recognition of the threat posed by infectious diseases has compelled political leaders to raise the need for effective responses to a higher position on the agenda. Yet, while once much could be achieved with what might now be considered relatively simple measures, the complexity of the environments in which people now live has made the design and implementation of effective responses much more difficult. Health systems in particular have become much more complex, yet this complexity has not always been accompanied by an improved understanding of how they interact with communicable diseases, whether by offering opportunities for control or, in the case of nosocomial infection, facilitating spread. The need for such an understanding is now pressing.

International initiatives, such as the declaration of TB as a global emergency, the subsequent advocacy of Directly Observed Treatment, Short-course (DOTS), the advance of the 3 by 5 initiative to provide Highly Active Anti-Retroviral Therapy (HAART) to 3 million HIV-positive people by 2005, and subsequent international efforts in further expanding access to HAART, have demonstrated the potential to galvanize broad support. Yet, for their potential health benefits to be achieved in full and beyond externally supported, often donor-driven, initiatives, health care systems must support them in ways that are effective, efficient and equitable. Furthermore, if such programmes are to offer durable benefits, vertical, disease-specific programmes need to be embedded more firmly in broader domestic health and social care systems.

We now examine briefly key changes affecting microbes, the host, health systems and the broader context within which these systems are situated, as well as discussing the challenges these changes bring.

Humans and microbes: a never-ending struggle

As the preceding paragraphs remind us, early in the 21st century infectious diseases continue to pose a profound global public health challenge. They have afflicted mankind ever since the emergence of *Homo sapiens* and, despite advances in science and the social environment in much of the world, continue to do so.

The earliest humans, originating in the tropical climate of Africa, would have been affected by the same parasites as the other primates among whom they lived, and from whom they descended. As these early hunters migrated into more temperate zones, the infectious agents to which they were exposed changed. As hunting gave way to agriculture, populations grew and stabilized. The development of agriculture and the domestication of animals led to a closer proximity between animals and humans, creating the opportunity for many zoonotic infections to spread to humans (Diamond 1997). Increases in population size and density provided the ideal conditions for person-to-person spread of infectious agents.

As civilizations developed further, trade routes became established, conflicts developed between neighbouring communities, and the movements of people and goods carried new pathogens to susceptible populations (McNeal 1976). Epidemics of infectious diseases such as plague, smallpox, and typhus devastated communities, shattered armies, and generated widespread terror. In some cases, epidemics changed the course of history (Box 1.1 and Box 1.2). Social and political responses, with varying degrees of success, were conceived and implemented. These responses often focused on individuals or groups of individuals perceived as the originators of disease. History is replete with examples of people being subjected to severe measures to protect the wider population. The conflation of minority populations, disease, and irrational fear has been a common feature of responses to infectious diseases for many centuries (Kraut 1994; McNeal 1976; Risse 1988; Watts 1997).

Humanity's proximity and changing relation to animals means that it has continued to be exposed to novel pathogens, experience novel diseases, and in a shrinking world as Gro Harlem Brundtland noted whilst Director General of WHO, experiences the consequences of a ". . . microbial [that] sea washes all of humankind. There are no health sanctuaries. Diseases cannot be kept out of even the richest of countries by rearguard defensive action" (Brundtland 2000).

Box 1.1   The plague of Athens

The Athenian city state was devastated by an epidemic that struck in 430 BC, the second year of the Peloponnesian war. The city's population had been swollen greatly by the movement of people from the countryside seeking protection from the Spartans behind its walls. The crowded conditions created the ideal circumstances for spread of disease and up to a third of the population died. The Greek writer Thucydides has described in detail how the disease affected society. Faced with a high probability of death from an invisible agent, the normally law-abiding Athenian citizens rejected authority. They spent money indiscriminately, as they saw little chance of living to enjoy any savings. Women cast aside the constraints on their roles and behaviour that characterized traditional Athenian society. The death of the Athenian leader Pericles, a victim of the plague, ushered in a series of weak and often incompetent leaders. It took at least 15 years for Athens to recover anything like its earlier status, by which time the balance of power in the region had changed, paving the way for the emergence of major powers of the Macedonians, including Alexander the Great, and in due course the Romans. In this way, a relatively confined outbreak of disease changed the course of history. Identification of the agent responsible for the plague of Athens remains contentious, although there is some evidence to suggest that it was typhus.

Box 1.2 The Black Death, the reformation, and the division of Europe

In 1347, Caffa, a Genovese trading outpost in the Crimea, was besieged by the Mongols, whose armies were afflicted by a plague. In October of that year, a Genovese fleet fleeing from the siege reached Sicily. All of its crew were either dead or unwell. During 1348 the disease spread rapidly throughout much of western Europe, following trade routes such as the River Rhone. Within a few years between one third and one half of the population of western Europe was dead and a quarter of all villages were abandoned. The scale of the tragedy led people to question their religious beliefs. The church was unable to offer an explanation for what was happening and the priests, who ministered to the dying, were dying in disproportionate numbers. Those who followed them into religious orders often lacked the vocation of their predecessors, creating widespread popular cynicism about the church and its status, circumstances that provided a basis for the reformation.

The depopulation that resulted from the Black Death had profound consequences for social structure. The much reduced peasantry was in a far stronger position compared to the ruling class. A series of peasants' revolts contributed to the end of serfdom across much of western Europe. In contrast, in eastern Europe, which because of its low population density was much less affected by the Black Death, serfdom continued until it was finally abolished in Russia in 1861 by Tsar Alexander II. It has been suggested that the difference in status of agricultural workers contributed to some degree to the economic differences in Europe that remain to this day.

During the late 19th century, through the work of Robert Koch and Louis Pasteur, amongst others, the isolation and identification of aetiological agents became possible, thus furthering scientific understanding of the causes of infectious diseases. An understanding of the "germ theory", first plausibly articulated in the 1870s, began to develop. This made it possible for the epidemiology of infectious diseases to be described, measures to support control to be introduced, and the impact of these measures determined. By the 1920s, the hygiene movement had emerged as a powerful force in the West. New public health infrastructures were established in many cities, exemplified by the large sanatoria built for the isolation of tens of thousands of people with TB. The incidence of diseases such as diphtheria and typhoid fever fell dramatically, and cholera epidemics – once a fearful scourge – became rare.

By the 1940s the advent of effective antimicrobial agents, along with the establishment of the principles and practice of immunization, hailed a new era. Famously, in 1948, George Marshall, then United States Secretary of State, captured this spirit of optimism when he proclaimed that the conquest of all infectious diseases was imminent. This confidence persisted for several decades, at least in the West. It later became clear that this sentiment was both misconceived and simplistic, as it was realized that relationships between man, the microbial world, and his environment are complex and ever changing.

Over recent decades the nature of public health has changed. The 1970s and 1980s were decades of considerable economic and political instability. Public health, it could be argued, focused on technological interventions but disregarded in large part the broader contextual social environment of emerging public health challenges. This neglect, it has been suggested, led to the failure of many control campaigns for major diseases. A simplistic view by health service planners and health reformers of the context within which they worked led them to believe that the task ahead required little more than the introduction of a new technology (such as vaccination). Yet this somewhat narrow thinking was occurring at the same time as, although quite separately from, an increasing recognition of the complex relations between disease, social environment, and public health systems. The concept of social medicine (that is, public health that acknowledges and responds to the social dimension of health) gained traction. This is not to say that there had not been advocates of this notion before. Public health professionals had been persuaded of the importance of the "social" dimension to "health" since the 19th century, and many of the reforms during that century implicitly acknowledged this. Indeed, in the mid-1880s Virchow had eloquently argued that medicine was a social science, and that politics was medicine on a large scale (Taylor and Rieger 1985).

Perhaps the apotheosis of this new way of thinking was the adoption by the World Health Assembly (WHA), in 1977 of the resolution on "Health for All by the Year 2000". The resolution envisaged that, by the year 2000, people should be using new ways to prevent and control diseases and to alleviate unavoidable illness and disability. The "new ways" would include a more equitable and efficient distribution of health resources, equitable provision of essential health care for all, and a greater recognition of the widening and now unacceptable gap between the "haves" and the "have nots". The Alma-Ata Declaration the following year advocated a primary health care approach that incorporated the principles of equity, community involvement, appropriate technology, and the necessity of a multisectoral approach. Alma-Ata was seen by many policy-makers as an opportunity to restructure their health systems (WHO 1978).

A second notable public health initiative emerged during the 1970s and 1980s to inform contemporary thinking on public health and communicable diseases. The global expanded programme of immunization, initiated by the World Health Organization (WHO) and the United Nations Children's Fund (UNICEF), was launched in 1974. At this time fewer than 5% of children under the age of five years in developing countries were being immunized against major childhood diseases. Following the successful smallpox eradication campaign, the expanded programme of immunization achieved remarkable results, and by 1990, 80% of all children in the world were protected against six major vaccine-preventable diseases before they were two years old.

These successes have not, however, been replicated in global responses to all communicable diseases. Successful control demands that the complex relationship between host, pathogen and environment is understood; that the determinants of disease are modified and alleviated; and that responses are appropriately and sustainably embedded in health and social care systems. The examples of TB, HIV/AIDS, and the scourge of drug-resistant microbes illustrate par excellence the complexity of the environment and profound nature of the challenges we face, as do other emergent diseases discussed below.

The changing face of infectious diseases

Infectious diseases are today a major cause of ill health and death. In 2002 they caused 14.9 million deaths, accounting for 26% of total global mortality and also accounted for almost 30% of the total disability-adjusted life years (DALYs) lost worldwide (Table 1.1 and Table 1.2).

Mortality from infectious diseases is highest in Africa, with both the highest number of deaths in absolute terms and the highest mortality rate for infectious and parasitic diseases (837 deaths per 100 000 population). The proportion of all deaths due to infectious diseases is also highest in Africa, where more than 60% of all deaths are due to infectious or parasitic diseases (compared with only 5% in Europe). Yet within Europe, marked differences exist. Death rates from infectious diseases in the former Soviet Union are approximately five times higher than in western Europe. A pattern similar to that for mortality is seen with the burden of disease attributable to infectious diseases. Over 187 million DALYs are lost yearly in Africa due to infectious or parasitic diseases. This compares with only 5.7 million in Europe. Yet again, the number of DALYs lost in the former Soviet Union due to infectious diseases is approximately five times that estimated for western Europe. This gradient in mortality and morbidity is replicated when one looks at Latin and North America, with high number of DALYs lost in the former due to infectious diseases (Monaghan 2002).

The global face of infectious diseases is changing in terms of magnitude, geographic scope, and the inability of science to provide all the answers, but also for other reasons. There are "new" diseases, most notably HIV/AIDS, SARS and variant Creutzfeldt-Jakob Disease (vCJD) (and its associated form bovine spongiform encephalopathy (BSE)), resulting from apparently new pathogens (Table 1.3), while "ancient" diseases such as TB and diphtheria are re-emerging as serious threats to public health. Novel agents are being implicated in the causation of a number of clinical syndromes, for example, parvovirus, human T-cell lymphotropic viruses I and II (retroviruses), human papilloma virus and a number of human herpes viruses. With advances in scientific investigation, causative agents are also being better defined – examples include Legionella pneumophila in Legionnaires' disease, *Borellia burgderfori* in Lyme disease, and Helicobacter pylori in stomach and duodenal ulcers, all age-old diseases where the causative organisms have only been defined in recent years (Table 1.4).

Weak health systems are contributing to the emergence of disease. Drug-resistant organisms, unresponsive to antimicrobial agents, have become a major global public health challenge in recent decades. Strains of resistant *Mycobacterium tuberculosis* have been reported from all countries in the world, with some now resistant to all first-line and many second-line drugs. Outbreaks of resistant *Staphylococcus aureus*, including methicillin-resistant *Staphylococcus aureus* (MRSA), threaten health care provision in many developed countries, with potentially huge economic costs. The emergence of HIV strains resistant to

Table 1.1 Deaths by cause in WHO Regions, 2002 estimates

	Total	% of total	Africa	The Americas	South-east Asia	Europe	Eastern Mediterranean	Western Pacific
Population (000)	6 224 985 (000)	100*	672 238 (000)	852 551 (000)	1 590 832 (000)	877 886 (000)	502 824 (000)	1 717 536 (000)
Total number of deaths	57 029	100*	10 664	5 962	14 657	9 564	4 152	11 940
Infectious and parasitic diseases	10 904	19.1	5 625	397	2 922	195	953	804
Respiratory infections	3 963	6.9	1 118	226	1 474	288	354	498
Maternal and perinatal conditions	2 972	5.2	785	191	1 184	68	370	370
Nutritional deficiencies	485	0.9	143	61	189	12	53	27
Neoplasms	7 270	12.7	419	1 145	1 178	1 871	296	2 347
Diabetes mellitus, nutritional/endocrine disorders	1 354	2.4	116	303	306	290	118	219
Neuropsychiatric disorders	1 112	1.9	90	240	267	256	89	167
Cardiovascular diseases	16 733	29.3	1 036	1 928	3 911	4 927	1 079	3 825
Respiratory diseases	3 702	6.5	257	398	874	404	155	1 609
Digestive diseases	1 968	3.5	157	284	502	389	152	480
Other noncommunicable diseases	1 521	2.7	187	237	389	188	175	342
Injuries	5 168	9.1	741	540	1 467	792	392	1 229

Source: (Adapted from) WHO 2004.

Note: *Percentages may not equal exactly 100% as a result of rounding.

Table 1.2 Burden of disease in disability-adjusted life years by cause in WHO Regions, 2002 estimates[1]

	Total	% of total	Africa	The Americas	South-east Asia	Europe	Eastern Mediterranean	Western Pacific
Population (000)	6 224 985 (000)		672 238 (000)	852 551 (000)	1 590 832 (000)	877 886 (000)	502 824 (000)	1 717 536 (000)
Total number of DALYs	1 490 125 643	100	361 376 478	145 586 527	426 572 902	150 321 605	139 079 337	264 879 260
Infectious and parasitic diseases	350 332 571	23.5	187 448 845	11 890 388	88 952 900	5 665 026	32 410 088	23 671 157
Respiratory infections	94 603 349	6.3	35 595 347	3 315 928	33 026 019	3 115 191	10 818 791	8 653 688
Maternal and perinatal conditions	130 966 679	8.8	33 104 006	9 319 806	50 542 629	3 554 015	16 654 594	17 602 104
Nutritional deficiencies	34 416 632	2.3	9 573 867	2 124 420	12 127 757	1 703 909	4 490 404	4 360 317
Neoplasms	77 293 663	5.2	4 914 205	11 405 860	14 070 924	17 445 197	4 183 809	25 151 663
Diabetes mellitus & nutritional/ endocrine disorders	24 155 400	1.6	2 404 904	5 753 643	5 893 601	3 169 056	2 095 680	4 751 614
Neuropsychiatric disorders	193 278 495	13.0	17 897 036	35 787 391	48 313 777	29 348 996	15 019 744	46 533 897
Cardiovascular diseases	148 190 083	9.9	10 910 418	15 173 288	42 987 030	34 417 792	12 059 668	32 413 230
Respiratory diseases	55 153 199	3.7	5 482 583	7 968 078	15 630 419	6 735 413	3 719 707	15 535 384
Digestive diseases	46 475 768	3.1	5 103 566	5 543 889	14 205 642	7 396 276	4 031 778	10 111 155
Other noncommunicable diseases	153 268 686	10.4	18 138 712	17 440 027	45 275 063	16 825 972	16 113 431	39 121 304
Injuries	181 991 119	12.2	308 02 990	19 863 809	55 547 140	20 944 762	17 481 643	36 973 747

Source: (Adapted from) WHO 2004.

Notes: DALY(s): disability-adjusted life year(s).
[1] Figures computed by WHO to assure comparability, they are not necessarily the official statistics of WHO Member States, which may use alternative rigorous methods.

Table 1.3 Examples of newly recognized pathogenic microbes and the diseases they cause, 1973–2003

Year	Microbe	Type	Disease
1973	Rotavirus	Virus	Infantile diarrhea
1977	Ebola virus	Virus	Acute hemorrhagic fever
1977	Legionella pneumophila	Bacterium	Legionnaires' disease
1980	HTLV1	Virus	T-cell lymphoma/leukaemia
1981	Toxin-producing Staphylococcus aureus	Bacterium	Toxic shock syndrome
1982	Escherichia coli O157:H7	Bacterium	Hemorrhagic colitis; hemolytic uremic syndrome
1982	Borrelia burgdorferi	Bacterium	Lyme disease
1983	HIV	Virus	AIDS
1983	Helicobacter pylori	Bacterium	Peptic ulcer disease
1989	Hepatitis C	Virus	Parentally transmitted non-A, non-B liver infection
1992	Vibrio cholerae O139	Bacterium	New strain associated with epidemic cholera
1993	Hantavirus	Virus	Adult respiratory distress syndrome
1994	Cryptosporidium	Protozoa	Enteric disease
1995	Ehrlichiosis	Bacterium	Severe arthritis?
1996	nvCJD	Prion	New variant (v)CJD
1997	H5N1	Virus	Influenza
1999	Nipah	Virus	Severe encephalitis
2003	Coronavirus	Virus	SARS

Notes: HTLV1: Human T-lymphotrophic virus; HIV: human immonodeficiency virus; AIDS: acquired immunodeficiency syndrome; CJD: Creutzfeldt-Jakob Disease: severe acute respiratory syndrome.

anti-retroviral (ARV) agents threatens, some believe, the sustainability of global efforts to control the disease (Brenner and Turner 2002; Doualla-Bell and Turner 2004).

The economic costs of communicable disease outbreaks are increasingly becoming a global concern (Table 1.5). The epidemic of BSE, which decimated the British beef industry, is estimated to have cost approximately €30 billion. Estimates of the cost of the SARS outbreak range from €8 billion to €24 billion, mostly due to behavioural changes from a perceived risk of SARS and loss of economic confidence in countries where SARS emerged; direct health care costs were marginal. This can be compared to the locally contained outbreak of plague in Surat, India, in 1994, estimated to have cost approximately €1.5 billion and the 1997 avian influenza outbreak in Hong Kong, estimated to have cost hundreds of millions of euros in lost poultry production, commerce and tourism. A study by the United States National Center for Infectious Diseases in 1999

Table 1.4 Diseases associated with infectious agents

Disease/syndrome/disorder	Agent
Chronic gastritis	H pylori
Peptic ulcer	H pylori
Guillain-Barre syndrome	Campylobacter jejuni
Bell's palsy	Borrelia burgdorferi, Herpes simplex virus
Tropical spastic paraparesis	HTLV-1
Haemolytic uraemic syndrome	E coli 0157
Throbotic thrombocytopenic purpura	E coli 0157
Polyarteritis nodosa	Hepatitis B virus
Insulin dependent diabetes	Enterovirus
Atherosclerosis	Chlamydia pneumoniae, CMV
Reactive arthritis	Salmonella spp., Yersinia spp., Chlamydia trachomatis
Human T-cell leukaemia	HTLV-1
Hairy cell leukaemia	HTLV-2
Hepatocellular cancer	Hepatitis B and C
Cervical cancer	HPV
Burkitt's lymphoma	EBV
AIDS-related CNS lymphoma	EBV
Kaposi's sarcoma	HHV8
AIDS-related body cavity lymphoma	HHV8
Castleman's disease	HHV8

Notes: HTLV1: Human T-lymphotrophic virus; CNS: central nervous system; CMV: Cytomegalovirus.

Table 1.5 Examples of economic impact of major infectious disease outbreaks

Year	Country	Disease	Cost (US$)
1979–1994	New York City	Tuberculosis	Over 1 billion
1990–1998	Malaysia	Nipah virus	540 million
1991	United Kingdom	BSE	38 billion
1994	India	Plague	2 billion
1997	Hong Kong	"Bird flu"	22 million
1998	Tanzania	Cholera	770 million
1999	New York	West Nile Fever	Almost 100 million
1999	Russian Federation	TB	Over 4 billion
2003	China, Hong Kong, Canada	SARS	15 billion

Source: (Adapted from) selected WHO reports.

Notes: BSE: Bovine Spongiform Encephalopathy; TB: tuberculosis; SARS: severe acute respiratory syndrome.

estimated that the economic impact of an influenza pandemic in the United States would range from US$ 71.3 billion to US$ 166.5 billion (Meltzer and Cox 1999). The economic toll of the epidemic of HIV is beyond comprehension.

Challenges to control

As noted above, factors beyond the immediate relationship between the pathogenic agent and the host influence communicable diseases and efforts to control them, in complex ways. Control is particularly challenging as the pathogens, the host, the context and the health systems (which interact with each other) are changing simultaneously.

The changing agent: microbial adaptation

Microorganisms are continually evolving. Resistant microbial agents and new strains of viral agents are emerging by mutation, often as a response to inappropriate use of antibiotics. In turn, immunological responses of hosts to these changes vary.

Briefly, in viral agents the change can take two forms. Antigenic drift is a gradual change in the genetic structure of a microorganism. This is what happens when successive strains of influenza appear, which can then spread to partially immune hosts. Antigenic shift, in contrast, occurs when two different strains of a microbe (typically influenza A, which infects humans and other animals) combine to create a new strain to which there is little immune protection, thus enabling the disease to spread very rapidly. This is what has happened with the H5N1 strain of influenza, explaining the potential for a global pandemic.

The changing host

Population growth

The world's population is growing at an average rate of approximately 1.5% per annum. Yet this growth is unequal, as some countries, such as the Russian Federation, are witnessing population shrinkage. Moreover, the age structure of populations is changing in dramatic ways. Some nations, such as many in the West, have ageing populations, while many in developing countries have relatively young populations. These demographic changes will have consequences, many unforeseen, for patterns of disease and corresponding control efforts. For example, while overcrowding is likely to promote the spread of infectious diseases, population shrinkages (especially when associated with an ageing population) may result in reduced economic growth or a shrinking tax base, increased pension obligations, higher demands on the health system and human resource constraints on provision of care, with serious implications for the sustainability of health systems.

Population movements

Globally some 150 million people live outside their country of birth – one out of every 40 people. Approximately 2 million people cross international borders every single day. People cross national borders for many reasons, including migration, seeking refuge and asylum, for trade, education and employment, and for tourism. The increased movement of people and the speed with which they can now traverse the globe mean that the potential for infectious microbes to be carried globally in a matter of days is very real. The SARS epidemic, affecting within days countries separated by thousands of miles graphically highlighted this potential.

Human behaviour

Changes in behaviour, including sexual behaviour and injecting drug use, are associated with changes in the incidence of several infectious diseases. However, other, less obvious behaviours also impact upon communicable diseases. For example, "non-compliance" by health care workers, patients, pharmaceutical producers, and health care systems has the potential to promote drug resistance in microorganisms. The collapse of health systems in the former Soviet Union and non-compliance with international norms of care for TB resulted in high rates of MDR-TB (Atun et al. 2005; Coker, Atun and McKee 2004).

Changing health systems and public health functions

In the 1980s it was hoped that the eradication of smallpox would presage the eradication of other communicable diseases, thus heralding the dawn of a new era of public health. The global smallpox campaign illustrated what could be achieved when a safe, effective, and affordable vaccine was allied to a comprehensive public health infrastructure that extended, even if only transiently, to the most remote corners of the world and was directed at a communicable disease with sufficiently favourable transmission dynamics. Importantly, eradication (zero cases and zero risk) demands the sustainability of a public health system only for the duration of the campaign. Elimination (zero cases but continuing risk), or sustained control, on the other hand, demand more, including the ongoing maintenance of capacity and performance, and long-term political and strategic focus and commitment. The experience of eradicating or eliminating many communicable diseases since the 1980s has been mixed. Leprosy elimination, for example, has been a relative success story. In 1991, the world community resolved to eliminate leprosy by the year 2000. From approximately 10 million cases globally in 1985, a decade later it was estimated that this had fallen to only one million cases. On the other hand, improving vaccine coverage for poliomyelitis has been patchy. The focus of an eradication campaign initiated in 1988, poliomyelitis vaccine coverage rates have improved markedly in many regions of the world but, to some extent reflecting the mistaken concerns of certain religious leaders, there are pockets where it has not been possible to achieve the high immunization rates needed.

Public health systems are susceptible to fashions, political vagaries, and economic cycles. The epidemic of TB that New York City responded to in the 1990s had its roots in the fiscal crisis of the 1970s and the withdrawal of funding by city, state and federal institutions (Coker 2000). Similarly, public health institutions in the former Soviet Union, rooted in Soviet traditions, are struggling to respond effectively to the challenges of resurgent infectious diseases such as TB, and newly emergent challenges such as HIV (Coker, Atun and McKee 2004). In the transition years, many post-Soviet countries with health systems rooted in the Semashko model prematurely embraced health insurance and privatization (in spite of evidence about the dangers of such changes) with the belief that this would solve all ills of the health system, only to realize that without structural changes to care delivery, improving quality and strengthening public health functions, little could be achieved. Many of these countries, which have had limited success in addressing public health challenges, have yet to undertake the structural reforms necessary for their health systems to improve system responsiveness and address effectively the burden of communicable disease.

The changing context: a new and uncertain world

Economic development, globalization, poverty and inequity

Since the mid-1970s there has been sustained global economic development. During this period, the world has become wealthier. However, this development has not benefited all equally. Inter- and intra-country differences in economic wealth have increased.

Approximately one quarter of the world's population still live in extreme poverty, surviving on less than US$ 1 per day, with most living in Asia and sub-Saharan Africa. However, there is also growing impoverishment in many transitional economies such as those of the former Soviet Union, where gross inequalities have emerged since the early 1980s. In the Russian Federation the mean income of those in the top 10% of the distribution of wealth was 13.8 times that in the bottom 10%, compared with an estimated 3.5 times during the Soviet period. Mortality from infectious and parasitic diseases nearly doubled in the first half of the 1990s and while it has largely stabilized now, it remains considerably higher than in western Europe.

Politics, warfare, terrorism and conflict

As global initiatives address age-old scourges, novel and re-emergent diseases continue to pose challenges. In a changing world where political imperatives shift, relations between nations and international agencies change, populations and goods cross borders in ever larger quantities and diverse ways, and unanticipated forces impel policies in new directions.

Wars and conflicts create environments that microorganisms exploit. The movements of large numbers of people, unhygienic living conditions, malnutrition, and the destruction of public infrastructures encourage diseases and their spread. Conflict also influences political focus and patterns of investment. With the "war on terror" the international community, and in particular the United States, has invested substantial political and financial capital in combating bio-terror, with important consequences for communicable disease control (Beaglehole 2003; Coker 2000; Levy and Sidel 2003). Thus, when faced with outbreaks of anthrax, perpetrated almost certainly by someone with access to American military facilities, a few days after Al Qaeda hijacked four airplanes on 11 September 2001, the United States mounted an unprecedented response, devoting vast resources to a perceived threat from chemical and biological weapons. In this way, the control of communicable disease moved from the public health to the national security agenda.

This discourse on health and security has been driven by a relatively small number of linked strategic concerns. The first is political recognition that in an era of increasing interconnections, diseases spread more readily from one region to another. The second is that disease may threaten economic interests. The third is that, through its undermining of the social, political and economic fabric and its disproportionate effects on governance and military institutions, disease may have destabilizing implications for state sovereignty and international security (Coker and Ingram 2006).

In these ways, infectious diseases are beginning to shape political discourse. This is seen in an alignment of the three traditional models of national interest: narrow self-interest; enlightened self-interest; and global engagement (Kassalow 2001). Yet this ideological alignment is not matched by adequate governance tools (a fact recognized by the adoption of the new International Health Regulations). As Brower and Chalk have noted, "Statecentric models of security are ineffective at coping with issues, such as the spread of diseases that originate within sovereign borders, but have effects that are felt regionally and globally. Human security reflects the new challenges facing society in the 21st century" (Brower and Chalk 2003).

New technologies

The development and application of new technologies may have both beneficial and deleterious consequences for communicable disease control. While technologies may enhance economies and support diagnostic and treatment capabilities, they may result in modifications to practices that have untoward effects. The epidemic of BSE, the almost certain cause of vCJD in humans, had by 2001 afflicted over 179 000 cows in Great Britain. It has been ascribed to technological changes in the animal and human food chain which dated from the 1980s.

A major challenge faced by the countries of eastern Europe and Latin America is access to medicines. Although investment in research and development is increasing globally, research outputs, in terms of new chemical entities approved, are declining. A very small amount of investment is directed to discovering or developing medicines for neglected conditions that predominantly affect the poorer countries. Recently, the WHA noted ". . . of 1400 new products developed between 1975 and 1999, only 13 were for tropical disease and just three for tuberculosis" (Kapp 2003). The WHA also recommended the establishment of an intergovernmental working group open to all interested countries to draw up a global strategy and plan of action in order to provide a medium-term strategy which aims, among other things, to secure "an enhanced and sustainable basis for needs-driven, essential health research and development relevant to diseases that disproportionately affect developing countries, proposing clear objectives and priorities for research and development, and estimating funding needs in this area."[1]

High prices deter access to innovative medicines. A lack of transparency in pricing of medicines and unexplained variation in prices internationally makes it difficult to ascertain whether value for money is achieved when procuring medicines. Currently, the new WHO recommended first-line regimen for HIV (TDF/3TC or FTC/EFV or NVP) is estimated to cost between US$ 321 and US$ 708 per month, which is simply unaffordable in most eastern European or Latin American countries.

In addition to high prices, access to pharmaceuticals is hampered by weak health systems and poor application of information technologies. In many cases, countries in the former Soviet Union lack the ability to effectively manage the supply logistics to distribute any medicines received.

Climate change

Global warming can be expected to result in massive changes that will affect communicable diseases. While low-lying areas will lose agricultural potential and fresh water reserves because of flooding and contamination of supplies, other areas may benefit from increased agricultural productivity. Large population movements are likely to ensue, as people seek economic security. Approximately 500 million people currently live at or near sea level. Changes in temperature and water distribution will result in different distributions of vectors.

Managing complexity: making connections

The examples of outbreaks of diphtheria and human cases of avian influenza in recent years illustrate some of the interconnected challenges to control and the complexities of causal relationships (Box 1.3 and Box 1.4).

Health systems and communicable disease control

The book is divided into 15 chapters. Following this introductory chapter, two chapters address the contextual environment of societies in transition. Chapter 2 describes the sociodemographic changes that have occurred in these transitional economies, and explores the public health consequences since the 1990s. Chapter 3 examines the purpose of government in the realm of public health and considers the functions entailed in controlling communicable diseases, paying particular attention to the challenges raised when capacity and political commitment are weak.

---

[1] WHA resolution 59/24. Public health, innovation, essential health research and intellectual property rights: towards a global strategy and plan of action (59th WHA).

Box 1.3 Diphtheria epidemics in the former Soviet Union: what were the causes?

Paul Farmer argues for a more profound understanding of causation when he asks: "Why, for example, were there 10 000 cases of diphtheria in Russia from 1990 to 1993? It is easy enough to argue that the excess cases were due to a failure to vaccinate. Yet only in linking this distal (and, in sum, technical) cause to the much more complex socioeconomic transformations altering the region's illness and death patterns will compelling explanations emerge. Standard epidemiology, narrowly focused on individual risk and short on critical theory, will not reveal these deep socioeconomic transformations, nor will it connect them to disease emergence" (Farmer 1999).

In reflecting upon the causes of the diphtheria epidemic witnessed in the former Soviet Union, Farmer raises a number of issues. Briefly, diphtheria had been well controlled in the Union of Soviet Socialist Republics (USSR) for more than two decades after universal childhood immunization was implemented from 1958. Until 1980, the immunization policy had been focused on children. However, in response to the emergence of some cases in adults, from the mid 1980s changes were made to the immunization schedule. Fewer doses of lower antigenic content were scheduled for children. In addition, an increasing number of contraindications to vaccination were identified by health professionals, resulting in a decline in coverage. Moreover, public confidence in the vaccination programmes had decreased both due to loss of trust in authority and the state functions and because the public experience of communicable disease epidemics was less immediate with the decline in incidence (Vitek and Wharton 1998).

One consequence of this decline in uptake and content was the development of a cohort of adults, born before 1958, who lacked immunity both because they had not been immunized, and were more likely to be exposed because herd immunity was also declining with the change in immunization policies and practices from the 1980s.

In 1990 epidemic diphtheria re-emerged in the Soviet Union with the highest incidence rates in adolescents and adults aged 40–49 years reaching a peak in 1994–1995.

The causes behind the diphtheria epidemics in the former Soviet Union can, thus, be viewed as a consequence of failing immunization policies. But, as Farmer notes, more distal and complex causes were likely also playing important roles. The social transformation is but one. Others probably include the urbanization of populations and overcrowding, increased mobility of populations following the collapse of the USSR (the epidemic spread rapidly across states and across the Russian Federation), and the fact that areas of conflict disrupted health systems and also impacted on population movements (Georgia, Armenia, Azerbaijan,

Tajikistan). The high militarization of populations is another cause proposed (recruits were not routinely vaccinated against diphtheria until 1990), as well as microbial adaptation.

In advancing this perspective, Farmer suggests that a greater understanding is needed in a number of areas, including the forces that determine and drive social inequalities, the impact of transnational forces on disease, and the "differentially weighted factors that promote or retard the emergence or re-emergence of infectious diseases" (Farmer 1999). Farmer also asks us to critically question what makes some epidemics visible whilst others remain invisible, whether motivations arise from narrow self-interest or because of an emerging sense of global solidarity. In doing so he raises questions of power and control.

Box 1.4 Endemic avian influenza in Asia: what are the causes?

Avian influenza is now endemic in many parts of East Asia. The possibility of bird-to-human transmission due to genetic changes to sustained human-to-human transmission is real. In December 2003, outbreaks of avian influenza (H5N1) in poultry populations occurred in seven countries (Cambodia, China, Indonesia, the Republic of Korea, Lao PDR, Thailand and Vietnam) in the East Asia and Pacific region. A new outbreak began in July 2005, with an outbreak in Malaysia. The outbreaks in Indonesia, Thailand, Vietnam and China expanded. Despite aggressive control measures involving the culling of more than 140 million birds since September 2005, outbreaks have continued in the region. The first cases of human infection of H5N1 were confirmed in Vietnam in late 2003. As of May 2006, WHO has confirmed a total of 207 cases of bird flu with 115 fatalities. Some 172 cases (and 99 deaths) occurred in East Asia.

The economic impact of avian influenza on economies in the region has been limited in the main to those who rely on agriculture and poultry, including, to a significant degree, the poor. The deaths of 140 million birds from culling and disease have resulted in losses for the poultry industry of over US\$ 10 billion, with some countries seeing a depletion of poultry stocks by 20%. As with SARS, there is also a risk that tourism will be affected by concerns about human infections.

Kennedy Shortridge has written that China is special as a potential source of pandemic influenza because the region has a permanent gene pool of avian influenza viruses year round. This is the result of domestication of the duck as a source of these viruses 4500 years ago in the southeastern region of the country and, during the Ching Dynasty, from 1644, the intensification and spread of duck production as an adjunct to rice farming. The high human population density in the countryside and preference of the population generally for its food to be as fresh as possible has provided ongoing possibilities for exposure of humans (and pigs) to avian influenza viruses. He asserts, therefore, that the influenza gene pool in southern China is already established and probably not dependent upon introductions from migratory birds. Southern China, unlike anywhere else in the world, therefore, has this substantial avian gene pool and poses an almost unique public health challenge in respect of zoonoses (Shortridge 1992; Shortridge 2003). From this perspective, the causes of the next pandemic of human influenza are multiple and include: the long-standing domestication of poultry and the nature of the existing gene pool; the high and growing density of humans associated with China's economic growth and urbanization; the increasing proximity of both poultry and humans (and pigs) and therefore the increased potential for exposure; and domestic and international economic forces related to demand for cheap food, driving the growth of the regional poultry industry.

Chapter 4 details the changing pattern of communicable diseases, from prehistory through to the present, while Chapters 5 and 6 describe in some detail the contemporary epidemiological situations in eastern Europe and Latin America.

Chapter 7 explores contemporary thinking about health systems as it relates to communicable disease. This is an issue that is intrinsically difficult because the determinants of "success" and the mechanisms by which these "successes" are achieved are multiple and varied. Programmes to tackle infectious disease sit within complex multidimensional settings. This complexity has, in the past, deterred systemic and multidimensional evaluations of communicable disease programmes so that current approaches to evaluation tend to be highly vertical, focusing principally on disease-specific elements of the programme and often disregarding the broader health system aspects (Atun et al. 2004). On the other hand, methods for assessing health systems often focus on a narrow aspect of the system, such as financing, and are too generic to offer useful insights to support specific disease challenges. This chapter provides a critique of the current approaches and suggests ways of moving beyond them.

Chapter 8 examines the international agencies and the tools at their disposal to support global and European control of communicable disease and documents the profound changes to structures that have occurred in recent years following SARS. The next five chapters which follow examine the challenges posed for transitional economy health care systems by HIV and TB, attempt to distil lessons from the mid-1990s onwards, and reflect on the role of external agencies and the political environment in which they act, in support of control efforts. The authors, writing from different perspectives, assert that if control efforts are to be assured, there is a need to address fundamental functions of the health system such as stewardship and governance, financing and resource allocation, organization and delivery, and strengthening surveillance, monitoring and evaluation, whilst implementing medical care based on a firm evidential foundation. Two countries in particular receive attention, the Russian

Federation and Brazil, as illustrative examples of the challenges currently being faced.

The penultimate chapter examines in detail the critically important issue of financing in support of communicable disease control and reflects on analyses conducted in a number of transitional economies in order to draw lessons in support of effective and sustainable reform.

In the final chapter Coker, Mensua, Atun and McKee address the conundrum laid out memorably by a United States politician when he recently said: "... there are known knowns; there are things we know we know. We also know there are known unknowns; that is to say we know there are some things we do not know. But there are also unknown unknowns – the ones we don't know we don't know" (Rumsfeld 2002). Here, the editors summarize what is known, posit what is unknown, and argue for what should be known.

References

Atun, R. A., Lennox-Chhugani, N., Drobniewski, F., Samyshkin, Y. and Coker, R. (2004). A framework and toolkit for capturing the communicable disease programmes within health systems: Tuberculosis control as an illustrative example, *European Journal of Public Health*, 14: 267–273.

Atun, R. A., Baeza, J., Drobniewski, F., Levicheva, V. and Coker, R. (2005). Implementing WHO DOTS strategy in the Russian Federation: stakeholder attitudes, *Health Policy*, 74 (2): 122–132.

Beaglehole, R. (2003). *Global public health: a new era*. Oxford: Oxford University Press.

Brenner, B. G. and Turner, D. (2002). HIV-1 drug resistance: can we overcome? *Expert Opinion on Biological Therapy*, 2(7): 751–761.

Brower, J. and Chalk, P. (2003). *The global threat of new and re-emerging infectious diseases: reconciling U.S. national security and public health policy*. Santa Monica, Calif.: Rand.

Brundtland, G. H. (2000). *ReithLecture. http://news/bbc.co.uk/hi/english/static/events/reith_2000/lecture4.stm*. London: British Broacasting Corporation.

Coker, R. (2000). *From chaos to coercion: detention and the control of tuberculosis*. New York: St. Martin's Press.

Coker, R. J., Atun, R. and McKee, M. (2004). Health care system frailties and public health control of communicable diseases on the European Union's new eastern border, *Lancet*, 363: 1389–1392.

Coker, R. J. and Ingram, A. (2006). Passports and pestilence: migration, security and border control, in A. Bashford (eds) *Medicine at the border: disease, globalization and security, 1850 to the present*. New York: Palgrave Macmillan.

Diamond, J. M. (1997). *Guns, germs and steel: the fates of human societies*. London: Jonathan Cape.

Doualla-Bell, F. and Turner, D. (2004). HIV drug resistance and optimization of anti-viral treatment in resource-poor countries, *Medical Science (Paris)*, 20(10): 882–886.

Farmer, P. (1999). *Infections and inequalities, the modern plagues*. Berkeley: University of California Press.

Kapp, C. (2003). WHA acts on health regulations and intellectual property. *The Lancet Infectious Diseases*, 3(7): 392.

Kassalow, J. S. (2001). *Why health is important to US foreign policy*. New York: Milbank Memorial Fund.

Kraut, A. M. (1994). *Silent travellers: germs, genes, and the "immigrant menace"*. Baltimore: Johns Hopkins University Press.

Levy, B. S. and Sidel, V. W. (2003). *Terrorism and public health: a balanced approach to strengthening systems and protecting people*. Oxford: Oxford University Press.

McNeal, W. H. (1976). *Plagues and peoples*. Middlesex: Penguin.

Meltzer, M. I. and Cox, N. J. (1999). The economic impact of pandemic influenza in the United States: priorities for intervention, *Emerging Infectious Diseases*, 5(5): 659–671.

Monaghan, S. (2002). *The state of communicable disease law*. London: The Nuffield Trust.

Risse, G. B. (1988). Epidemics and history: ecological perspectives and social responses, in E. Fee and D. M. Fox (eds). *AIDS: the burdens of history*. Berkeley: University of California.

Rumsfeld, D. (2002). *Department of Defence Press Briefing, 12 Feb*. Washington DC: Department of Defence.

Shortridge, K. F. (1992). Pandemic influenza: a zoonosis? *Seminars in Respiratory Infections*, 7: 11–25.

Shortridge, K. F. (2003). Severe acute respiratory syndrome and influenza: virus incursions from southern China, *American Journal of Respiratory and Critical Care Medicine*, 168: 1416–1420.

Taylor, R. and Rieger, A. (1985). Medicine as social science: Rudolf Virchow on the typhus epidemic in upper Silesia, *International Journal of Health Services*, 15: 547–559.

Vitek, C. R. and Wharton, M. (1998). Diphtheria in the former Soviet Union: re-emergence of a pandemic disease, *Emerging Infectious Diseases*, 4: 539–50.

Watts, S. J. (1997). *Epidemics and history: disease, power and imperialism*. New Haven: Yale University Press.

WHO (1978). Primary Health Care. Report of the International Conference on Primary Health Care, Alma-Ata, USSR, 6–12 September 1978. "Health for All" Series, No 1. Geneva: World Health Organization.

WHO (2004). *World Health Report 2004 – changing history*. Geneva: World Health Organization.

chapter two

The changing face of transitional societies

Martin McKee, Jane Falkingham

Introduction

In the continual evolutionary struggle between humans and microorganisms, microorganisms are constantly poised to take advantage of any change that will give them the slightest advantage (Diamond 1997). This book explores the two-way relationship between these two combatants, focusing on two regions of the world where the pace of social, political, and economic change has provided so many opportunities for microorganisms and where human ingenuity has, at best, been only just ahead of the game.

The first of these regions comprises the countries of central and eastern Europe and the former Soviet Union. These countries experienced a seismic transition in the years after 1989, as communist regimes fell like dominoes. The consequences varied. In many cases the authoritarian communist regimes gave way to democracy, culminating in the accession in 2004 of eight central and eastern European countries (including three former Soviet republics) into the European Union (EU), followed in 2007 by two more (McKee, MacLehose and Nolte 2004). In others, however, one authoritarian regime was simply replaced by another, with the labels changing but the political leaders and systems remaining relatively unscathed. In many cases, the transition was peaceful, exemplified by the term "Velvet Revolution" to describe Czechoslovakia's democratic transition. In others, as in the former Yugoslavia and the Caucasus, it was characterized by extreme violence, on a scale not seen in Europe since the Second World War (Rechel and McKee 2004).

The political changes led rapidly to economic and social changes. A severe economic depression affected many countries in the aftermath of transition, as the manufacturing sector was unable to compete in global markets and existing trading links were fractured (Rosefielde 2005). However, during the mid to late 1990s this gave way to high levels of economic growth, although especially in parts of the former Soviet Union this has been dominated by growth in income from extractive industries such as oil and gas, often yielding little benefit for ordinary citizens. As a consequence, in many parts of this region, income inequalities have risen considerably. Borders that were once closed have opened, making possible large-scale movement of both people and commodities, exemplified, on the one hand, by the growing numbers of eastern Europeans now working in countries such as the United Kingdom and Ireland and, on the other, by the vastly greater diversity of goods available in the shops of eastern Europe.

The other region is Latin America and the Caribbean. This is an enormously diverse region and there is no single event, such as the collapse of communism, characterizing its transition. Yet it too has been changing rapidly over the past few decades. Throughout the 20th century, many countries in Latin America were ruled by totalitarian regimes, frequently installed by the military (Williamson 1992), themselves supported by economically powerful countries to protect their geo-strategic and economic interests. Although it never exerted the same degree of control that the Union of Soviet Socialist Republics (USSR) did over its satellite states under the terms of the Brezhnev Doctrine, the United States set out, in the Monroe Doctrine, a clear statement that it had a special responsibility for the entire continent of the Americas (Smith 1994). Five years after the USSR invaded Czechoslovakia to extinguish the emerging Prague Spring, the United States intervened to overthrow the democratically elected Salvador Allende, president of Chile. Slowly, however, during the 1980s and 1990s, military regimes were replaced by elected civilian administrations. In the early 20th century, several countries, including Venezuela, Bolivia, Brazil and Chile, elected presidents with strong reforming agendas, pursuing policies that marked a dramatic change from the past (Gott 2005).

Economically, the continent has experienced mixed fortunes. Many countries are, like those of the former Soviet Union, highly dependent on income from extractive industries such as oil, iron ore or copper. The continent suffered greatly in the late 1970s, in the aftermath of the 1974 Middle East war and subsequent oil crisis. This led a number of countries to default on their debts (Kaufman 1988). The subsequent economic depression in the 1980s, when only Colombia and Chile recorded positive economic growth, has been characterized as the "lost decade". Subsequent recovery in some countries was halted during the 1990s by a series of economic crises, for example in Mexico in 1994 and Argentina in 1998.

The Caribbean nations, although geographically distinct from Latin America, have much in common with their neighbours and so are also considered in this book. They have also experienced rapid change in recent decades. Many gained independence from colonial powers in the 1970s (Hart 1998). Their economies have benefited from the growth of mass tourism but they have also suffered from the dependence of their agricultural sectors on a few crops, especially bananas, where they have found it difficult to compete with low-wage production on the Central American mainland (Godfrey 1998). Some have done relatively well overall but others, such as Haiti, have not.

In summary, therefore, these two regions, although geographically separate and superficially very different, have had many similar experiences, with periods of political instability and rapid economic change. Many countries are characterized by high levels of income inequality. Latin American countries have some of the highest levels of inequality recorded anywhere and these are particularly long standing, typically dating back to the colonial period. Central and eastern Europe and the former Soviet Union were, in contrast, rather more equal for much of the post-war period but in many countries inequalities are widening rapidly. Countries in both regions are suffering from environmental degradation, exemplified by the disappearances of the Aral Sea, in central Asia (Zavialov 2005), and large parts of the Amazon rain forest (Faminow 1998). Some are also exhibiting evidence of loss of the social capital that is increasingly understood as being important for health. This is exemplified by the fact that these regions include all 10 of the countries with the highest recorded homicide rates in the world (WHO 2002).

Of course, the world as a whole is changing, as technological developments, economic growth, the global exchange of information, and easier international travel, among many other factors, change the way that people lead their lives. These two regions are not immune to these changes; it is just that the specific political and economic transitions that they have experienced have been superimposed on these more general trends.

It would be surprising if microorganisms were not to take advantage of the opportunities created by these changing circumstances. Inevitably, they have. Thus, the discarded car tyres that symbolize both the growth of personal mobility and a disposable society now contain the pools of water in which mosquitoes can breed, so driving the spread of dengue fever far beyond its previous distribution (Shaw 2002). Faster travel has fuelled the spread of many infectious diseases, as it has throughout history. The most obvious example is HIV/AIDS, the prevalence of which is now increasing rapidly in the former Soviet Union, the Caribbean, and some parts of Latin America.

Humans are, of course, responding to these changes, as is catalogued in subsequent chapters. Those common infectious diseases of childhood that are susceptible to immunization have been coming under increasing control, with polio now eliminated from both of these regions. Yet disease control remains vulnerable to changing circumstances, with the history of malaria control in both regions characterized by both advances and setbacks. There are, however, some responses that risk making things worse. The widespread use of antibiotics, once seen as a panacea for many common bacterial infections, has led to the emergence of resistance.

The phenomenon of antibiotic resistance goes to the heart of this book. It is intrinsically linked to the emergence of health systems. Whether or not it occurs is, to a considerable extent, an indication of how well those systems are performing. Health systems that are carefully regulated and well managed, providing accurate diagnosis, appropriate treatment, continuous pharmaceutical supplies and careful follow-up are unlikely to experience high rates of resistance. In contrast, where treatment is poorly coordinated and erratic there is a risk of high levels of resistance. It is no coincidence that the two regions included in this book have some of the highest rates of MDR-TB in the world.

The remainder of this book looks in detail at the changing nature of communicable diseases in this region. Before doing so, however, this chapter briefly reviews contemporary economic trends in these regions as a means of providing some context for what follows. For convenience, it divides the European and central Asian (ECA) countries into four broad groups: those that joined the EU in 2004 and 2007; the countries of South-eastern Europe still outside the EU; the Russian Federation and its Slavic neighbours; and the countries of the Caucasus and central Asia. The countries in the Americas are divided into those in the Caribbean and those in South and Central America. Inevitably, given the enormous diversity in both regions, there are many countries that do not fit neatly into these groupings. Nonetheless, it is hoped that it will still provide some useful insights that will help to understand the transition that is taking place in these regions.

Clearly, in the space available, it would be impossible to cover in detail all the countries in these two regions, or to provide a comprehensive assessment of their situation. Instead, a small number of key indicators are presented and discussed from selected countries, representing the diversity within each grouping. The majority of the indicators are taken from the World Bank's 2006 World Development Indicators (World Bank 2006). Two indicators capture the level of economic development, a snapshot of the contemporary situation, per capita gross national product (GDP) in 2000 US$, and a measure of recent progress, the annual percentage growth in gross domestic product (GDP). These measures provide an indication of the resources available to combat infectious disease. A second set of indicators captures the extent of poverty and inequality, here expressed as the percentage of the population living on under US$ 2 per day and the Gini index of the income distribution, where 0 is equivalent to perfect equality and 100 is equivalent to perfect inequality. These indicate the extent to which available resources are distributed within the population. A third set of measures captures the countries' current and future human capital; the projected population growth between 2004 and 2020 (reflecting the combined effects of birth, death, and migration rates) and the percentage of children of the appropriate age enrolled in secondary education. The last of these reflects living standards and thus provides some indication of the vulnerability of the population to infectious disease.

Finally, two indicators have been taken from the World Bank's Investment Climate Surveys, which examine the conditions for investment (World Bank 2007a). These are the percentage of senior managers reporting corruption as a major or very severe constraint and the ease of doing business. These latter indicators are relevant as they indicate the functioning of institutions. Thus, agencies responsible for infectious disease control can easily take advantage of a climate that tolerates corruption, for example taking bribes from food outlets for hygiene certificates or as payment to prevent enforcement of regulations. Public health agencies often have to react rapidly in the event of outbreaks. They may be inhibited in doing so where there are lengthy bureaucratic procedures, reflected by the difficulty of opening a small business.

New European Union Member States

Eight former communist countries in eastern Europe joined the EU in 2004, with a further two, Romania and Bulgaria, joining in 2007. Summary statistics for selected countries are presented in Table 2.1.

The first eight countries can be thought of as falling into three groups. Slovenia was the only one to have been outside the Soviet sphere of influence. Formerly the wealthiest part of Yugoslavia, its economy was already well connected with those of its western neighbours. At the time it acceded to the EU its GNP per capita was about twice the average for the other acceding countries. The second group comprises the Czech Republic, Slovakia, Poland, and Hungary. These countries had been part of the COMECON system, which regulated trade between the USSR and its satellite states. At the time of independence, all had weak economies with obsolete infrastructure but made rapid economic progress during the immediate post-transition period in the early 1990s. The third group comprises the three Baltic states. Occupied during the Second World War, they regained independence in 1991 with the break-up of the USSR. With economies much more closely linked into that of the USSR, they suffered from the disruption of trading links in the early 1990s, experiencing an initial steep fall in output, before recovering to achieve rapid economic growth in the latter part of the decade. Between 2000 and 2004 all three achieved growth in GNP of over 7% per annum.

The two countries that joined in 2007, Romania and Bulgaria, experienced very little growth in the 1990s, only recovering after about the year 2000. They remain very much poorer than their neighbours, with obsolete infrastructure. They have, however, achieved relatively rapid economic growth subsequently.

Widening gaps in income in the immediate post-transition period have generally been reversed, with most of these countries now experiencing Gini indices comparable to those in western Europe (for example, the value for Germany is 28.3), and with all achieving much lower values than the United States (40.8). The greatest degree of inequality is in Poland and the three Baltic states, with indices comparable to those of the United Kingdom (36.0).

Throughout this region, levels of absolute poverty are low, except in Romania, where one in eight of the population subsists on under US$ 2 per day, the three Baltic states, where the figures are between 4 and 7%, and Slovakia (under 3%), but recent data are unavailable from Bulgaria, which is likely to resemble Romania in this respect. Low national poverty rates may, however, mask important differentials between different groups, and when considering poverty and social exclusion in this region, it is important to be aware of a large ethnic minority, the Roma (Fonseca 1995). Originally from northern India, they travelled overland to Europe approximately 1000 years ago. They are now concentrated in Romania, Bulgaria, Hungary and Serbia, with smaller numbers in all countries of Europe. For at least the past few centuries they have been subject to high levels of discrimination, often living in extremely substandard conditions and denied access to employment and welfare services (European Roma Rights Centre 2006). Large numbers perished in the Nazi concentration camps and, although their conditions improved slightly during the communist era, the post-transition period has seen the re-emergence of racist campaigns against them in several

Table 2.1 Summary of economic and social statistics for 8 of the European Union Member States joining the EU since May 2004, selected years

	Per capita GDP (2000 US$) (2006)	Annual per capita GDP growth 2006	Gini index 2003 or *2002	% living on under US$ 2 PPP per day 2003 or *2002	Secondary education net enrolment rate 2005	Annual population growth rate 2006	Ease of doing business index (1 = most business-friendly regulations) 2006	Corruption % major constraint 2005
Bulgaria	2 256	7	29	n/a	88	−0.5	54	18
Czech Republic	7 040	6	n/a	n/a	n/a	−0.2	52	20
Estonia	6 945	12	36	8	91	−0.4	17	4
Hungary	6 126	4	27*	2*	90	−0.3	66	10
Latvia	5 683	13	38	5	n/a	−0.6	24	9
Poland	5 521	6	35*	2*	93	−0.1	75	15
Romania	2 443	8	31	13	80	−0.4	49	28
Slovenia	12 047	5	n/a	n/a	94	−0.2	61	4

Source: World Bank 2007b.

Notes: GDP: gross domestic product; PPP: purchasing power parity; n/a= not available.

countries. In several countries laws on citizenship and identity cards have been used in ways that further exclude them, for example denying them access to health insurance (Ringold and Orenstein 2003). There are, however, major initiatives to improve their situation, with Roma rights being a core element of the accession negotiations for several of the new EU Member States (EC and DG for Employment and Social Affairs 2004). In addition, heads of government in this region have signed up to the Decade of Roma Inclusion, which also involves several international agencies, such as the World Bank, and nongovernmental agencies, such as the Open Society Institute (Open Society Institute 2006).

Across all of this region educational participation rates are high, although there was evidence of falling attendance in some countries during the 1990s (UNICEF 2003). This region is characterized by a highly skilled workforce, a factor that has contributed to a high rate of emigration, especially since EU accession. This is apparent from the data on projected population growth. All are expected to experience continuing population declines. However, this also reflects a dramatic fall in the birth rate; despite some recovery in birth rates since the end of the 1990s, all have total fertility rates well below replacement rate. In terms of overall health, while there is still a substantial gap in life expectancy compared to western Europe, and there are many problems that need to be addressed, in particular risk factors for noncommunicable diseases, in global terms this region fares relatively well.

Efforts to eliminate corruption featured strongly in the process of EU accession. In many parts of the region, perceived levels of corruption are now at a low level that is comparable to what is seen in western Europe. In others, there is still some way to go, in particular in Romania and Bulgaria (EUMAP 2002), although reducing it further remains a priority for these governments and for the EU.

South-eastern Europe

The countries in this region comprise Albania and the countries that emerged from the break-up of Yugoslavia, with the exception of Slovenia which joined the EU in 2004. Summary statistics for selected countries are presented in Table 2.2. In the aftermath of the Second World War, Yugoslavia, which unlike its northern neighbours had not been occupied by the Red Army, broke away from the Soviet bloc, playing an important role in the non-alignment movement that emerged from the 1955 Bandung Conference. Although the extent and nature of post-war reprisals and suppression of opposition were similar to those in other parts of the Soviet bloc, Yugoslavia opened up to the West during the 1960s, with mass tourism and active engagement in the international economy.

This contrasted markedly with the situation in Albania. Long isolated from the rest of Europe by high mountains on its land borders and malaria-infested marshes on its coast, it became even more isolated in the post-war period. Like Yugoslavia, it broke its links with the USSR, instead briefly aligning itself with Maoist China. During the 1980s it was by far the least developed country in Europe, with only a few motor vehicles, non-mechanized agriculture, and almost complete isolation from international developments. Significant

Table 2.2 Summary of economic and social statistics for selected countries in South-eastern Europe, selected years

	Per capita GDP (2000 US$)	Annual per capita GDP growth 2006	Gini index 2003; † 2001; * 2004	% living on under US$ 2 PPP per day 2003; † 2001; * 2004	Secondary education net enrolment rate 2005; † 2003; * 2004	Annual population growth rate 2006	Ease of doing business index (1 = most business-friendly regulations) 2006	Corruption % major constraint 2005
Albania	1604	5	31*	10*	74*	0.2	120	31
Bosnia & Herzegovina	1741	6	26†	n/a	n/a	0	95	23
Croatia	5461	5	29†	2†	85†	-0.1	124	17
The former Yugoslavian Republic of Macedonia	1940	3	39	2	82	0.2	92	32
Serbia	1157	6	n/a	n/a	n/a	0	68	24

Source: World Bank 2007b.

Notes: GDP: gross domestic product; PPP: purchasing power parity; n/a = not available.

quantities of its limited resources, both financial and labour, were used to construct tens of thousands of concrete gun emplacements that surrounded even the smallest settlements (Pearson 2006). The communist regime was overthrown following popular demonstrations in 1990, after which multi-party elections took place. Many thousands of Albanians quickly took advantage of the opportunity to leave, in some cases crowding on to ancient ships to make the short passage to Italy. The limited economic progress of the early 1990s was cruelly reversed in 1997 when the country was beset by a series of pyramid selling scandals, in which many people lost their life savings. Rioters stormed police stations, removing weapons which fuelled widespread criminality (Jarvis 2000). Albania suffered further when it absorbed large numbers of refugees following the conflict in neighbouring Kosovo, and this is reflected in the high rates of absolute poverty with nearly one in eight of the population living on less than US$ 2 per day. However, since 2000, economic growth has averaged over 5% per annum and Albania's long-term prospects look positive.

The break-up of Yugoslavia came in stages, with Croatia and Slovenia first declaring independence. While conflict in Slovenia lasted only a few days, the conflict in Croatia was much more serious, with widespread destruction in Western Slavonia, still one of the poorest parts of Croatia, and large-scale displacement of population, including the movement of several hundred thousand Serbs to other parts of former Yugoslavia from the Krajina region. This was, however, only a prelude to the war in Bosnia, which saw the city of Sarajevo besieged for several years and the emergence of the phenomenon that came to be termed "ethnic cleansing" (Glenny 1996). Although spared the epidemics that accompanied earlier wars, this conflict did contribute to the emergence of Hanta Virus infection, as soldiers dug into rodent-infested lands (Markotic et al. 1996).

In due course, further conflicts broke out in The former Yugoslav Republic of Macedonia, between the two main ethnic groups, Macedonians and Albanians, and in Kosovo, which led to the involvement of the North Atlantic Treaty Organization (NATO) and, subsequently, the overthrow of the regime in Belgrade. What had been a Federation of Serbia and Montenegro split up in 2006, creating Montenegro as an independent country. Future options for Kosovo, historically a province of Serbia but under international administration, were set out in a 2007 report by the then United Nations Special Envoy, Martti Ahtisaari, in February 2007 (Ahtisaari 2007). One year later the Kosovan authorities declared independence, an act that divided the international community. Kosovo has inherited a communicable disease and response system that reported to the WHO (McKee and Atun 2006).The countries of this region all receive support from the Stability Pact for South-eastern Europe, an organization funded by a number of western countries that seeks to promote democratization, economic reconstruction, and security (WHO/Council of Europe Bank 2006).

Given these events, economic statistics from this region in the 1990s are largely meaningless. These countries are, however, now at various stages of rebuilding their economies. Croatia and The former Yugoslav Republic of Macedonia are both candidate countries for EU membership, although only

Croatia has begun negotiations. The remaining countries have association agreements with the EU and are deemed to be potential candidate countries.

Within this region, Croatia is by far the wealthiest country, with a GNP per capita of approximately three times that of its neighbours. However, several of these countries (but not all) are now achieving a high level of economic growth.

In many respects, these countries, with the exception of Croatia, experience conditions that are similar to those in Romania and Bulgaria. Reported levels of income inequality are comparable to those in western Europe and levels of absolute poverty (living on under US$ 2 per day) are almost negligible, except in Albania. Participation in secondary education is high, although lower in Albania than in its neighbours. Looking ahead, in the western part of this region, such as Croatia, populations are expected to decline further, while the high birth rates in the eastern countries, such as Albania, are expected to sustain population growth despite large-scale migration.

Finally, this region scores rather badly by comparison with most of the new EU Member States in terms of governance, with between a quarter and a third of senior managers in most countries identifying corruption as a major or severe problem, while those seeking to establish new businesses face significant delays everywhere except Serbia.

The Russian Federation and its neighbours

The Russian Federation, Ukraine, Belarus and the Republic of Moldova form a natural geographic and cultural grouping within the countries that emerged as independent states following the break-up of the USSR. Summary statistics for each country are presented in Table 2.3. However, when interpreting the summary statistics it is important to recognize the geographical scale involved, with the Russian Federation extending from the Baltic to the Pacific. Consequently, there is enormous diversity within several countries.

Each country experienced a painful transition in the 1990s. The economy of the USSR had been highly integrated, with, for example, a tractor completed in Ukraine being assembled from components manufactured in other republics from raw materials mined in yet other republics. The creation of new international frontiers seriously disrupted these processes while domestically manufactured products could not hope to compete with the much higher quality goods from abroad. People working in obsolete factories increasingly found themselves being paid many months in arrears or in goods rather than cash. In due course many large industrial plants closed, with huge social implications as, in addition to the resultant loss of wages, employees had depended on them for health care and many other benefits. Life expectancy across this region plummeted in the early 1990s (Leon et al. 1997), with the largest declines seen in the regions experiencing the greatest amount of economic restructuring (Walberg and McKee 1998). By 1994, in the Russian Federation, male life expectancy had fallen below 58 years, a level comparable with that in some developing countries. This was followed by a brief recovery but was again reversed following a fiscal crisis in the Russian Federation in 1998, with repercussions that extended to its neighbours. As of 2005, life

Table 2.3 Summary of economic and social statistics for the Russian Federation and selected neighbouring countries, selected years

	Per capita GDP (2000 US$)	Annual per capita GDP growth 2006	Gini index 2003; * 2002	% living on under US$ 2 PPP per day 2003; * 2002	Secondary education net enrolment rate 2005	Annual population growth rate 2006	Ease of doing business index (1 = most business-friendly regulations) 2006	Corruption % major constraint 2005
Belarus	2070	11	30*	2*	89	-0.6	129	6
Moldova	492	5	33	21	76	-0.9	103	20
Russian Federation	2621	7	40*	12*	n/a	-0.5	96	15
Ukraine	1040	8	28	5	80	-1.1	128	21

Source: World Bank 2007b.

Notes: GDP: gross domestic product; PPP: purchasing power parity; n/a = not available.

expectancy across this region was either stagnating or continuing to deteriorate.

Mortality in the USSR had long been substantially worse than that of its western neighbours. There were several reasons for this, at different stages in the pathway that leads to premature death, including poor nutrition (with a diet high in animal fat and low in fruit and vegetables), smoking (with very high rates among men and rapidly increasing rates among women) (Bobak and Gilmore 2006), and inadequacies in the delivery of health care, in particular for chronic disorders such as hypertension (Andreev et al. 2003). However, the most important factor underlying the fluctuations since the mid-1980s has been the almost ubiquitous heavy alcohol consumption, in particular of surrogate alcohols, such as aftershaves, that are ostensibly produced for other purposes but in reality are sold to be drunk. Research in the Russian Federation found that these substances, many of which contain approximately 95% ethanol, were being drunk by almost 8% of men of working age (McKee et al. 2005). Consumption of these substances dramatically increases the risk of death from many causes, including cardiovascular disease, alcohol poisoning, and cirrhosis (Leon et al. 2007).

As discussed later, this rapid transition had implications for infectious disease. An early breakdown in public health systems contributed to an epidemic of diphtheria in the early 1990s (Markina et al. 2000), while societal problems contributed to a rapid increase in the incidence of TB (McKee and Atun 2006). The reopening of pre-revolutionary trade routes from South Asia to Europe provided a conduit for the spread of narcotics, which accelerated when the overthrow of the Taliban in 2001 created the conditions for an upsurge in poppy cultivation in Afghanistan.

The industrial collapse that took place in this region during the early 1990s was accompanied by a deep economic recession that only came to an end in 2000. Since then, however, economic growth in all countries has been strong, to a considerable extent driven by high revenues from extractive industries in the Russian Federation, in particular oil, gas, and precious metals. Inevitably, there have been winners and losers, with increasing income inequality especially in the Russian Federation (Shkolnikov et al. 2006). However, the reported Gini index is unlikely to reflect the full extent of the inequality, which might be better reflected by the large share of the world's output of prestige cars now being sold in the Russian Federation, at a time when one in eight Russians is subsisting on under US$ 2 per day.

The Republic of Moldova is by far the poorest country in the region. Linguistically and historically linked to Romania, the Republic of Moldova lacks natural resources and has little modern infrastructure. Almost two thirds of its population subsist on under US$ 2 per day. Its problems were compounded following independence by the secession of its Trans Dneistria region, which remains beyond the control of the Moldovan Government. It declared independence in 2006 but this is not recognized internationally. In the present context, the importance of this lies in its non-participation in the global health surveillance and customs systems. The Moldovan authorities do obtain some information from this region but flows of such information are erratic (McKee and Atun 2006). Both Trans Dneistria and the Republic of Moldova have experienced large-scale people trafficking. The Republic of Moldova's precarious position is apparent in its lower level of participation in secondary education compared to its neighbours.

In contrast, social protection systems and access to health care, have been protected in Belarus, where President Lukashenko has resisted political and economic reform, at the cost of increasing international isolation (Korosteleva and Lawson 2003).

All countries in this region are experiencing severe declines in population, with low birth rates, high death rates and large-scale migration. This has profound consequences, especially for the Russian Federation, where there is a risk of depopulation of many regions. Looking ahead, there are concerns in the Russian Federation about whether there will be enough conscripts for the armed forces, especially given evidence that many recruits fail to achieve the necessary health standards (Twigg 2005). A recent World Bank study highlighted the importance of investing in better health to secure future economic growth in the Russian Federation (World Bank 2005).

Across this region there are concerns about the quality of governance. Belarus is an especially difficult country in which to start a new business, although, compared to its neighbours, senior managers there report relatively low levels of corruption. These problems are compounded by a weak public health infrastructure. Although the Soviet era sanitary-epidemiological service is extensive, it is poorly equipped and lacks expertise in modern public health methods. It also suffers from the legacy of Soviet science, which prioritized ideology over evidence (McKee 2007).

Life expectancy across this region plummeted in the early 1990s, with the largest declines seen in the regions experiencing the greatest amount of economic restructuring. By 1994, in the Russian Federation, male life expectancy had fallen below 58 years, a level comparable with that in some developing countries. This was followed by a brief recovery but was again reversed following a fiscal crisis in the Russian Federation in 1998, with repercussions that extended to its neighbours. As of 2005, life expectancy across this region was either stagnating or continuing to deteriorate.

Caucasus and central Asia

The countries of the Caucasus and central Asia were always the poorest regions in the USSR (McKee, Healy and Falkingham 2002). Most of the region that they now occupy was only absorbed into the Russian Empire in the second half of the 19th century. The central Asian countries, in particular, were viewed by the Soviet planning system mainly as sources of primary products such as hydrocarbons, minerals, and agricultural products, while manufactured goods, with their greater added value, were mostly produced in the western parts of the USSR. Summary statistics for selected countries are shown in Table 2.4.

In economic terms, these countries can be divided into those with extensive natural resources, in particular hydrocarbons, and those without. The former include Kazakhstan and Azerbaijan (oil), and Turkmenistan (natural gas). These countries are currently experiencing rapid economic growth, although as is

Table 2.4 Summary of economic and social statistics for selected countries in the Caucasus and central Asia, selected years

	Per capita GDP (2000 US$)	Annual per capita GDP growth 2006	Gini index 2003; * 2001	% living on under US$ 2 PPP per day 2003; * 2001	Secondary education net enrolment rate 2005; * 2004	Annual population growth rate 2006	Ease of doing business index (1 = most business-friendly regulations) 2006	Corruption % major constraint 2005
Azerbaijan	1576	33	36*	33*	78	1.0	99	19
Georgia	1070	10	25	25	81*	−0.8	37	19
Kazakhstan	2164	9	34	16	92	1.1	63	11
Tajikistan	247	6	33	43	80	1.5	133	15
Uzbekistan	724	6	37	2	n/a	1.4	147	7

Source: World Bank 2007b.

Notes: GDP: gross domestic product; PPP: purchasing power parity; n/a = not available.

often the case when growth is based on extractive industries, these gains are not being shared equally, with high Gini indices in several countries. The gaps that are opening up have major consequences for health, exemplified by the situation in Kazakhstan and Kyrgyzstan. These neighbouring countries had similar levels of economic development during the Soviet period but Kazakhstan's oil wealth has given it a GNP per capita that is almost six times higher than in Kyrgyzstan. This has allowed Kazakhstan to pay its health workers much higher wages, leading to large-scale migration from Kyrgyzstan.

The historically low levels of economic development in this region are apparent in the high levels of poverty (Falkingham 1997), with a quarter of people living in Georgia subsisting on under US$ 2 per day. This rises to over 40% in Tajikistan, always the poorest country in this region. Tajikistan is a mountainous country with poor internal transport links and very weak infrastructure. It suffered badly from the effects of a civil war during the years immediately following independence. Although World Bank survey-based measures of corruption suggest that this is not a great problem, there is considerable evidence from other sources that it is in reality a major issue, driven to a considerable extent by the major role played by illicit drugs trafficking in the Tajik economy. There are significant concerns about governance throughout this region, with several countries scoring very poorly in Transparency International's rankings (Transparency International 2006).

It is impossible to isolate public health from political developments. Consequently, it is necessary to recognize the tenuous hold that democracy has taken in this region. An exception is Georgia, where the Rose Revolution brought about regime change in the aftermath of electoral fraud (Wheatley 2005). However, elsewhere, elections have been judged not to comply with international norms. The most extreme example has been Turkmenistan, ruled by President Niyazov from independence until his death in 2006. He developed a unique personality cult, renaming months of the year and prominent landmarks after himself and his family and making it compulsory to study the Ruhnama, a collection of his writings, with examinations on it required even to acquire a driving licence. In his final years he fired several thousand health professionals, replacing them with untrained conscript labour. Credible accounts relate how many nurses turned to prostitution. Turkmenistan ceased submission of health statistics to WHO after 1998 but even then the reported two cases of AIDS in the country were widely considered to be a gross underestimate. News of outbreaks of communicable diseases was also suppressed, including an outbreak of plague that was reported, by unofficial sources, to have led to 10 deaths (Rechel and McKee 2005).

Unlike other parts of the former Soviet Union, the population of the region is projected to grow over the coming few decades, particularly in the southern, overwhelmingly Muslim, countries of Uzbekistan and Tajikistan, reflecting their high birth rates. In contrast, falling populations in Georgia and Armenia reflect, in part, large-scale migration, as well as falling birth rates.

The education system inherited from the USSR ensures that participation rates in secondary education are still relatively high, although lower than in the past. Poor living conditions persist for many people, especially in rural areas.

Any consideration of the ability to respond to communicable disease in this region must take account of the existence of several enclaves outside the control of the governments in the states of which they are formally part, as was the case with Trans Dneistria and Kosovo, mentioned in the previous sections. Thus, in Georgia, separatist groups control South Ossetia and Abkhazia, while Nagorno-Karabakh is a territory inhabited by ethnic Armenians but surrounded entirely by Azerbaijan (McKee and Atun 2006). Communication between Armenia and Nagorno-Karabakh is via a single road passing through Azerbaijani territory. The Georgian authorities do obtain some information on threats to health arising inside the two enclaves on their territory, a process facilitated by nongovernmental organizations (NGOs) and the Organisation for Security and Co-operation in Europe (OSCE). The Armenian authorities also obtain some information from Nagorno-Karabakh but here the flow of information is much less satisfactory.

Central America

The countries of central and eastern Europe and the former Soviet Union, described in the previous sections, all shared the common experience of a transition from communism at the end of the 1980s or the beginning of the 1990s. There is no such common factor affecting the countries in the three subregions that will be covered in the remainder of this chapter, although there are some similarities among them. For example, many have had long periods of one ruling party or of dictatorship but, as in many other parts of the world, multi-party democracy is now becoming established. Thus, in Mexico the *Partido de la Revolución Democrática*, which held power almost continuously from 1929 was finally defeated in 2000 (Suchlicki 2001). In Nicaragua, Daniel Ortega's election victory in 2006 led to a peaceful transition of power, in marked contrast to his first election in 1984, which led to sanctions and covert military action by the United States (Walker and Walker 2003).

Clearly, it is beyond the scope of this book to describe the situation in each country individually; instead some general patterns are discussed. Summary statistics for selected countries are shown in Table 2.5.

The countries of Central America include one large country, Mexico, and several smaller ones situated on the isthmus connecting North and South America. Since gaining independence from Spain in the aftermath of the Napoleonic wars (with the exception of Belize, formerly a British colony), their history has been shaped to a considerable extent by the United States. In 1823 the United States President James Monroe established the doctrine – that bears his name – that the European powers should no longer have influence in the entire Americas and, by inference, the United States should become the dominant power. Most recently, this role was played out in the conflicts during the 1980s, when the United States supported an insurgency against the left-wing Government in Nicaragua. Civil conflict and internal repression has characterized many of the smaller countries of central America during the 20th century; the exception has been Costa Rica that, exceptionally, does not have an army, has invested heavily in its health and social welfare system, and has long had a life expectancy substantially higher than would be expected given its level of economic development (Hertz, Hebert and Landon 1994).

Table 2.5 Summary of economic and social statistics for selected countries in Central America, selected years

	Per capita GDP (2000 US$)	Annual per capita GDP growth 2006	Gini index 2003; † 2001; * 2002; ** 2004	% living on under US$ 2 PPP per day 2003; † 2001; * 2002; ** 2004	Secondary education net enrolment rate 2005	Annual population growth rate 2006	Ease of doing business index (1 = most business-friendly regulations) 2006	Corruption % major constraint 2005; * 2003; † 2006
Costa Rica	4723	6	50	10	n/a	1.4	105	40
Guatemala	1771	2	55*	32*	34	2.4	118	81*
Honduras	1024	4	54	36	n/a	2.1	111	63*
Mexico	6387	4	46**	12**	65	1.1	43	18†
Nicaragua	904	2	43†	80†	43	1.9	67	66*

Source: World Bank 2007b.

Notes: GDP: gross domestic product; PPP: purchasing power parity; n/a = not available.

The wealthiest country in the region is Mexico, followed by Costa Rica, with GNPs per capita in excess of US$ 4000 PPP (purchasing power parity). In marked contrast, the GNP per capita in Nicaragua is only US$ 904. There are correspondingly high levels of poverty, with almost 80% of Nicaraguans living on under US$ 2 per day. Within this region, poverty levels are especially high among the indigenous Amerindian populations. All countries in this region exhibit levels of income inequality that are substantially greater than in central and eastern Europe or the former Soviet Union, although per capita incomes are somewhat higher than in central Asia and the Caucasus.

Long beset by financial crises, the countries in this region have enjoyed sustained, although relatively modest, economic growth in recent years. Mexico experienced a major financial crisis in 1994 when a series of political miscalculations led to a run on foreign exchange reserves and devaluation of the peso. Since then the country has put in place a number of measures that have achieved macroeconomic stability and economic growth, providing the resources needed for sustained investment in infrastructure, although in recent years it has suffered from a deceleration in growth, in large part due to its close integration with the United States economy, by virtue of its membership of the North American Free Trade Agreement (NAFTA).

The poorest countries in the region, Honduras and Nicaragua, have also experienced growth in recent years, although both are hindered by their dependence on agriculture, and are thus vulnerable to fluctuations in commodity prices, as well as having very weak transport and financial infrastructures.

Unlike the countries of central and eastern Europe and the former Soviet Union, these countries were never able to put in place universal education and health services, as illustrated by the much lower levels of secondary school enrolment. In recent years, however, there are some more promising signs. This is exemplified by the situation in Mexico, where major investments, focused particularly on people in rural areas, have led to dramatic improvements in child survival and access to health care (Sepulveda and Bustreo 2006). However, in many parts of this region, access to basic amenities remains extremely poor, especially in rural areas.

Although all countries in this region have continued to experience high levels of migration, largely to the United States, populations are predicted to continue to grow, reflecting high birth rates.

Governance is clearly a matter of great concern in this region, with most senior managers perceiving corruption to be a major concern, while those seeking to achieve change face many bureaucratic obstacles.

South America

The countries of South America are as almost diverse as those in Central America. However, many of them share with some of their northern neighbours a history of military or one-party rule, which has given way to democracy only in recent decades. Several, such as Peru and Colombia, have also experienced widespread civil conflict in recent years. An exception was Chile, which for many decades was a bastion of parliamentary democracy until the overthrow, in an American supported coup, of President Allende in 1973 (Constable and Valenzuela 1991).

The contemporary population of South America has been shaped by, among other factors, the combined effects of historic patterns of migration and epidemics of infectious disease. The earliest settlers crossed the Bering Strait from Siberia at least 12 000 years ago, taking several thousand years to occupy the entire land mass of the Americas (Hey 2005). With none of the animals domesticated by the early farmers in Eurasia, they were isolated from the many animal infections that transmuted into human diseases in Eurasia, where humans lived in close proximity to dogs, cattle and sheep, among others. As a consequence, when the first European settlers arrived in the Americas, in the wake of Columbus' voyage of 1492, the indigenous population had no immunity to many by now common European infections (Diamond 1997). As many as 90% or more of many societies perished, allowing European settlers to occupy large swathes of by now depopulated territory with ease. Subsequent settlement patterns, and in some cases political developments across all of the Americas, have also been shaped by infectious diseases, in particular yellow fever. Thus, an attempt by the French authorities to suppress an uprising among slaves in Haiti in 1802 foundered when half of their army succumbed to yellow fever (James and Walvin 2001). The construction of the Panama Canal only became possible once the aetiology of the disease had been established by Carlos Finlay and Walter Reed, allowing control measures to be put in place (Chaves-Carballo 2005).

The earliest European settlements were determined by the 1494 Treaty of Tordesillas, which divided the Americas between Spain and Portugal, which gave rise to the division between Portuguese-speaking Brazil and its Spanish-speaking neighbours. Subsequently, smaller colonies were established on the north-east coast of South America by France (now French Guiana, the only part of the EU on the American continent), the Netherlands (Surinam) and the United Kingdom (Guyana). However, subsequent waves of migration brought communities from many nations, especially Italians and Germans in the 19th century, followed by the Japanese, and Arabs in the early 20th century following the break-up of the Ottoman Empire.

In economic terms, this region is very mixed. Summary statistics for selected countries are given in Table 2.6.

Overall the region is experiencing slow but sustained economic growth, but progress for many countries has been erratic. Thus, Argentina experienced a severe economic shock in 2001, leading it to default on its debts the following year (Romero 2002). The peso was devalued by 75%, wiping out savings. Since then, however, it has shown signs of rapid recovery, with a surge in exports and a cessation of capital flight. In 1999 Colombia experienced a recession, which took rather longer to overcome. Many countries are susceptible to changes in commodity prices. Thus, Chile, which along with many other countries in the region suffered in the 1999 global slowdown, experienced a boost to its growth subsequently from record copper prices. Ecuador has similarly benefited from substantial revenue from oil, despite having major structural weaknesses in its economy. In contrast, during the 1980s, Bolivia suffered from the downturn in world prices for silver.

Table 2.6 Summary of economic and social statistics for selected countries in South America, selected years

	Per capita GDP (2000 US$)	Annual per capita GDP growth 2006	Gini index 2003; † 2002; * 2004	% living on under US$ 2 PPP per day 2003; † 2002; * 2004	Secondary education net enrolment rate 2005; * 2004; † 2002	Annual population growth rate 2006	Ease of doing business index (1 = most business-friendly regulations) 2006	Corruption % major constraint 2005; † 2003; * 2004; ** 2006
Argentina	8695	7	51*	17*	79*	1.0	101	4**
Bolivia	1091	3	60†	42†	73*	1.8	131	8**
Brazil	4055	2	57*	21*	78*	1.2	121	67†
Chile	5846	3	55	6	n/a	1.0	28	13*
Colombia	2317	5	58	18	55†	1.3	79	3
Ecuador	1597	3	n/a	n/a	52*	1.4	123	49†
Venezuela	5427	8	48	40	63	1.7	164	n/a

Source: World Bank 2007b.

Notes: GDP: gross domestic product; PPP: purchasing power parity; n/a = not available.

This region is characterized by very high levels of inequality and, in many countries, of absolute poverty. This inequality is vividly illustrated by the juxtaposition of *favelas*, or shanty towns, and luxury high-rise apartments in Brazilian cities. There are also large economic gaps between many capital cities, which display the trappings of wealth associated with high-income countries, and rural areas that often lack even basic amenities. Once again, indigenous populations are often especially disadvantaged.

Concerns about the distribution of resources have contributed to a series of political changes in which left-leaning (in terms of their political orientation) governments have been elected across the continent (Petras and Veltmeyer 2005). Thus, in 2005 Bolivia elected its first ever president from among its indigenous population and President Morales has subsequently pursued a policy of renationalizing foreign-owned assets in the energy sector as well as challenging United States policies of coca eradication which has failed to provide alternative employment opportunities for the coca farmers. In Venezuela, President Chávez has also taken many private enterprises under state control. In Brazil, President Lula has not pursued a policy of nationalization but has instituted major anti-poverty and hunger-eradication programmes.

The Caribbean

The countries of the Caribbean also form a very diverse group, whether they are considered in terms of size, economic development, or political complexion. Cuba, the largest, has a population of over 11 million, while Anguilla has a population of only 7500.

As in South and Central America, the contemporary political and demographic context has been shaped by a history of colonization, although here the situation is rather more diverse. Spain was the dominant power in the northern Caribbean, occupying Dominican Republic, Cuba and Puerto Rico. The first of these gained independence in 1865, while Spanish rule ended in the others during the 1902 Spanish–American war, when Cuba became independent and Puerto Rico became an unincorporated territory within the United States. As noted earlier, Haiti achieved independence from France in the aftermath of the French Revolution. Some of the smaller territories were colonized by Sweden and Denmark but the dominant colonial powers in the remainder of the Caribbean were the British, French and Dutch, with some islands changing hands several times.

Most of these territories became independent in the 1970s and 1980s, although the three European colonial powers have retained a presence, in differing forms. Some of the very small islands, such as Anguilla and Montserrat, have remained as British Dependent Territories, Martinique and Guadeloupe are overseas Departments of France (and thus part of the EU), and the Netherlands Antilles is an autonomous entity within the Kingdom of The Netherlands. Currently outside the EU, it is proposed that in 2008 the Netherlands Antilles will be dissolved and some of the separate islands (Bonaire, Saba and Sint Eustatius) will join the EU as "outermost regions", a status shared with France's overseas Departments.

The economic status of the countries of the Caribbean is extremely diverse. Statistics for selected countries are shown in Table 2.7. Some have developed strong economies, with tourism and financial services playing an important role. Some, such as the Bahamas and the Virgin Islands, have long-established tourist industries, while in others it has developed more recently. Some, such as St Kitts and Nevis or St Maarten, have opted for lower volume, high-value tourism, while others, such as Dominican Republic, have chosen lower-cost mass tourism.

In marked contrast to those that have developed their economies successfully, Haiti is the poorest country in the western hemisphere, with an estimated per capita GNI of just over US$ 400 in 2006. At one stage more developed than Dominican Republic, which occupies the remainder of the island of Hispaniola, it suffered over centuries from overpopulation, deforestation and environmental degradation (Diamond 2005). Subsequently, it suffered under a long period of dictatorship which gave way to a series of unstable governments and widespread civil conflict, eventually necessitating the intervention of a United Nations peacekeeping force.

Cuba is in a unique position. *De facto* part of the Soviet bloc until 1991, it benefited from guaranteed purchases by the USSR at above-market prices of its sugar cane crop, while obtaining subsidized supplies of oil. Although now establishing a thriving tourist industry, the country is handicapped by the persistence of United States sanctions, which provide the American courts with powers to act against enterprises in other jurisdictions, preventing them from dealing with Cuba, as well as by the end of support from the USSR. Unfortunately no economic data are available for Cuba.

Several of the larger countries of the region benefit from supplies of natural resources, such as aluminium in Jamaica and oil in Trinidad and Tobago, although as with their South American neighbours this can render them vulnerable to fluctuating commodity prices. Thus, many of the smaller islands suffered when several countries in the EU, under pressure from the World Trade Organization (WTO), were forced to abandon previous preferential terms for banana producers.

The very wide variation in economic development is apparent in the statistics on poverty levels, with negligible levels in some countries but almost four out of every five Haitians subsisting on under US$ 2 per day. As in South and Central America, there are high levels of inequality throughout this region.

Standards of governance also vary. While many countries have well-functioning legal systems, property rights, and active and free mass media, in a few there is a high level of corruption or, as in Haiti, government failure. The finding that someone wishing to start a new business legally in Haiti would require 203 days to do so is an indication of the difficulty involved in making anything happen.

Summary

This book brings together two regions of the world that are rarely considered together yet have some features in common. This commonality is exemplified

Table 2.7 Summary of economic and social statistics for selected countries in the Caribbean, selected years

	Per capita GDP (2000 US$)	Annual per capita GDP growth 2006	Gini index 2003; † 2001; * 2004	% living on under US$ 2 PPP per day 2003; † 2001; * 2004	Secondary education net enrolment rate 2005; † 2003; * 2004	Annual population growth rate 2006	Ease of doing business index (1 = most business-friendly regulations) 2006	Corruption % major constraint 2005
Dominican Republic	2 694	9	51*	17*	53	1.5	117	n/a
Haiti	443	1	59†	78†	n/a	1.4	139	n/a
Jamaica	3 367	2	45*	14*	79	0.4	50	46
Trinidad and Tobago	10 268	12	n/a	n/a	69	0.3	59	n/a

Source: World Bank 2007b.
Notes: GDP: gross domestic product; PPP: purchasing power parity; n/a = not available.

by one of the few topics where they are brought together, in discussions on the global spread of MDR-TB; some of the highest rates anywhere in the world are seen in the Russian Federation and in Peru (Farmer and Reichman 1999). However, the most important commonality between them is the experience of political and economic transition. Many of the countries of central and eastern Europe and of Central and South America have undergone a transition to democracy, although in both regions there are some countries that have yet to make this change. Both regions have experienced major economic changes, largely for the better but again not everywhere. A significant number of countries have experienced civil conflict and in a few this still continues. In both regions, recent transitions in many countries have been accompanied by widening inequalities.

As was noted in this and other chapters of this book, microorganisms exploit change. The events in these regions have given them many opportunities to do so, as is described in detail in the remainder of this book.

References

Ahtisaari, M. (2007). *The comprehensive proposal for Kosovo status settlement*. Pristina: United Nations Office of the Special Envoy for Kosovo.

Andreev, E. M. and Nolte, E. (2003). The evolving pattern of avoidable mortality in Russia, *International Journal of Epidemiology*, 32 (3): 437–446.

Andreev, E. M., Nolte, E., Shkolnikov, V. M., Varavikova, E. and Mckee, M. (2003) The evolving pattern of avoidable mortality in Russia, *International Journal of Epidemiology*, 32(3): 437–446.

Bobak, M. and Gilmore, A. (2006). Changes in smoking prevalence in Russia, 1996–2004. *Tobacco Control*, 15(2): 131–135.

Chaves-Carballo, E. (2005). Carlos Finlay and yellow fever: triumph over adversity, *Military Medicine*, 170(10): 881–885.

Constable, P. and Valenzuela, A. (1991). *A nation of enemies: Chile under Pinochet*. New York; London: Norton.

Diamond, J. M. (1997). *Guns, germs and steel: the fates of human societies*. London: Jonathan Cape.

Diamond, J. M. (2005). *Collapse: how societies choose to fail or survive*. London: Allen Lane.

EC and DG for Employment and Social Affairs (2004). *The situation of Roma in an enlarged European Union*. Brussels: Commission of the European Communities.

EUMAP (2002). *Monitoring the EU accession process: corruption and anti-corruption policy*. New York: Open Society Institute.

European Roma Rights Centre (2006). *Ambulance not on the way: the disgrace of health care for Roma in Europe*. Budapest: European Roma Rights Centre.

Falkingham, J. (1997). *Household welfare in central Asia*. Basingstoke: Macmillan; New York: St. Martin's Press.

Faminow, M. D. (1998). *Cattle, deforestation, and development in the Amazon: an economic, agronomic and environmental perspective*. Wallingford, Oxon: CAB International.

Farmer, P. E. and Reichman, L. B. (1999). *The global impact of drug-resistant tuberculosis*. Boston MA: Harvard Medical School/Open Society Institute.

Fonseca, I. (1995). *Bury me standing: the gypsies and their journey*. London: Chatto & Windus.

Glenny, M. (1996). *The fall of Yugoslavia: the third Balkan war*. London: Penguin.

Godfrey, C. (1998) A *future for Caribbean bananas: the importance of Europe's banana market to the Caribbean*. Oxfam, Policy Department.

Gott, R. (2005). *Hugo Chavez and the Bolivarian revolution: Richard Gott*. London: Verso.

Hart, R. (1998). *From occupation to independence: a short history of the peoples of the English-speaking Caribbean Region*. London: Pluto Press.

Hertz, E., Hebert, J. R. and Landon, J. (1994). Social and environmental factors and life expectancy, infant mortality, and maternal mortality rates: results of a cross-national comparison, *Social Science and Medicine*, 39(1): 105–114.

Hey, J. (2005). On the number of New World founders: a population genetic portrait of the peopling of the Americas, *Public Library of Science Biology*, 3(6): e193.

James, C. L. R. and Walvin, J. (2001). *The black Jacobins: Toussaint L'Ouverture and the San Domingo revolution*. London: Penguin.

Jarvis, C. (2000). The Rise and Fall of Albania's Pyramid Schemes, *Finance & Development*, March: 46–49.

Kaufman, R. R. (1988). *The politics of debt in Argentina, Brazil, and Mexico: economic stabilization in the 1980's*. Berkeley: Institute of International Studies.

Korosteleva, E. A. and Lawson, C. W. (2003). *Contemporary Belarus: between democracy and dictatorship*. London: Routledge Curzon.

Leon, D. A., Chenet, L., Shkolnikov, V. M. et al. (1997). Huge variation in Russian mortality rates 1984–94: artefact, alcohol, or what? *Lancet*, 350(9075): 383–388.

Leon, D. A., Saburova, L., Tomkins, S., et al. (2007). Hazardous alcohol drinking and premature mortality in Russia (The Izhevsk Family Study): a population-based case-control study, *Lancet*, 369: 2001–2009.

Markina, S. S., Maksimova, N. M., Vitek, C. R., et al. (2000). Diphtheria in the Russian Federation in the 1990s, *Journal of Infectious Diseases*, 181 Suppl 1: 27–34.

Markotic, A., LeDuc, J. W., Hlaca, D., et al. (1996). Hantaviruses are likely threat to NATO forces in Bosnia and Herzegovina and Croatia, *Nature Medicine*, 2(3): 269–270.

McKee, M. (2007). Cochrane on communism: the influence of ideology on the search for evidence, *International Journal of Epidemiology*, 36: 269–273.

McKee, M. and Atun, R. (2006). Beyond borders: public-health surveillance, *Lancet*, 367(9518): 1224–1226.

McKee, M., Healy, J. and Falkingham, J. (2002). *Health care in central Asia*. Buckingham: Open University Press.

McKee, M., MacLehose, L. and Nolte, E. (2004). *Health policy and European Union enlargement*. Maidenhead: Open University Press.

McKee, M., Szûcs, S., Sárváry, A., et al. (2005). The composition of surrogate alcohols consumed in Russia, *Alcohol Clin Exp Res*, 29(10): 1884–1888.

Open Society Institute (2006). Decade of Roma inclusion [web site] (http://www.romadecade.org/, accessed 27 November 2007). Budapest: Open Society Institute.

Pearson, O. (2006). *Albania as dictatorship and democracy: from isolation to the Kosovo war, 1946–1998*. London: Centre for Albanian Studies in association with I.B. Tauris.

Petras, J. F. and Veltmeyer, V. (2005). *Social movements and state power: Argentina, Brazil, Bolivia, Ecuador*. London: Pluto Press.

Rechel, B. and McKee, M. (2004). *Learning lessons from the experience of the Task Force on Communicable Disease Control in the Baltic Sea Region*. London: European Centre on Health of Societies in Transition, London School of Hygiene & Tropical Medicine.

Rechel, B. and McKee, M. (2005). *Human rights and health in Turkmenistan*. London: London School of Hygiene & Tropical Medicine.

Ringold, D. and Orenstein, M. A. (2003). *Roma in an expanding Europe*. Washington, D.C.: World Bank.

Romero, L. A. (2002). *A history of Argentina in the twentieth century*. University Park, Pa.: Pennsylvania State University Press; London: Eurospan.

Rosefielde, S. (2005). *The Russian economy: from Lenin to Putin*. Oxford: Blackwell.

Sepulveda, J. and Bustreo, F. (2006). Improvement of child survival in Mexico: the diagonal approach, *Lancet*, 368(9551): 2017–2027.

Shaw, T. (2002). Once nearly eliminated, dengue now plagues all of Latin America, *Bulletin of the World Health Organization*, 80: 606.

Shkolnikov, V. M., Andreev, E. M., Jasilionis, D., et al. (2006). The changing relationship between education and life expectancy in central and eastern Europe in the 1990s, *Journal of Epidemiol and Community Health*, 60(10): 875–881.

Smith, G. (1994). *The last years of the Monroe doctrine, 1945–1993*. New York: Hill and Wang.

Suchlicki, J. (2001). *Mexico: from Montezuma to the fall of the PRI*. Washington, D.C.: Brassey's.

Transparency International (2006). Corruption Perceptions Index [web site] (http://www.transparency.org/policy_research/surveys_indices/global/cpi, accessed 27 November 2007). London: Transparency International.

Twigg, J. (2005). *PONARS Policy Memo 360 – National Security Implications of Russia's Health and Demographic Crisis*. Washington, D.C.: Center for Strategic and International Studies.

UNICEF (2003). *Social monitor 2003: the MONEE Project, CEE/CIS/Baltic states*. Florence, Italy: United Nations Children's Fund.

Walberg, P. and McKee, M. (1998). Economic change, crime, and mortality crisis in Russia: regional analysis, *British Medical Journal*, 317(7154): 312–318.

Walker, T. W. and Walker, T. W. (2003). *Nicaragua: living in the shadow of the eagle*. Boulder, Colo: Westview Press.

Wheatley, J. (2005). *Georgia from national awakening to Rose Revolution: delayed transition in the former Soviet Union*. Aldershot; Burlington, Vt.: Ashgate.

WHO (2002). *World report on violence and health: summary*. Geneva: World Health Organization.

WHO/Council of Europe Bank (2006). *Health and economic development in South-eastern Europe*. Paris: Council of Europe Bank.

Williamson, E. (1992). *The Penguin history of Latin America*. London: Allen Lane.

World Bank (2005). *Dying too young*. Washington, D.C.: World Bank.

World Bank (2006). *2006 World Development Indicators*. Washington, D.C.: World Bank.

World Bank. (2007a). Investment Climate Surveys [web site] (http://iresearch.worldbank.org/InvestmentClimate/, accessed 9 March 2007). Washington, D.C: World Bank.

World Bank (2007b). World Development Indicators [online database]. Washington, D.C.: World Bank (www.worldbank.org/data/, accessed November 2007).

Zavialov, P. (2005). *Physical oceanography of the dying Aral Sea*. New York, NY: Springer.

chapter three

Effective governmental responses to communicable disease challenges in transitional societies

Kelley Lee, John Wyn Owen

Introduction

Reforms that have swept across health care systems worldwide in recent decades, profoundly affecting how health care is financed and delivered, have also challenged long-held notions about the appropriate roles of the State and the market. From the first half of the 19th century, governments began to play a more active and direct role in protecting and promoting public health. Epidemics during the industrial revolution, spread by migration, trade and conflict, led to the adoption of new public policies to address water and sanitation, housing, nutrition and working environments. During the 20th century, the State grew to play an even bigger role in many countries, including the creation of national health systems (Lee 2003). The unprecedented improvements in health status since the early 1900s have largely been due to these efforts to address the broad determinants of health (Sen and Bonita 2000).

Health sector reforms sweeping the globe since the 1980s have again raised the question of the appropriate role of government. Initial reforms shifted many health systems back towards a more "minimalist" state in terms of health financing and service provision. Since the mid-1990s, the ideological pendulum has begun to swing back again towards recognition that governments must invariably play a lead role in providing certain essential functions. The challenge facing all societies today is defining and agreeing what essential functions governments must provide to best protect and promote health.

This chapter examines the role of government in providing effective responses to communicable diseases, with a particular focus on transitional societies. It begins by arguing that key functions concerned with communicable diseases fall within the realm of a "public good", thus requiring collective action led by governments. A brief discussion of what these functions entail is provided, with a focus on the principles of resilience in dealing with public health emergencies. The chapter then discusses the particular challenges faced by societies in transition where governments can face weak capacity, political and economic instability, and even conflict. The chapter concludes with recommendations on how transitional societies might be supported within the context of global health.

Why the role of government?

By definition, communicable diseases pose a shared risk to more than one individual within a society and, as such, must be dealt with by a combination of individual and collective action. Communicable diseases encompass "any disease that can be transmitted from one person to another" (Martin 1998). Depending on the specific disease, the risk can be limited to a discrete population group or be more "democratic" (i.e. indiscriminately affecting entire populations). Moreover, communicable diseases can pose a risk to populations locally or much further afield.

It is the shared nature of the risk that makes efforts to prevent, control and treat communicable diseases a "public good". A pure "private good" (e.g. cake) is one whereby consumption can be withheld until payment is made and, once consumed, cannot be consumed again. A pure public good (e.g. lighthouse) has two important characteristics: (a) consumption is non-rival, meaning that use by one individual does not limit use by others of the same good; and (b) consumption is non-excludable, meaning that once provided it is available to all others. In reality, most goods fall between pure private and pure public goods – there are a range of private goods with externality effects and public goods with private benefits (Woodward and Smith 2003). Traditionally, governments are expected to play an active role in providing public goods as, left solely to the market, such goods would be undersupplied.

In recent years, the concept of public goods has been applied to the health field in an effort to distinguish what functions can best be fulfilled by the State versus the market. The prevention, control and treatment of communicable diseases can be usefully understood in this way, with certain key functions characterized as public goods. All individuals within a society benefit from minimizing the spread of communicable diseases, and such a "good" (a reduced risk and health burden from communicable disease) can be seen as both non-rival and non-excludable.

Furthermore, there are certain market failures that would lead to the undersupply of many goods concerned with communicable diseases. First, there is little incentive for individuals to privately invest in such goods. Benefits from the creation of a disease surveillance system are shared by all within a society and cannot be withheld until payment is received. Individuals benefit from disease surveillance whether or not they have paid. Second, and as a related point, the problem of "free riders" will arise if certain functions, such as immunization programmes, are left to the market. While a population's collective risk from measles, for example, declines at a given rate of vaccination, there may be an individual incentive to "free ride" on the compliance of others. If sufficient numbers acted in this way, and immunization coverage declined sufficiently, this could lead to a disease outbreak that would pose a risk to all non-immunized individuals. Third, there are many communicable diseases that, because they affect limited numbers or disadvantaged populations, do not offer a sufficient economic return to entice the market into action. So-called neglected diseases attract inadequate attention by pharmaceutical companies, for example, because of the small numbers affected or the inability of sufferers to pay for treatment. In such cases, governments are required to mobilize alternative resources or create additional incentives to address such diseases. Fourth, increased risk from communicable disease can be a negative externality from the individual or collective behaviour of others within society. Regulatory measures are needed to ensure that such behaviours are minimized. Fifth, situations where action leads to collective benefits rather than individual gain require governments to pool costs across all individuals. The overall benefit to society of, for example, a disease surveillance system, far exceeds its cost, but only if this cost is collectively shared. Similarly, the cost–effectiveness of disease eradication (e.g. polio) cannot be realized unless governments invest in such campaigns. Overall, if left to the market alone, public goods are not produced in sufficient quantity and it becomes necessary for governments to act.

While there are clearly situations where governments must act to provide public goods related to communicable diseases, given limited resources and capacities, governments must invariably make decisions about priorities. There are two factors that might influence the role of government. First, while communicable disease poses a collective risk, diseases vary in the type of risk they pose. Some pose a potential risk to all individuals within a society (e.g. influenza, measles), albeit some members of society are at relatively greater risk than others (e.g. elderly, infants). Other diseases may be confined to certain population groups due to geography (e.g. tropical region), engagement in certain "risk behaviours" (e.g. injecting drug user), or other factors (e.g. genetic make-up, occupation) that lead to increased exposure to a pathogen. Diseases also vary in their acuity and severity. The pneumonic plague continues to evoke great fear because of the acute nature of the disease if left untreated and its high mortality rate. Other communicable diseases pose less serious risks to health (e.g. herpes simplex virus type 1). In determining its role, governments must consider the nature of the risks to society from specific diseases and the relative benefits of allocating scarce resources.

Second, the role of government will vary according to specific prevention, control, treatment and recovery activities available. While perhaps ideal, it is impossible for any government to prevent all communicable diseases from occurring. Causation is sometimes unknown (such as newly emerging diseases); some may lie beyond the direct control of governments (e.g. migration of wild birds); others may require the cooperative actions of many governments (e.g. meningococcal disease outbreaks during Haj pilgrimage). In seeking to respond effectively to communicable diseases, existing public health infrastructure will determine capacity to act. Affected populations may be geographically isolated, or diagnostics may be scientifically unavailable (e.g. vCJD) or politically sensitive (e.g. HIV/AIDS) to apply. For treatment, pharmaceuticals and other treatment regimes (e.g. prophylaxis, anti-virals) may or may not be available, due to the state of medical science, economic affordability or scarcity of supply.

The role of government in communicable disease outbreaks

While the role of government, in relation to a specific communicable disease, will be determined by a complex mixture of policy considerations, it is possible to identify six core principles that all governments may seek to fulfil in building their capacity to respond effectively (Table 3.1). These principles can be usefully understood in relation to the concept of "resilience", defined as "the ability at every level of the system to detect, prevent, control and recover from disruptive challenges", an ability dependent on establishing "a well planned, carefully orchestrated and fully integrated emergency management response" (SARS Expert Committee 2003). While the performance of these functions may or may not be fulfilled by governmental bodies (e.g. laboratory services, training of health workers), it is government that necessarily plays a lead role in ensuring the principles of resilience serve as the guiding framework for action.

One example is the Health Protection Agency (HPA), the lead statutory agency in the United Kingdom, established in 2005, with responsibility for advising and supporting the Government's response to major infectious disease incidents and outbreaks and with significant powers to provide a nationally consistent, effective and expert response to health threats. Since its inception, the HPA has had to respond to several new challenges, including the SARS outbreak, pandemic influenza preparations, major chemical incidents, and training and scenario testing. As such, one important role is to promote resilience and to look ahead, scanning the horizon for potential new threats to prepare for them, prevent them from happening and, should they arrive, help protect the public and reduce their impact. This resilience approach of preparation, prevention and protection to current and potential health threats is embedded in an integrated health protection service at all levels.

There is thus a clear role for government in ensuring effective responses to communicable disease challenges. As a public good, strengthening resilience to disease outbreaks (and other public health emergencies) offers shared benefits to all members of society. Building capacity, based on the six principles mentioned above, is a useful framework for understanding the operational challenges faced by governments.

The role of public health law

Public health law is critical to underpinning the role of government. Gostin (2004a) defines public health law as "the study of the legal powers and duties of the State to assure the conditions for people to be healthy (e.g. to identify, prevent and ameliorate risks to health in the population) and the limitation on

Table 3.1 Basic principles for ensuring public health resilience to communicable disease outbreaks

Principle	Activities
Surveillance and reporting	Provision of epidemiological training and supervision; development of surveillance standards; tracking of disease trends geographically and temporally; identification of new disease threats; detection of outbreaks; notification of suspected and confirmed cases to relevant authorities at local, national, regional and global levels; design of appropriate prevention and control measures; evaluation of effectiveness of interventions.
Comprehensive contingency planning	Development and implementation of incident plan for dealing with major outbreaks; agreement of protocols for declaring outbreak, forming outbreak control team and initiating control actions; specification of roles and responsibilities of outbreak team members and other relevant bodies; arrangements for resource mobilization (pooling and sharing of resources); arrangements for communication among outbreak control team and with public; evaluation of incident plan after outbreak events.
Clear command and control structures	Operational command and control structures to manage front-line decisions and actions; tactical command and control structures to determine priorities for obtaining and allocating resources, and to plan and coordinate overall response; strategic command and control structure to establish strategic objectives and overall management framework, and to ensure long-term resourcing and expertise; creation of necessary legislative framework to enable an appropriate public health response.
Integrated response	Review of relationships among various organizations and levels of the health system to ensure a combined and coordinated response at local, national, regional and global levels.
Sufficient surge capacity	Investment in adequate facilities at primary and tertiary levels of the health system including facilities for isolation and infection control; recruitment and training of personnel in required clinical specialties and skills; basic training of other health personnel in infectious disease control measures.
Transparent and effective communication	Provision of clear, timely and factually accurate information to public; training of senior officials in working with media; development of public education programme on public health issues.

Source: (Adapted from) SARS Expert Committee 2003.

the power of the State to constrain the autonomy, privacy, liberty, property or other legally protected interests of individuals for the protection or promotion of community health." In most countries, current public health legislation can be described as untidy, not comprehensive and in need of updating and streamlining. It is at its worst in relation to communicable disease, where there can be ambiguity about where leadership and authority lie. Consequently, there is a serious risk of confusion of roles and responsibilities, of wasted effort and duplication, and a dangerous vacuum between different levels of government. Much existing public health law was originally drafted in the 19th century as a result of crisis measures taken to respond to a particular event rather than a comprehensive body of legislation. Public health law thus often lags behind general reforms in both the health service and local government.

The need for an appropriate legislative framework for effective responses to communicable disease outbreaks extends beyond individual countries. Communicable diseases are perhaps the classic example of where cooperation across countries is essential, given the potential for diseases to spread across national borders. Individual countries can act collectively, much as individuals within society, to more effectively address a shared risk. The focus of such cooperation is WHO, which cooperates on communicable diseases with designated public health institutions within each member country. This relationship is governed by international harmonization of nomenclature and disease classification systems, as well as evolving International Health Regulations which, until recently revised, requires mandatory outbreak reporting of only three diseases – plague, yellow fever and cholera. A government may also collaborate regionally, through one of six WHO regional offices or through the EU. These functions may include surveillance and reporting, cross-border cooperation, scenario planning and resource mobilization.

Recognition of the existing weaknesses of public health law has led to "a renaissance", and "signs of revitalization can be seen in diverse national and global context international agencies, national governments are initiating broad reforms of antiquated public health laws and calling for effective public governance systems at all levels – local, national and global." Gostin identifies five essential characteristics of public health laws at the national level:

- government – public health is a special responsibility of government, with partners in the community, business, the media and academia;
- populations – public health focuses on the health of populations rather than individual patients;
- relationships – public health addresses the relationship between the individual and the State and the population (or between the State and individuals who place themselves or the community at risk);
- services – public health deals with the provision of population-based services founded on the scientific methodologies of public health (biostatistics and epidemiology); and
- power – public health authorities posses the power to regulate individuals and business for the protection of the community, rather than relying on a near universal ethic of voluntarism.

Public health law therefore places special responsibility on governments to secure the health needs of the population. It should be recognized that it is a highly political process and, to be effective, public health advocates must engage in energetic and ongoing action, working with affected communities.

Global governance of communicable diseases

As governments reflect on the adequacy of public health institutions within their domestic spheres, there have been corresponding efforts to strengthen an even weaker framework at international level. International law represents the body of rules and principles that regulates the conduct of and relationships amongst states; the operation of international organizations; the relation between states and natural or juridical persons; and in some cases the conduct of persons towards each other. Historically, law has been a central mechanism in the governance of international relations. In this context, international law serves as a critical process that allows states to coordinate their behaviour and cooperate on problems of mutual concern. Over time, international law has evolved to regulate not only interstate relations but also the relationship between states and their citizens, as in the case of human rights and obligations that persons owe each other as human beings.

For public health, important areas of international law include trade, environment, humanitarian, labour and arms control laws. International laws on specific health problems have largely been developed in the second half of the 20th century and outside of WHO. WHO's reluctance to adopt international legal instruments or "hard law" demonstrates a preference for using "soft law" or non-binding conventions and agreements with states on how they should approach international health problems. The two notable exceptions are the Framework Convention on Tobacco Control and the International Health Regulations (IHR), administered by WHO, which, in the context of this analysis, remain the key legal mechanism for dealing with infectious disease outbreaks. Originating from the International Sanitary Conferences of the 19th century, held to minimize the impact of selected epidemic diseases on trade and commerce, the International Health Regulations have long been recognized as narrowly defined in scope and authority. These shortfalls have become especially evident as globalization processes have greatly intensified flows of people, other life forms, trade and finance, and knowledge and ideas across national borders. Within this increasingly globalized context, revision of the International Health Regulations has sought to address various problems, including: adherence due to state sovereignty; reliance on border controls rather than "globally established health rules that require, for example, strong national public health capacities"; and power imbalances in setting the global health agenda, resulting in inadequate technical assistance and resources for improving health in low and middle-income countries (Gostin 2004b). Amid a degree of foot-dragging over the revision process, the SARS crisis highlighted the need for renewed effort to update the International Health Regulations. Adopted in May 2005, the revised International Health Regulations constitute a radically new international legal regime designed to strengthen global health security against public health emergencies of international concern (including biological, chemical and radionuclear). They establish a new basis for collaboration in the event of international public health emergencies by defining the circumstances under which health events should be reported in terms of their potential risk to international health. As well as an enhanced surveillance system, the International Health Regulations recommend health measures and national "core capacities" for disease surveillance and response. These measures are, in turn, located within the framework of human rights protections and good governance principles (Gostin 2004c). They also require states to maintain capacity to monitor and respond to such circumstances, with assistance and support from WHO, other states or agencies such as the United States or European Centers for Disease Control.

Challenges for transitional societies

Each society under transition facing rapid and significant changes to their political, economic and social institutions faces specific challenges, depending on their historical, political and economic context. One shared concern is with the inability or unwillingness of government institutions to perform certain essential functions and provide adequate public goods to their peoples, including safety and security, public institutions, economic management and basic social services such as health care, education and water supplies. In some cases, this may be due to weak capacity to carry out territorial control and presence; to effectively exercise political power; to exert competent economic management; or to provide sufficient administrative capacity to implement public policies. In other cases, there may be an unwillingness by the State, in the form of an explicit political commitment, to fulfil certain essential functions for selected (e.g. poor, ethnic minorities, regional groups) or entire population groups (Moreno Torres and Anderson 2004).

The specific communicable diseases challenging societies in transition are covered elsewhere in this book. On the role of government, a notable starting point is recognition that high-level political commitment to disease control under the Soviet system facilitated an epidemiological transition in the region. Similar to western countries, acute infections are no longer a leading cause of death in the former Soviet Union, given the development of a pervasive system of monitoring and use of compulsion (McKee and Zatonski 2003). However, since the end of the Cold War, there has been a sharp decline in state capacity in many countries as a consequence of political and economic instability. Particularly hard hit have been countries in central Asia and the Caucasus, but there have also been major challenges faced by the Russian Federation and eastern Europe. A rising incidence of certain communicable diseases has followed suit.

There are major challenges faced by the State in transitional societies that impact on the effectiveness of government action on communicable diseases. First, there has been a significant decline in spending on public services, including health, in many transitional societies. World Bank data on 118 developing and transition countries show that, since the mid-1980s, real per capita spending on education and health has increased, on average, in developing countries, but decreased in the transition economies (Gupta, Clements and Tiongson 1998).

This has included a lack of sufficient investment in public health infrastructure, as well as a shrinking of the scope and scale of government's role in carrying out additional supporting functions concerned with communicable diseases, as described above. For example, in many former socialist countries in Europe, the index of real per capita health spending dropped dramatically during the early years of transition (with the exception of Hungary and the Czech Republic). Based on an index of 100 in 1990, real per capita health spending in 1993 was 37.7 in Albania, 44.9 in Lithuania, 98.2 in Slovenia (up from 65.7 in 1991) and 42.2 in Turkmenistan (ILO 1999). In Latin America and the Caribbean, macroeconomic reforms adopted in the 1980s led to reduced public spending on health associated with declines in health indicators (Franco-Giraldo, Palma and Álvarez-Dardet 2006).

In large part, this has been due to economic instability during transition. This can take the form of institutional weaknesses in raising revenue to finance public sector activities and spending revenue productively. As Tanzi (1999) writes,

> The transformation to a market economy is not complete until functioning fiscal institutions and reasonable and affordable expenditure programs, including basic social safety nets for the unemployed, the sick, and the elderly, are in place. Spending programs must be financed from public revenues generated – through taxation – without imposing excessive burdens on the private sector. Because the level of taxation of a country depends on, among other criteria, the extent of its economic development and the sophistication of its tax systems and administration, these constraints must be considered in discussions of public spending. . . . When a public employee is not paid or when pensioners do not receive pensions to which they are legally entitled, something is fundamentally wrong with the whole political budgetary process.

However, insufficient political commitment may also explain declines in public health spending. Transitional societies face many demands on limited public resources, made more problematic by the demands of transition itself. Priorities may be placed elsewhere, such as creating new economic and political institutions necessary for a market economy. Historically, public health has been seen as a low priority even in high-income countries and this can become the case in transitional societies. For example, an evaluation of the Task Force on Communicable Disease Control in the Baltic Sea Region, established by the heads of government in 2000 to strengthen communicable disease control in the region, found the need for greater political and financial commitment (Rechel and McKee 2004). Similarly, 10 000 cases of diphtheria occurred in the Russian Federation during 1990–1993 due to failures in vaccination programmes (CDC 1993).

Second, in some transitional societies, political authority has faced direct challenge, in turn, affecting the capacity of governments to set and implement public policies. There have been demands for greater democratic rights by ethnic groups in the Russian Federation, Ukraine, Chechnya, Kazakhstan, Uzbekistan and other countries, suggesting a widening of what the Commission on Weak States and the United States National Security Agency calls a "legitimacy gap": "where the State is failing to maintain institutions that protect the basic rights and freedoms of its citizens. An absence of legitimacy provides an opening for violent political opposition, as well as creates greater opportunities for corruption" (Commission on Weak States and US National Security 2004). Governments cannot act effectively where they are unable to command political authority over their citizens and social institutions. Given the collective risk posed by communicable disease, governments must represent the needs of all populations, including minority, marginalized or disenfranchised populations.

Third, governments in transitional societies are struggling with the technical and operational capacity to deal effectively with communicable disease. Along with hospitals and health centres, research institutions, higher education institutions and medical colleges have faced resource constraints and increasing migration of skilled personnel to other countries. The "brain drain" has been a notable feature of the early phases of transition as the best and brightest have left the region to pursue education and careers elsewhere (Berglöf 2001). The accession of 10 countries to the EU in 2004 granted their workers freer movement across the 15 existing Member States, many of which have severe health worker shortages. Migration of health workers has become a global chain of supply and demand.

Among industrialized countries, too, there is an ever-shifting pattern of movement. The United Kingdom has replaced its health professionals who have emigrated to North America with entrants from Germany. Germany, in turn, hosts a significant and growing number of physicians from the Czech Republic. In anticipation of a mass exodus after EU expansion in May 2004, Czech health systems identified recruitment from neighbouring Slovakia as a coping strategy. The downstream effects of such recruitment strategies have a profound effect on source countries (Hamilton and Yau 2004).

There are hopes that transitional societies, as sources of skilled workers will benefit positively through training opportunities and remittances. In reality, too few migrants return to their home countries resulting in a chronic weakening of public health systems.

Fourth, transitional societies may face additional difficulties due to wider changes that impact on the broad determinants of communicable disease. It is no coincidence that communicable diseases thrive where there is greater political and economic instability. In the Russian Federation, for example, there has been a dramatic rise in both cases of and deaths from TB since the early 1990s up to the high levels that were last seen in the late 1970s. The death rate from TB among men aged 20–24 is now twice what it was in 1965. Causal factors include deepening poverty and unemployment, homelessness and migration. The growth in the prison population living in overcrowded and squalid conditions and the alarming increase in drug-resistant TB also illustrate the close link between social context and communicable disease (Stern 1999). Similarly, increased economic insecurity of individuals due to unemployment, non-payment of wages and lack of welfare safety nets, alongside social isolation and fragmentation, have contributed to a rise in so-called risk behaviours, such as injecting drug use and commercial sex work. Both have contributed to an alarming rise in HIV infections in the countries of the former Soviet Union (Schwalbe and Harrington 2002). When rising incidence is coupled with deteriorating health systems, this has meant that the Government of the Russian

Federation has been sorely stretched to mount an effective public health response. The impacts on public health have been an afterthought, rather than integrated as a central part of the large-scale transition policies undertaken.

In summary, it is no coincidence that the political and economic instability experienced by transitional societies has been accompanied by the increased incidence of many communicable diseases. For many countries, the throwing out of old forms of governance has coincided with ongoing struggles to create new ones that can effectively carry out core functions of the State. Amid this institutional vacuum, governments have been weakened in their capacity and willingness to act effectively. This clear link between able governments and effective communicable disease control offers important lessons for supporting such countries.

Supporting effective governmental responses in transitional societies

The imperative to support transitional societies, to respond effectively to communicable disease challenges, begins with the goal of protecting and promoting population health within the region. The role of government is essential to providing this public good, and ensuring collective efforts to build resilience to communicable disease outbreaks. In addition, good health is a fundamental prerequisite to the functioning of a peaceful and stable society. Successful "transition" is dependent, in short, on how well governments can fulfil such responsibilities (core functions).

Moreover, efforts made in transitional societies cannot be separated from wider efforts to protect and promote global health. Globalization has enabled many communicable diseases, which have historically never respected national borders, to become more mobile in terms of speed and distance. The collective risk to the global community from acute epidemic diseases has long been recognized, and cooperation embodied in agreed measures such as the International Health Regulations. Efforts to revise and implement the International Health Regulations, to give them greater relevance in a changing world, remain a key challenge. It is hoped that the shift from disease-specific measures to public health emergencies of international concern will bring greater attention to health systems, and even societies as a whole. As Mills and Shillcutt (2004) write, ". . . sustainable health improvement requires some combination of a strengthened and accessible health service plus focused efforts to strengthen the control of priority diseases." Much global cooperation on communicable diseases remains focused on disease surveillance and reporting. Far less attention is given to the development of treatments and vaccines and, perhaps the biggest challenge, deploying appropriate and adequate resources to build up the capacity of weak health systems.

Another difficulty lies in the fundamental contradiction between the collective interests of the global community and the limited powers currently available to regulate the actions of sovereign states. At the national level, public health laws backed by punitive measures are available to most governments, to be used when necessary to ensure compliance by individuals to measures that reduce or minimize collective disease risks. At the national level, non-compliance by individual citizens to public health law should carefully balance likely risks to the broader community with the human rights of individual citizens. Extrapolated to the global level, intergovernmental cooperation can be prevented by fierce protection of state sovereignty and disincentives to comply with the International Health Regulations. In the absence of a supranational authority (i.e. a world government), how can compulsion be reconciled with recognized norms regarding human rights?

Foreign intervention in countries failing to comply with the International Health Regulations is likely to be highly problematic. More promising are efforts to diversify data sources on disease outbreaks. For example, the Global Outbreak Alert and Response Network (GOARN) draws on information from both governmental and nongovernmental sources. While WHO remains the coordinating body, the success of GOARN lies in its ability to detect and verify outbreaks using multiple data sources. Exploitation of global information and communication technologies, supported by a combination of hard and soft law (i.e. mediation, adjudication and incentives), offers a new framework for building global health governance (Gostin 2004a).

A different challenge, although with similar effect, involves governments unable to cooperate effectively due to weak capacity. There is a need for individual governments to think globally, recognizing that helping to achieve a minimum level of domestic capacity in each individual country is vital to the collective interests of all countries. In this context, transitional societies need support in strengthening their resilience to communicable disease outbreaks. Appropriate investment is likely to yield substantial benefits to society as a whole (Mills and Shillcutt 2004), as well as reduce potential cross- and transborder risks. As Barrett et al. (1998) write, "The recent resurgence of infectious disease mortality marks a third epidemiologic transition characterized by newly emerging, re-emerging, and antibiotic-resistant pathogens in the context of an accelerated globalization of human disease ecologies." Thus, all governments have an interest in investing in "global public goods" defined as "goods exhibiting a degree of publicness (i.e. non-excludability and non-rivalry) *across national boundaries*" (Woodward and Smith 2003).

Given these challenges, what recommendations can be made to support the effective functioning of governments in transitional societies? First, *it is recommended that minimum standards for national public health systems be agreed.* These standards may be organized, for example, around the concept of resilience as described in this book. Core functions, such as capacity for surveillance and response, should be "uniformly strong [across] national public health systems" to enable them to "rapidly detect and respond to health threats at their source" (Gostin 2004c). Incorporated within these standards should be an obligation by governments to maintain such core capacities as citizens of an increasingly global health community.

Second, it is recommended that the allocation of resources for strengthening public health capacity be understood as a cost-effective investment to support preparedness and resilience. Analysis of the direct and indirect financial costs of major disease outbreaks reveals that impacts can be widespread, and in some cases debilitating, for national and regional economies. Investment in ensuring that minimum standards for national public health systems are met within transition societies enables countries to better respond to and recover from such events. Where governments require support in fulfilling public health obligations, appropriate technical and financial assistance must be provided from the global community. High-income countries must recognize this as an investment in a global public good, and that supporting resilience at the national level strengthens the global community's capacity to respond to and recover from public health emergencies.

Third, it is recommended that branches of government beyond the health sector be incorporated in efforts to build resilience to communicable diseases challenges. Building resilience requires close coordination among all four pillars of the State – legislature, executive, judiciary and bureaucracy. Recognizing the importance of the broad determinants of health, in turn, means that building public health capacity cannot be separated from the challenges facing transition societies in grappling with fundamental political and economic change. Recent public health emergencies have shown that "joined-up" government is essential for ensuring that all relevant sectors are tasked with the six principles of resilience. And there is a need to recognize that the consequences of communicable disease outbreaks reach far beyond the health sector, and coordinated action is essential for minimizing such impacts.

Fourth, while governments must take a lead role in ensuring effective responses to communicable disease challenges, it is recommended that transition societies recognize the important contribution of the private sector and civil society in health governance. Achieving an appropriate balance between state and non-state institutions is an enduring challenge for all health systems worldwide. In transition societies, state institutions have been eroded without due attention to the strengthening of other institutional actors.

Fifth, it is recommended that transition societies give due attention to strengthening public health law in relation to communicable diseases. Existing domestic laws should be reviewed to take account of the changing domestic and global contexts. This legal framework should articulate the State's duties and responsibilities in protecting and promoting public health, outlining both the State's power to act and limitations to this power (i.e. human rights). Furthermore, this framework must extend to support more effective public health law at the global level. The revised International Health Regulations are likely to form a core pillar of this framework. Global health governance, in the absence of supranational authority, will need to grapple more directly in future with the invariable tension between public health rights and responsibilities.

References

Barrett, R., Kuzawa, C., McDade, T. and Armelagos, G. (1998). Emerging and re-emerging infectious diseases: the third epidemiologic transition, *Annual Review of Anthropology*, 27: 247–271.

Berglöf, E. (2001). Reversing the brain drain in transition economies, *Beyond Transition, Newsletter about Transition Economies*. World Bank, (May–August) pp. 29–31 (http://

www.worldbank.org/html/prddr/trans/May-Aug2000/pgs29-31.htm, accessed 27 November 2007).

CDC (1993). Diphtheria outbreak – Russian Federation, 1990–1993, *Morbidity and Mortality Weekly Report*, 42(43): 840–847.

Commission on Weak States and US National Security (2004). *On the brink: weak states and US National Security*. Washington, D.C.: Center for Global Development.

Franco-Giraldo, Á., Palma, M. and Álvarez-Dardet, C. (2006). The effect of structural adjustment on health conditions in Latin America and the Caribbean, 1980–2000, *Pan American Journal of Public Health*, 19(5): 291–299.

Gostin, L. (2004a). "Health of the people the highest law", Conference Proceedings, Nuffield Trust, London, 8 January.

Gostin, L. (2004b). The International Health Regulations and beyond, *Lancet Infectious Diseases*, 4: 606–607.

Gostin, L. (2004c). International Infectious Disease Law, revision of the World Health Organization's International Health Regulations, *Journal of the American Medical Association*, 291(21): 2623–2627.

Gupta, S., Clements, B. and Tiongson, E. (1998). Public spending on human development, *Finance & Development*, 35(3): 10–13.

Hamilton, K. and Yau, J. (2004). *The global tug-of-war for health care workers*. Washington, D.C.: Migration Policy Institute (www.migrationinformation.org/Feature/print.cfm?ID=271, accessed 27 November 2007).

ILO (1999). *Decent work, report of the International Labour Conference*. Geneva: International Labour Organization Conference.

Lee, K. (2003). Globalization and health: an historical perspective, in K. Lee (ed.) *Globalization and health, an introduction*. London: Palgrave Macmillan, 30–60.

Martin, E.A. (1998). *Oxford concise colour medical dictionary*. Oxford: Oxford University Press.

McKee, M. and Zatonski, W. (2003). Public health in eastern Europe and the former Soviet Union, In: R. Beaglehole (eds) *Global public health: a new era*. Oxford: Oxford University Press: 87–104.

Mills, A. and Shillcutt, S. (2004). Communicable diseases, in B. Lomborg (ed.) *Global crises, global solutions*. Cambridge: Cambridge University Press: 62–114.

Moreno Torres, M. and Anderson, M. (2004). *Fragile states: defining difficult environments for poverty reduction. Poverty reduction in difficult environments team*. Working Paper 1. London: Department for International Development.

Rechel, B. and McKee, M. (2004). *Learning lessons from the experience of the Task Force on Communicable Disease Control in the Baltic Sea Region*. London: European Centre on Health of Societies in Transition, London School of Hygiene & Tropical Medicine.

SARS Expert Committee (2003). *SARS in Hong Kong: from experience to action*. Hong Kong: Office of the Chief Executive (www.sars-expertcom.gov.hk, accessed 27 November 2007).

Schwalbe, N. and Harrington, P. (2002). HIV and tuberculosis in the former Soviet Union, *Lancet*, 360: 19–20.

Sen, K. and Bonita, R. (2000). Global health status: two steps forward, one step back. *Lancet*, 356: 577–582.

Stern, V. (1999). *Sentenced to die, the problem of TB in prisons in Eastern Europe and central Asia*. London: Kings College.

Tanzi, V. (1999). Transition and the changing role of government, *Finance & Development*, 36(2) (http://www.imf.org/external/pubs/ft/fandd/1999/06/tanzi.htm, accessed 27 November 2007).

Woodward, D. and Smith, R. (2003). Global public goods and health: concepts and issues, in R. Smith, R. Beaglehole, D. Woodward and N. Drager (eds) *Global public goods for health*. Oxford: Oxford University Press.

chapter four

A continuing evolutionary struggle: microbes and man

Anthony McMichael

"There will come yet other new and unusual ailments, as time brings them in its course . . . And this disease of which I speak, this syphilis too will pass away and die out, but later it will be born again and be seen again by our descendants – just as in bygone ages we must believe it was observed by our ancestors."

Girolamo Fracastoro, De Contagione, 1546

Introduction

Since the mid-1970s there has been much discussion about the apparent "emergence and resurgence" of infectious diseases around the world (Weiss and McMichael 2004). At issue is not only the emergence of new infectious diseases such as Ebola virus, HIV/AIDS and SARS, but also the concurrent increases in various major ancient infectious diseases such as TB, malaria and cholera. Meanwhile, others (such as cryptosporidiosis, Lyme disease and hepatitis C) that have been quietly circulating for some time, sometimes perhaps only locally, may have recently increased to the point of being noticed. Lurking in the background is the increasingly ominous problem of the rise of antimicrobial-resistant infectious agents.

These several recent changes in the landscape of human infectious diseases are a consequence of the continuing interplay of co-evolution between microbes and humans. Humans, as large multicellular organisms, are a potential source of energy and nutrients for single-celled bacteria and multi-celled protozoa and a source of molecular genetic assistance for viruses. An infected human therefore enables the infecting microbe to reproduce itself. That process of parasitism often causes biological dysfunction or damage in the host human. This we refer to as "infectious disease". The microbe's interest is in surviving and reproducing. The human host's interest lies in minimizing loss of nutrients and energy and in averting dysfunction or disease. This accounts for the continuing co-evolutionary struggle between microbes and humans whereby natural selection, dispassionate as ever, favours the most effective genetic variants, in both parasite and host.

The modern human species *Homo sapiens* has acquired its infectious disease microbes from two general sources. First, there are ancient parasites that have been passed down the mammalian and, latterly, the primate line. These have been referred to as "heirloom" infections (Karlen 1995) and include the various staphylococcal and streptococcal bacteria and the coliform bacteria that, respectively, cause routine wound infections, throat infections and diarrhoeal diseases. Some recent evidence suggests that TB may also be an heirloom infection, passed down via the primate line.

Second, many other infectious disease pathogens have directly entered the human species from animal and environmental sources. Most of these emerging infectious diseases have come from animals; a minority comes from soil (e.g. legionellosis, melioidosis) or water sources (e.g. cholera). The initial animal-to-human cross-species infection is often facilitated by cultural, social, behavioural, or technological changes – as happened, in the best-known example, when hunter-gatherers changed to settled living and animal husbandry. Approximately 60% of the almost 1500 species of infectious organisms known to be pathogenic in humans come to us from animals (Taylor, Latham and Woodhouse 2001). For those zoonotic organisms, however, we humans usually turn out to be a dead-end host – no onwards transmission can occur.

Sometimes a microbe that makes an incidental "jump" between animal and human is, by chance (perhaps as a serendipitous mutant strain), suited to infecting and reproducing in humans as a new host species. If the microbe also has the capacity for human-to-human transmission, it may graduate to becoming an endemic and exclusively human infectious disease. Alternatively, if the exploratory infective agent finds an effective assisted passage between humans (as with the flea-borne plague bacterium *Yersinia pestis*, or the mosquito-borne Ross River virus in Australia) then it may retain its ecological base in other non-human "reservoir" species – e.g. ground-dwelling rodents as natural hosts for the plague bacterium – and only occasionally cause outbreaks in humans.

Infection and genetic promiscuity as a way of microbial life

Throughout prehistory and history, human populations everywhere have encountered new and resurgent infectious diseases (McNeill 1976). The microbial world is distinguished by great genetic lability, with the free exchange of genetic material unrestrained by the formalities of sexual reproduction, and by ecological opportunism. During aeons of existence, microbes have honed, through continuous genetic evolution, their adaptive responses to nature's antibiotics, nutrient shortages and hostile immune systems. We humans, in evolutionary terms, are newcomers.

Consider the recent concern over the H5N1 strain of avian influenza. Avian influenza ("bird flu") viruses naturally infect many wild bird species. They can readily infect chickens and ducks and various mammals – including pigs and humans. Presumably, then, avian influenza viruses have caused zoonotic infections in our human forebears for many millennia, and have occasionally acquired, via the vicissitudes of reshuffled genes, the capacity for human-to-human spread.

The opportunities for avian influenza viruses to enter human populations has been increased over the centuries by the crowding together of pigs, poultry and humans and by the increases in their absolute numbers (Weiss and McMichael 2004). In southern China the traditional intimate pig/duck farming culture creates a particularly efficient environment in which several strains of avian influenza viruses, coming from wild bird, poultry and human sources, may infect the same pig. Pigs have cell-surface receptors for both avian and human-adapted strains of influenza virus. Any such multiply-infected pig may then act as a "mixing vessel", yielding new recombinant-DNA strains of influenza virus, some of which may then be able to infect the pig-tending humans (Box 4.1).

Further, each such new viral variant may also acquire, via this genetic reassortment process within the infected pig, various genes from the prevailing (endemic) human strain of influenza. Some of these newly formed viral strains may then be capable of human-to-human transmission. This is a prerequisite to the occurrence of a major new influenza pandemic – and has understandably been the particular focus of recent public health concern.

Three such influenza pandemics occurred during the 20th century: the catastrophic "Spanish" flu pandemic of 1918–1919, when approximately 30–40 million people died; the "Asian" flu of 1957, and the "Hong Kong" flu of 1968. Those pandemic strains of the virus were characterized as the H1N1, H2H2, and H3N2 strains, respectively. This refers to the genetically determined molecular variant strains of the two key antigens haemagglutinin (H) and neuraminidase (N) which confer a distinctive capacity for infectivity and virulence, respectively.

Box 4.1 Genetic profile of the avian influenza A virus

- The avian influenza A virus is a very simple virus – and is therefore readily adaptable.
- The virus contains only 10 genes (the human genome contains approximately 25 000).
- The virus needs more than 10 genes to replicate, and gets access to these by hijacking the molecular DNA machinery of the host's cells.
- Viral adaptability is further enhanced because the 10 genes are carried on 8 separate gene segments. These segments can be swapped between viruses, thereby producing new viral strains.
- This genetic reassortment requires two different strains of influenza virus to infect one cell. Such double infection is a rare event. However, when millions of people, chickens and pigs (pigs can be infected by both human and bird influenza viruses) live close together, as in China, rare events are more likely to happen.

The most recent (and threatening) variant, H5N1, combines an H5 antigen from wild geese or quail with the pre-circulating N1 antigen. Evidence that the Spanish flu variant (H1N1) may have acquired its human-to-human transmission capacity by spontaneous mutation within an avian viral variant has heightened concerns that a similar genetic step could occur with the H5N1 strain without having to draw on the genetic repertoire of human-adapted strains (Taubenberger et al. 2005; Tumpey et al. 2005).

Major transitions in the relationship between microbes and humans

The co-evolution of humans and infectious agents has a long history (Cockburn 1977; McNeil 1976). The primate line and its 7 million year-long hominin branch, extending through the australopithecines (from approximately 4 million to 2 million years ago) to the *Homo* genus, and on to modern humans, has its own set of heirloom infections. These include, in addition to the still-familiar staphylococcal and streptococcal infections, various flukes and helminths. The story of human infections becomes more interesting and specific to the human line as dietary behaviours and then cultural practices began to change during the past 2 million years – a period of progressive global cooling, with the onset of recurring glaciations and great changes in the peri-equatorial landscape of eastern Africa as drying caused rain forests to recede and woodlands and savannahs to extend (McMichael 2001).

In prehistory, as early humans gradually became regular meat-eaters from approximately 2 million years ago, they would have been exposed increasingly to various animal (enzootic) pathogens. Much later, from approximately 70 000 years ago when *Homo sapiens* spread out of Africa into new environments and climates, those migrating bands of pre-modern humans encountered unfamiliar microbes. Various new human infectious diseases must have resulted – and presumably often involved, initially, great virulence since the newly infected human population would have had no immunological and genetic defences against these unfamiliar microbial predators.

This story has gathered pace since the hunter-gatherer way-of-life began to be replaced by farming, herding and animal husbandry. The advent of agriculture and, later, animal husbandry occurred approximately 11 000 years ago and 7000 years ago, respectively – in each case apparently in the "fertile crescent" regions of the Eastern Mediterranean. Since that time, and the ensuing dawn of "history" via written records from approximately 5000 years ago, three other great transitions have occurred in the human–microbe relationship (McMichael 2001).

First, the early civilizations of the Middle East, Egypt, South Asia, East Asia and Central and South America each acquired their own distinct repertoire of locally evolving "crowd" infectious diseases. These infectious diseases had arisen on a local basis as a consequence of the increasing contact between humans and animals in settled agrarian communities following the advent of agriculture and animal husbandry, from approximately 7000–8000 years ago, and the attainment of larger, denser human populations (Cockburn 1977). Thus, the measles virus emerged very early on, probably from the rinderpest virus of cattle, and, via genetic change, was able to become an exclusively human infection when population size and density became sufficient to maintain the virus without the need for an animal reservoir. Likewise, smallpox appears to have become epidemic approximately 4000 years ago, possibly evolving from camelpox or a close relative. The historian Alfred Crosby remarks that farmers and herdsmen could drive away wolves and pull up weeds, but there was little they could do to stop infections raging through their densely packed fields, flocks and cities (Crosby 1986).

Second, over the course of a thousand years or so the ancient civilizations of greater Eurasia, especially Rome, China and India, made contact, swapped infectious diseases and underwent a painful microbiological equilibration. Approximately 2000 years ago, the Roman Empire and China's Imperial Han Dynasty, at opposite east–west poles of Eurasia, began to make contact via overland trade through central Asia. Subsequently, epidemic convulsions emerged as virulent newly exchanged epidemics ravaged both populations. Meanwhile, most of the Middle East and India, however, with their longer history of regional trade and germ-swapping, appear to have experienced fewer serious epidemics.

The records indicate that, in the 2nd century AD both Rome and China were overwhelmed and probably politically enfeebled by pestilence. Smallpox entered the Roman Empire in the 2nd century AD when Roman troops returned from quelling (in their usual unsubtle fashion) unrest in Syria. The Antonine plague of Rome in AD 165 was the initial dramatic result, after which smallpox spread widely in the western empire, depopulating many areas. The Antonine plagues brought the high-achieving era of the empire, overseen by Emperors Trajan, Hadrian and Antoninus, to a close. The empire failed to recover from the combined impact of epidemics and the southwards incursions of Germanic tribes. Meanwhile, the east–west trade linking Rome with China via the Silk Road periodically introduced smallpox and measles to China. This appears to have caused a catastrophic halving of the northern Chinese population during the third and fourth centuries AD.

This great Eurasian microbial pooling process thus climaxed with several devastating exchanges of infectious disease between the great empires of Rome and the Chinese Han Dynasty. Perhaps the most spectacular example was the arrival of bubonic plague in the Roman Empire and its subsequent regional and transcontinental spread. Bubonic plague, caused by *Yersinia pestis*, probably made its European debut as the frightful Justinian Plague of AD 542, which brought Constantinople (by then the capital of the Roman Empire) to a state of collapse.

The third of these great transitions occurred on a transoceanic scale. From the 15th century onwards, Europe, with its rapidly improving sea-faring capacity and motivated by a mix of exploratory curiosity, a search for overseas treasure and territorial ambition, inadvertently exported its lethal germs to the Americas, and later to the South Pacific, Australia and Africa.

The triumph of the Spanish conquistadors is widely attributed to a combination of smallpox and measles, both wholly unknown to the New World population (Crosby 1972). The "Columbian exchange" of infectious agents was, in reality, a one-way process – the one possible though still contentious exception being syphilis, perhaps taken back to Europe in the late 15th century. The New

World apparently had substantially fewer potentially epidemic infectious diseases and, further, infections that were vector-borne (like South America's Chagas disease) could not travel without an appropriate vector. This lack of microbes from the Americas was offset by an abundance of new food species – potatoes, tomatoes, corn, and many others – that greatly boosted Europe's agricultural output.

During the 18th and early 19th centuries, European explorations in the Australasian-Pacific region spread Old World infectious diseases to the native populations of that region. The story was, by now, becoming familiar. The Australian Aborigines, New Zealand Maori and countless Pacific island populations were decimated by these introduced infectious disease epidemics.

In 1836, Charles Darwin made a 2-month visit to the east coast of Australia, en route home after his famous stopover in the Galapagos Islands. Following his observations of diseases in Australian Aboriginals, in his *Journal* (1839) he wrote (Darwin 1839):

> Besides these several evident causes of destruction, there appears to be some more mysterious agency generally at work. Wherever the European has trod, death seems to pursue the aboriginal. We may look to the wide extent of the Americas, Polynesia, the Cape of Good Hope, and Australia, and we shall find the same result.

He continues:

> It is certainly a fact, which cannot be controverted, that most of the diseases that have raged in the islands during my residence there, have been introduced by ships; and what renders this fact remarkable is that there might be no appearance of the disease among the crew of the ship which conveyed this destructive importation.

Here, half a century before the elucidation of the germ theory, Darwin was making both clear-headed observation and ecological inference.

Today: a fourth, global, transition?

The recent and ongoing increase in lability in occurrence, spread and biological behaviour of infectious diseases suggests that, today, we are experiencing a Fourth Transition, and this one is on a worldwide scale. Box 4.2 lists the main new infectious diseases or their pathogens identified since the mid-1970s.

This transition reflects aspects of the scale and intensity of the modern human enterprise (Box 4.3). Overuse of antibiotics, increased human mobility, long-distance trade, intensification of food production, large dam and irrigation projects, urbanization, extended sexual contact networks, expanding numbers of refugees, and the exacerbation of poverty in inner-urban ghettos, shanty towns and in poor undernourished populations everywhere – all these trends have great consequences for the evolution and spread of infectious diseases (Weiss and McMichael 2004).

Consider the intensification of livestock production. The emergence in recent decades of various new infectious agents that have crossed from animals

Box 4.2   The recent procession of (apparently) emerging infectious diseases

Since the mid-1970s, the following infectious diseases or their pathogens have been newly identified:

2003   Severe Acute Respiratory Syndrome (SARS)
1999   Nipah virus
1997   H5N1 avian influenza virus ("bird flu")
       variant Creutzfeldt-Jakob Disease (human "mad cow disease")
       Australian bat lyssavirus
1995   Human herpes virus 8 (Kaposi sarcoma virus)
1994   Sabia virus (Brazil)
       Hendra virus
1993   Hantavirus pulmonary syndrome (Sin Nombre virus)
1992   Vibrio cholerae 0139
1991   Guanarito virus (Venezuela)
1989   Hepatitis C
1988   Hepatitis E
       Human herpes virus 6
1983   Human immunodeficiency virus (HIV)
1982   Escherichia coli O157:H7
       Lyme borreliosis
       HTLV-2 virus
1980   Human T-lymphotrophic virus
1977   Campylobacter jejuni
1976   Cryptosporidium parvum
       Legionnaires' disease
       Ebola virus (Central Africa)

to humans – such as "mad cow disease" (BSE) and its human variant, Nipah virus disease (from pig farming in Malaysia) and SARS – has often been viewed in episodic fashion, each as a "natural" disaster, by officialdom, general public and media. In fact, these outbreaks reflect a more generalized transformation of agriculture and livestock production, especially the intensification of factory farming. The greatest rise in industrialized crop and animal production is now occurring near the urban centres of Asia, Africa, and Latin America. The traditional relationships between small farmers, their animals and local environment are thus being broken, resulting in risks to environments, livelihoods, community stability and, by mobilizing "new" microbes, human health.

Meanwhile, and especially in the urban setting, the relaxation of traditional cultural norms is yielding newer, freer, patterns of human behaviour, including sexual activities and illicit drug use. Modern medical manoeuvres, including blood transfusion and organ transplantation, are creating new ecological opportunities for viruses to pass from person to person. In recent times, the

Box 4.3 Major factors affecting probabilities of infectious disease emergence and spread

- Population growth and density (often accompanied by peri-urban poverty)
- Urbanization: changes in social and sexual relations
- Globalization of travel and trade (distance and speed)
- Intensified livestock production
- Live animal food markets: longer, faster supply lines
- Changes to ecosystems (deforestation, biodiversity loss, etc.)
- Global climate change
- Biomedical exchange of human tissues (transfusion, transplantation)
- Misuse of antibiotics (humans and domestic animals)
- Increased human susceptibility to infection), due to population ageing, HIV infection, intravenous drug use.

estimated prevalence of Americans infected with the hepatitis C virus has been of the order of 4 million, mostly silently disseminated by blood transfusion prior to the early 1990s. Other hospitalization practices have opened up new ecological niches for various bacteria, such as those of the *Proteus* and *Pseudomonas* genuses.

Over the past half-century antimicrobials have been used widely, and often unwisely, including for livestock and agricultural purposes (Barnes 2005). It is estimated that approximately half of the antibiotics made in the United States are fed to livestock to enhance growth. A large portion of the antibiotics prescribed for humans have little or no benefit since they are ineffective against viral diseases. This overuse and frequent misuse of antibiotics has nurtured the rise of drug-resistant organisms on an increasingly broad scale. The threat posed by MDR-TB in the 1990s (Bloom and Small 1998) has more recently been heightened by the alarming emergence of "extremely drug-resistant tuberculosis" (XDR-TB). In hindsight, it is remarkable that we did not foresee more clearly that microbes would naturally and rapidly respond to the threat to their survival posed by antimicrobials via the processes of natural selection.

Long-distance trade is also contributing to the global dissemination of various infectious diseases. In the mid-1990s, several outbreaks of the potentially lethal toxin-producing E. coli 0157 in North America and Europe were caused by contaminated beef imported from infected cattle in Latin America. Large development projects, particularly dams, irrigation schemes and road construction, often potentiate the spread of vector-borne infectious diseases such as malaria, dengue fever and schistosomiasis.

Meanwhile, a new and longer shadow is being cast over the future of infectious disease risks by ongoing human-induced changes in the world's climate (Dobson et al. 2006; McMichael 2006), losses of local species (Dobson et al. 2006), and disruptions of ecosystems – along with entrenched poverty in an increasingly market-dominated world. These all tend to exacerbate infectious disease risks.

By destabilizing the natural checks and balances of ecosystems we potentiate the proliferation of small and opportunistic species (the so-called "r" species, with their high reproductive rates). Microbes, with their extraordinarily high reproduction rate, are exemplary species.

Establishing a foothold: the evolution of infectivity and virulence

Most microbes that have the opportunity to try out potential new host species, fail. Success, too, is often temporary. The mysterious "English Sweats" which ravaged the English population several times during the first half of the 16th century then simply disappeared. SARS may not reappear. However, over the long haul, there is a trickle of new infectious diseases in humans that succeed in the long term, and then become our "textbook" infections: measles, chickenpox, TB, typhoid, cholera, syphilis and so on.

Even so, all species have a high probability of becoming extinct, either by termination or by replacement through speciation. In nature there is no permanent success. Pinta, yaws, non-venereal syphilis, and, later, venereal syphilis display an intriguing evolutionary trail, in which each of the earlier forms has apparently evolved to the next. Smallpox, after several thousand years as a major infectious disease in humans has now been eliminated.

When the infecting agent and the host are relatively new acquaintances, evolutionarily, and have not yet fully come to terms with one another, the resultant infectious disease tends to be more severe because of greater "virulence" of the infecting agent (Anderson and May 1991). However, it is often to the advantage of the microorganism to minimize damage to the host, and it is always to the host's advantage to acquire some additional resistance (Ewald 1994). An excellent example of this biological evolutionary counterpoint comes from the experience in Australia in the 1950s, when scientists deliberately introduced viral myxomatosis into the rabbit population. The disease eliminated a very high proportion of rabbits, killing over 98% of all those infected. This created an intense selection pressure in favour of genetically resistant rabbits – and also in favour of less lethal strains of virus that were therefore more likely to have time to generate viral progeny. Myxomatosis-resistant rabbits and the less virulent strain of the myxomatosis virus now predominate in Australia (Fenner 1957).

The microbial world illustrates well the improvised ingenuity of biological evolution – the creative genius of nature in microcosm. Basically, anything goes if it works. Sometimes, in the course of pursuing their self-interest (survival, replication, dissemination) they disrupt the infected host's biology and so disease ensues. Sometimes the symptoms of disease – diarrhoea, sneezing, scratching – are essential to the dissemination of the microbe. The following are two fascinating examples:

- Chickenpox, like other acute and highly contagious infections, can exhaust the local population's supply of non-immune individuals. This puts the virus at risk of dying out within that population. Therefore, in a few infected individuals the virus surreptitiously takes cover within the nervous system, where it is beyond the routine surveillance of the immune system, and bides time for five to six decades (Barnes 2005). Then in later adulthood it migrates along peripheral nerves to colonize the filamentous neural network that sensitizes areas of skin. Inflamed blotches of skin called "shingles" are the result. Scratching these itching lesions disseminates the virus into a population which, by this time, has been replenished with young susceptible persons. And so the cycle repeats itself.

- The rabies virus, like the chickenpox virus, exploits the immunological sanctuary afforded by the nervous system (Barnes 2005). It achieves its survival goal by migrating to the animal's brain, inducing deranged aggressive behaviour, and so achieving transmission to other canines – or, inadvertently, to humans – via infected saliva from the bite of the rabid animal. Humans, of course, are a "dead end" for the virus since they do not then routinely bite one another.

Once a microbe has successfully colonized a new host species, the infectivity and virulence of the infectious agent evolves in favour of genotypic variants better able to achieve sustained transmission. These genetic adaptations are of various kinds. For example, evolution of the outer antigenic surface of the infecting pathogen usually occurs as a consequence of the selective culling of detectable strains by the immune surveillance system of the infected host.

While a lesser virulence may enhance the transmission probability of the microbe, because its current host can survive longer, in some situations this restraint may not apply. For example, there has been surprise at the unusual virulence of the H5N1 strain of avian influenza in the past several years. It has infected and killed populations of wild birds (normally unaffected by the avian influenza virus) and the case fatality rate in humans has been approximately 50% (much higher than the 5–10% figures of earlier influenza pandemics). A possible reason for this is that the virus has been able to evolve in an unprecedented situation of huge, crowded, stressed flocks of industrially farmed poultry. In that setting, virulence is no disadvantage since other susceptible hosts are crowded against the index host – and, indeed, if virulence were correlated with infectivity, then selection would operate in favour of increased virulence.

Achieving transmissibility is often a challenge for a microbe. A pathogen of low infectivity (reproduction number R less than 1.0) may only infect close contacts, and thus soon fade away. This has occurred with brief outbreaks of Lassa fever and Ebola virus. SARS almost became self-sustaining, but was brought under control within about six months of the first cases appearing. However, insidious new infections with long and silent incubation periods during which the person is infectious are less easy to identify and control. Hence, when a new disease is eventually recognized, as happened with AIDS in the early 1980s, the infection may have already spread extensively within the population and established a foothold. HIV/AIDS has, for the time being, thus become, in microbial terms, a huge success story. Time alone will confirm the durability of this viral infection.

There are some interesting biochemical and molecular "scars" that are left in host populations as a result of adaptive responses to infectious agent challenge. An example in European populations is the genetically based defect in some individuals in their cellular uptake of vitamin D. This may reflect an earlier successful coevolutionary defensive adaptation in cell surface architecture that denied the TB bacterium entry into host cells. The vitamin D molecule and the TB bacterium both use the same molecular cell receptor to gain entry to the cell.

Environmental change and emerging infectious diseases

We humans are, in ecologists' terminology, patch disturbers. We encroach on the natural environment and change its composition, structure and function. This process of human-induced environmental change has been amplified hugely over the past two centuries, as human numbers have surged from approximately 1 million to today's almost 7 billion and as mechanized power and increasing consumer wealth has intensified our economic activities. These increasingly large-scale, systemic changes to the natural environment have a wide range of consequences for the relationships between humans and the world of microbes.

A major conclusion of the recently completed Millennium Ecosystem Assessment (the "MA": a major international 5-year scientific assessment) is that, since around 1950, humans have changed ecosystems more rapidly and extensively than in any comparable period in human history (Millennium Ecosystem Assessment 2005). Many of these changes have achieved increases in carrying capacity, primarily via the extensification of food-producing agro-ecosystems, and have thus contributed to gains in human health. However, in addition to the widespread damage done to soils (salination, erosion, water-logging, chemicalization), this has also caused substantial and largely irreversible losses in the diversity of life on Earth. The MA reported that the rate of species loss in today's world is 3–4 orders of magnitude faster than the natural background rate. We humans are causing the Sixth Great Extinction since vertebrate life emerged half a billion years ago.

This disruption and simplification of ecosystems and associated losses of biodiversity can affect human well-being and health in many ways, reducing nature's various services such as the cleansing of water and air, climate regulation, provision of food, fibre and other essential materials, pollination, carbon sequestration, constraints on mosquito populations and many others.

At this still relatively early stage of our understanding of the problems and risks posed by human-induced ecosystem changes, there have been few studies of how these changes affect human health. Undoubtedly, there are many impacts on the probabilities of infectious disease transmission. For example, changes in ecological relationships and in biodiversity can influence infectious disease risks by altering the balance between reservoir hosts for the infectious agents and between vectors and their predators. Studies have shown how the depletion of certain mammalian species within complex ecological communities leads to an increase in the intensity and efficiency of replication and transmission of certain microbes that can infect humans (e.g. the spirochaete *B. burgdorferi* that causes Lyme Disease), or leads to a greater exposure of humans, no longer protected by other biteable targets, to disease-transmitting mosquitoes (Dobson et al. 2006).

As humans encroach further into previously uncleared or uncultivated environments, new contacts between wild fauna, insect vectors, domesticated livestock and humans increase the risk of cross-species infection. An example of such contact followed the establishment of piggeries close to the tropical forest in Perak, northern Malaysia, where, in 1997–1998, the Nipah virus first crossed over from fruit bats (flying foxes, *Pteropus* spp.) to pigs and thence to pig farmers (Daszak et al. 2006). That zoonotic infection illustrates how the conjunction of intensified animal husbandry in association with large-scale environmental change and ecosystem disruption can potentiate a new zoonotic infection. In that case, forest clearing and, perhaps, El Niño regional drying reduced the natural food supplies for forest fruit bats, the natural reservoir of the virus. The presence of pig farming, in cleared forest settings with associated fruit orchards, then acted as an alternative feeding site for the fruit bats that duly infected the pigs and, thence, the pig farmers.

More generally, the clearance and fragmentation of forests have increased the exposure of Third World rural populations to various infectious diseases, such as the several newly encountered arenaviruses that cause haemorrhagic fevers in South American rural populations (Barnes 2005). Other research has shown that progressively intensive levels of forest clearance in the Peruvian Amazon leads to a several orders of magnitude of increase in the abundance of *Anopheles darlingi* mosquitoes, the major local malaria vector.

Climate change and emerging infectious diseases

Many infectious diseases are sensitive to climatic conditions, particularly vector-borne infections that are transmitted by insects and those that are spread person-to-person via contaminated food and water. Natural climatic variations and events can influence infectious disease emergence. For example, unusually heavy summer rains due to an El Niño event in 1991–1992 stimulated the proliferation of rodent populations in the south-west United States, leading to an unexpected outbreak of the hantavirus infection in humans (Engelthaler 1999). In Australia, studies have shown that rainfall patterns (especially in association with the El Niño cycle), temperature, tidal movements and the ecology of vertebrate host species influence outbreaks of mosquito-borne Ross River virus, the major Australian arboviral infection.

The advent of human-induced climate change has focused new attention on this topic area, since climate change is widely anticipated to affect patterns of infectious disease occurrence. Globally, malaria, dengue fever, cholera, and foodborne infections are of particular concern. They occur widely and frequently around the world and are all sensitive to aspects of climate.

There have been a small number of documented changes in the geographic range and seasonality of several infectious diseases or their vector organisms, in association with observed local changes in climatic conditions. While it is not possible to attribute any one such change to climate change with confidence, when viewed together they constitute a pattern that suggests that climate change is beginning to influence some infectious diseases. Examples include the northwards extension of tick-borne encephalitis (TBE) in Sweden since the mid-1980s, associated with warming winters (Lindgren and Gustafson 2001); the ascent of highland malaria to higher altitudes in some parts of eastern Africa (Patz 2002); and, in the Shanghai region, the northwards drift of the water-snails that spread schistosomiasis (Yang 2005).

We can expect that as today's various global environmental changes (including climate change) continue, with increasing intensity in the immediate future, there will be a growing risk of infectious disease outbreaks and wider dissemin-ation. This unprecedented set of large-scale influences on infectious disease patterns is part of the Fourth Transition, discussed above. It represents yet another influence, pressure, on the ever-evolving relationship between popula-tions of humans and the myriad species and strains of microbes in the world around us.

Conclusion

The chapter title uses the word "struggle". The word is not intended to connote deliberate combat. Rather, it reminds us that the process of achieving and maintaining healthy life, and sustaining it across generations, is not easy. Reduced to essentials, life is necessarily predicated on self-interest, sometimes group-interest. As the physical and biotic environment undergoes change, often rapidly, even chaotically, so species are challenged. Life on Earth has evolved via the morally neutral and random processes of genetic mutation and reassort-ment, enabling the more viable offspring to thrive, reproduce and to occupy the available ecological niche(s). Those processes underlie the age-old and con-tinuing co-evolution of microbes and humans, as each party seeks to survive, remain healthy and reproduce.

After the surprising, chastening infectious disease experiences of the past several decades, we humans will do better in future in our response to infectious disease risks if we think and act in accordance with ecological processes and principles. Crude militaristic thinking and behaviour will not work.

References

Anderson, R. M. and May, R. M. (1991). *Infectious diseases of humans: dynamics and control.* Oxford: Oxford University Press.

Barnes, E. (2005). *Diseases and human evolution.* Albuquerque, NM: University of New Mexico Press.

Bloom, B. R. and Small, P. M. (1998). The evolving relation between humans and Mycobacterium tuberculosis, *New England Journal of Medicine*, 338: 677–678.

Cockburn, A. (1977). *Where did our infectious diseases come from? The evolution of infectious disease. CIBA Foundation Symposium 49.* London: CIBA Foundation.

Crosby, A. (1972). *The Columbian exchange.* Westport, CT: Greenwood.

Crosby, A. (1986). *Ecological imperialism. The biological expansion of Europe, 900–1900.* Cambridge: Cambridge University Press (Canto edition).

Darwin, C. (1839). Journal and remarks 1832–1836, in F. W. Nicholas and J. M. Nicholas (eds) *Charles Darwin in Australia.* Cambridge: Cambridge University Press.

Daszak, P., Plowright, R., Epstein, J. H., et al. (2006). The emergence of Nipah and Hendra virus: pathogen dynamics across a wildlife-livestock-human continuum, in S. K. Collinge and C. Ray (eds) *Disease ecology: community structure and pathogen dynamics*. Oxford: Oxford University Press: 186–201.

Dobson, A., Cattadori, I., Holt, R. D., Ostfeld, R. S. and Keesing, F. (2006). Sacred cows and sympathetic squirrels: the importance of biological diversity to human health, *Public Library of Science and Medicine*, 3: 231–245.

Engelthaler, D. M. (1999). Climatic and environmental patterns associated with hantavirus pulmonary syndrome, Four Corners region, United States, *Emerging Infectious Diseases*, 5(1): 87–94.

Ewald, P. (1994). *Evolution of infectious disease*. New York: Oxford University Press.

Fenner, F. (1957). Myxomatosis in Australian wild rabbits – evolutionary changes in an infectious disease, *Harvey Lecture*, 53: 25–55.

Karlen, A. (1995). *Plague's progress. A social history of disease*. London: Gollancz.

Lindgren, E. and Gustafson, R. (2001). Tick-borne encephalitis in Sweden and climate change, *Lancet*, 358: 16–18.

McMichael, A. J. (2001). *Human frontiers, environments and disease: past patterns, uncertain futures*. Cambridge: Cambridge University Press.

McMichael, A. J. (2006). Climate change and human health: present and future risks, *Lancet*, 3667: 859–869.

McNeil, W. H. (1976). *Plagues and peoples*. Middlesex: Penguin.

Millennium Ecosystem Assessment (2005). *Ecosystems and human wellbeing: synthesis*. Washington, D.C.: Island Press.

Patz, J. A. (2002). Regional warming and malaria resurgence, *Nature*, 420: 627–628.

Taubenberger, J. K., Reid, A. H., Lourens, R. M. and Wang, R. (2005). Characterization of the 1918 influenza virus polymerase genes, *Nature*, 437: 889–893.

Taylor, L. H., Latham, S. M. and Woolhouse, M. E. (2001). Risk factors for human disease emergence, *Philosophical Transactions: Biological Sciences*, 356: 983–989.

Tumpey, T. M., Basler, C. F., Aguilar, P.V., et al. (2005). Characterization of the reconstructed 1918 Spanish Influenza Pandemic Virus, *Science*, 310: 77–80.

Weiss, R. and McMichael, A. J. (2004). Social and environmental risk factors in the emergence of infectious diseases, *Nature Medicine*, 10: 70–76.

Yang, G. J. (2005). A potential impact of climate change and water resource development on the transmission of Schistosoma japonicum in China, *Parasitologia*, 47(1): 127–134.

chapter five

Communicable disease in Europe

**Shazia Karmali, Andrew Amato-Gauci,
Andrea Ammon, Martin McKee**

Introduction

This book is about the response to communicable disease in societies undergoing transition. This chapter, and the accompanying one on Latin America and
the Caribbean, describe the patterns and trends in communicable disease in ECA.
This is a region that has seen major transitions in recent years, as discussed by
McKee and Falkingham in Chapter 2. As McMichael makes clear, in Chapter 4,
microorganisms excel in their ability to adapt to changing circumstances. Consequently, as Europeans and the environments they inhabit change, so too do
the microorganisms that attack them. The changes driving this evolutionary
process include:

- an ageing population, with implications for the population's herd immunity,
  leading to increased susceptibility to certain infections;
- climate change, with global warming facilitating the spread of vectors of
  tropical diseases beyond their traditional habitats;
- increased travel and migration increasing contact with diseases not endemic
  in the EU;
- societal changes, such as urbanization, which increases the intensity of sustained interaction among individuals living in close proximity to one another,
  facilitating the spread of respiratory disease in particular;
- changing sexual mores, increasing the risk of sexually transmitted infections
  (STIs);
- resistance in response to overuse of antibiotics.

This chapter reviews the end result of these changes, looking at how the
epidemiology of some important communicable diseases is changing.

Brucellosis

Brucellosis is a disease whose epidemiology is changing. It is the most common zoonotic infection worldwide (Pappas et al. 2006) and is caused by bacteria of the genus *Brucella*. Variants have different animal reservoirs, including cattle (*B. abortus*), dogs (*B. canis*), sheep, goats and camel (*B. melitensis*), and pigs (*B. suis*) but *B. melitensis* is the most common species and is thought to be responsible for up to 90% of cases worldwide (Amato-Gauci and Ammon 2007; Memish and Balkhy 2004). Infection can occur through a myriad of exposures, including direct or indirect contact with animals or with contaminated animal products such as milk, cheese and other dairy products, as well as from the inhalation of aerosols. Thus, those at greatest risk are individuals working with domestic animals and animal products.

Clinical presentation of Brucellosis is as diverse as its modes of infection and, after an incubation period of 5 to 60 days, symptoms can appear either acutely or go unnoticed (Amato-Gauci and Ammon 2007). Without treatment, symptoms can become chronic, in some cases leading to death. However, many cases go unnoticed altogether.

Although no human vaccine is available, the disease can be controlled in animals by a combination of immunization, test-and-slaughter of infected animals, and pasteurization of milk and dairy products.

In the EU the incidence of Brucellosis has been declining, except in the Republic of Northern Ireland. Indeed, Sweden, Denmark, Finland, Germany, the remainder of the United Kingdom, Austria, the Netherlands, Belgium and Luxembourg are now "Officially Brucellosis-Free" (OBF) and re-emergence of human brucellosis is considered unlikely given the existence of effective surveillance systems (Pappas et al. 2006). The disease remains endemic in many parts of Spain, with occasional cases in neighbouring areas of France and Portugal, attributed to consumption of dairy products from across the border. It also remains endemic in Greece, with evidence of underreporting of cases along the Greek-Albanian border.

In marked contrast, there has been a resurgence in many parts of the former Soviet Union, where Pappas et al. (Pappas et al. 2006) have described "... a seemingly uncontrollable, constantly increasing incidence [which] poses a serious public health problem, especially in the context of inadequately developed health care networks".

A study of trends of infection in two districts in Kyrgyzstan identified exposure to aborted home-owned animals and consumption of home-made milk products obtained from bazaars or neighbours as probable sources of infection in humans (Kozukeev et al. 2006). Control of the disease in central Asia was always particularly fragile since a substantial percentage of the population is reliant on livestock for survival. However, it seems that the most important factor in its increasing incidence has been the transition from a socialist state to a free market economy, which has led to a reduction in support for state veterinary services.

Campylobacter

The campylobacters, consisting of *campylobacter jejuni* and *campylobacter coli*, are responsible for 5–14% of all diarrhoea worldwide (Ashbolt 2004). The most common risk factor for infection is the consumption of contaminated food and/or water (Amato-Gauci and Ammon 2007). Swimming in natural surface waters and direct contact with infected animals have also been identified as risk factors. Symptoms usually occur following an incubation period of 2–5 days and present with severe abdominal pain, watery and/or bloody diarrhoea and fever.

Campylobacter disproportionately affects children under four years of age in developed countries and children under two years in developing countries (Ashbolt 2004). Within the EU, notification of campylobacter infection has increased steadily, although this is likely to reflect more stringent reporting (Amato-Gauci and Ammon 2007). The highest incidence rates were reported by the Czech Republic, followed by the United Kingdom. In the Czech Republic, Lithuania and Slovakia, over 99% of cases were reported as being domestic in origin, compared with Sweden and Finland, where approximately 50% of cases were identified as imported (Amato-Gauci and Ammon 2007).

Many countries experience a seasonal peak in cases between June and September. One study hypothesized that these seasonal fluctuations in infection were due to a combination of changes in human behaviour that increase exposure and seasonal variations in the prevalence of campylobacter in reservoirs (Nylen et al. 2002), although it was not possible to obtain definitive evidence for either mechanism in the nine European countries studied.

Diphtheria

Diphtheria, once a common childhood infection, was brought under control in Europe by universal childhood immunization in the 20th century. It is transmitted by the direct projection of droplets containing the bacteria *corynebacterium diphtheriae* and is especially dangerous because of its production of a toxin that can potentially cause myocarditis, paralytic symptoms and nephritis. Thus, even with treatment, infection of non-immunized individuals can be fatal (Amato-Gauci and Ammon 2007).

As noted in Chapter 1, control of diphtheria broke down in the countries that had emerged from the Soviet Union in the early 1990s, initially among large urban centres such as Moscow, St Petersburg and Kiev, before spreading to other parts of the country (Dittman et al. 2000). This was attributed to six factors that characterized the sociopolitical situation in the region at the time:

- large-scale population movements
- socioeconomic instability
- partial deterioration of the health infrastructure
- delay in implementing aggressive measures to control the epidemic
- inadequate information for physicians and the public, and
- lack of adequate supplies for prevention and treatment in many countries.

A second central Asian epidemic was thought to have originated in Afghanistan, spreading through Tajikistan, Uzbekistan and Kyrgyzstan; however, outbreaks in Kazakhstan have been linked to the epidemic in the western part of the former USSR (Dittman et al. 2000).

Since then there has been a marked decrease in incidence since the mid-1990s, with Latvia reporting most cases since 1995. Most reported cases are among children between the ages of 0 and 4 primarily, followed by children aged 5–14 years. In total, 12 out of 25 EU countries have reported no cases in recent years, although it is believed that there is some failure to report what are now rare cases, making it difficult to gain a full picture of current trends (Amato-Gauci and Ammon 2007).

HIV/AIDS

The human immunodeficiency virus (HIV) is now well established within populations in ECA. Eastern Europe and central Asia are disproportionately affected, with an estimated 1.5 million people living with HIV at the end of 2005, 200 000 of whom were infected within that year. The corresponding numbers are lower in western and central Europe, where 720 000 persons were thought to have been living with HIV in the same year, with 20 000 new infections (UNAIDS 2006). In eastern Europe the incidence peaked in 2001, after which it declined but is once again rising. It is also rising steadily in western Europe.

Two types of HIV are known to exist: HIV-1 and HIV-2, of which HIV-1 is more virulent and produces a more severe infection. Most HIV infections are due to HIV-1. In other respects, HIV-1 and HIV-2 behave similarly. HIV is a retrovirus transmitted through the exchange of bodily fluids (infected blood, semen, vaginal fluid or breast milk) through sexual contact, the sharing of needles, syringes, or (less commonly) blood transfusions. Transmission can also occur from infected mother to newborn during birth or through breastfeeding.

Ultimately, progressive reduction in CD4 T lymphocytes and increased viral load leads to the development of the acquired immunodeficiency syndrome (AIDS). This is characterized by the presence of one or more opportunistic illnesses. It may take a very long time to progress from infection to the manifestation of disease. As a consequence, assessment of the spread and burden of the epidemic is no longer based on surveillance of cases of AIDS, but of HIV infection.

Availability of data on the prevalence of HIV infection is highly variable among countries, with surveillance programmes having varying degrees of coverage and having been in existence for varying periods.

In the EU, the predominant source of infection is through heterosexual transmission, with an increasing number of cases among migrants from high-prevalence countries outside Europe. Of all cases of heterosexual transmission, at least one partner was a migrant from a high-prevalence country in 47% of all newly diagnosed infections in the European Economic Area (EEA), ranging from 17% in Portugal to 80% in Iceland. Transmission among men having sex with men (MSM) appears to have declined around the year 2000, after which it began to rise again. Similarly, infections among injecting drug users has declined, although data are unavailable from Estonia, Italy, Spain and Portugal, so this observation should be treated with caution. Mother-to-child transmission accounts for less than 1% of all new HIV infections in the EEA.

The prevalence of HIV infection is unevenly distributed by age and gender. In general, HIV is more prevalent in men, who account for up to 63% of known cases, as well as those between the ages of 30–39 years, who account for 43% of known cases. However, these figures are based on diagnosed infections and it is estimated that undiagnosed infections may contribute anything from 15% of total cases in Sweden to up to 60% in Poland.

The HIV/AIDS epidemic in central Asia is driven predominantly by injecting drug use. The political, economic and social environment in the region following the collapse of the Soviet Union has given rise to conditions facilitating rapid transmission of HIV, a situation exacerbated by the location of these countries on the narcotic trafficking route between Afghanistan and Europe. Drivers of the epidemic in the region "... include a rapid increase in drug use and commercial sex, concurrent epidemics of sexually transmitted diseases, migration, poverty, stigma and a lack of awareness of safe behaviours ... exacerbated by the limited capacity to deliver effective responses, in part, due to weaknesses in health systems" (Mounier et al. 2007).

There is considerable diversity among countries in this subregion (Table 5.1). The overall increase in the years leading up to 2001 was due largely to what was happening in Kazakhstan, as was the subsequent decline. In contrast, infections are rising steadily in neighbouring countries. The virtual absence of recorded infections in Turkmenistan reflects the ban imposed by the Government, under the late President Niyazov, on notifying certain infectious diseases. This was a means of "*assur[ing] the international community of the absolute well-being and the complete non-existence of any contagious diseases and problems with medication and treatment in Turkmenistan*" (Rechel and McKee 2007). As a result, by 2004 only two cases of HIV/AIDS had been reported from Turkmenistan. However, the known existence of an epidemic of injecting drug use (with credible reports of involvement by senior politicians in the narcotics trade), along with widespread sex work (especially involving the many health workers removed from their

Table 5.1 Newly diagnosed cases of HIV infection, by year of report (rate/million population)

	Kazakhstan	Kyrgyzstan	Tajikistan	Turkmenistan*	Uzbekistan
1997	437 (27.0)	2 (0.4)	1 (0.2)	0 (0.0)	7 (0.3)
1998	299 (18.7)	6 (1.3)	1 (0.2)	0 (0.0)	3 (0.1)
1999	185 (11.7)	10 (2.1)	0 (0.0)	1 (0.0)	28 (1.1)
2000	347 (22.2)	16 (3.3)	7 (1.1)	0 (0.0)	154 (6.2)
2001	1175 (75.6)	149 (29.8)	37 (6.0)	0 (0.0)	549 (21.7)
2002	694 (44.9)	162 (32.0)	29 (4.7)	0 (0.0)	981 (38.2)
2003	747 (25.3)	130 (25.3)	42 (6.7)	0 (0.0)	1836 (70.4)
2004	157 (30.1)	157 (30.1)	198 (31.4)	0 (0.0)	2016 (76.1)

Source: Mounier et al. 2007.

Note: * Due to the political climate, data from Turkmenistan are not credible and believed to be a substantial underestimate.

posts) suggests a potentially large undiscovered epidemic. Turkmenistan is the only central Asian country not receiving support from the Global Fund (Rechel and McKee 2007).

Although 75% of infections in central Asia have been linked to injecting drug use, with many others among commercial sex workers and their contacts (Godinho et al. 2005), effective action has been constrained by limited access to harm-reduction strategies and punitive legal sanctions aimed at high-risk populations, leading to stigma, with infected and/or high-risk individuals facing many obstacles to obtaining support (Mounier et al. 2007).

It has been suggested that once HIV prevalence reaches 10–20% among a high-risk group, the epidemic is likely to become self-perpetuating (Friedman et al. 2000). Although strategies have been developed that propose multisectoral responses to the epidemic within a number of central Asian countries, legal and structural barriers, limited involvement of NGOs, low technical capacity and inadequately trained health professionals pose major challenges to the implementation of effective measures (Mounier et al. 2007).

Hepatitis A

Hepatitis A is caused by a small RNA virus belonging to the genus Hepatovirus, transmitted through the faecal-oral route, person-to-person contact, or by the ingestion of contaminated food or water (Amato-Gauci and Ammon 2007; Poovorawan, Chatchatee and Chongsrisawat 2002). Presentation is closely related to the age of the infected individual, with children below the age of six often asymptomatic and adults presenting with symptoms including jaundice and fever, loss of appetite, nausea and vomiting (Poovorawan, Chatchatee and Chongsrisawat 2002). Infections are most frequent in children under 15 years of age (Poovorawan, Chatchatee and Chongsrisawat 2002).

This differential presentation has implications for the epidemiology of Hepatitis A. Improvements in hygiene and environmental sanitation, particularly during food production mean that fewer children are being affected, leaving an increasing number of adults susceptible to the disease (Poovorawan, Chatchatee and Chongsrisawat 2002).

Overall, there has been a general decrease in incidence across Europe (Amato-Gauci and Ammon 2007) but considerable differences remain. Based on trends since the mid-1990s, central and eastern European countries within the EU have been divided into two groups, based on the degree of endemicity. Countries considered to be of intermediate endemicity include Slovakia, the Czech Republic, Poland and Bulgaria, reporting an incidence of approximately 10 per 100 000 population. Countries transitioning *towards* intermediate endemicity were Estonia, Lithuania, Latvia, the Russian Federation and Romania, some of which had reported an incidence of greater than 50 per 100 000 (Amato-Gauci and Ammon 2007; Poovorawan, Chatchatee and Chongsrisawat 2002). As of 2005, only Slovakia and Latvia continued to report more than 5 cases per 100 000 population.

As the traditional methods of transmission have declined in importance, other factors are accounting for a greater share of infections. These include migration of individuals from high-incidence regions and sexual transmission between MSM (Amato-Gauci and Ammon 2007).

Hepatitis B

Hepatitis B is caused by the hepatitis B virus and can cause either an asymptomatic or a symptomatic infection which can be acute or chronic, following an incubation period of up to six months. Chronically infected individuals are at a higher risk of developing complications such as liver cirrhosis and cancer, and act as reservoirs for the virus. The virus can be transmitted through contact with blood or bodily fluids of an infected individual (Amato-Gauci and Ammon 2007).

There are three common routes of transmission: sexual contact, injecting drug use, and nosocomial infection from contaminated instruments (including needles) in health care settings. All of these factors have been changing within Europe, in different ways in different places, with implications for the epidemiology of Hepatitis B.

The highest incidences tend to be among adults between the ages of 25 and 44, with men twice as likely to acquire the disease than women (Amato-Gauci and Ammon 2007). Within the EU, Austria and Belgium have reported increasing numbers of infections, while Estonia, Latvia, Lithuania and Luxembourg all have incidences significantly higher than the EU average (Amato-Gauci and Ammon 2007). There is, however, an overall decline in incidence in the EU.

The situation in South-eastern Europe and many parts of the former Soviet Union is much less clear. Data are difficult to obtain, but what information is available suggests that annual incidence rates may be between 20 and 100 per 100 000. Seroprevalence within central Asia has been found to be as high as 46.7% in Kyrgyzstan (Custer et al. 2004).

Hepatitis C

Caused by the hepatitis C virus, an RNA virus belonging to the Flaviviridae family, hepatitis C is most often manifest as a chronic illness; clinical evidence of acute infection is much less common (Amato-Gauci and Ammon 2007). Humans are the only reservoir. Infection occurs mainly through exposure to infected blood through blood transfusions, sharing of infected needles among injecting drug users, or occupationally, as with needle-stick injuries (Poovorawan, Chatchatee and Chongsrisawat 2002). Chronic infection can lead to liver cirrhosis and cancer over time, with hepatitis C the leading cause of liver cancer and the main indication for liver transplantation in Europe and the United States (Amato-Gauci and Ammon 2007).

Within Europe, the lowest prevalence rates are observed in north-western Europe, with intermediate rates in eastern European, Mediterranean and Asian countries. Wasley and Alter (2000) describes three patterns of infection, with implications for the future burden of liver disease. In many western countries the risk of transmission was highest in the recent past (10–30 years ago) among those who were then young adults (Wasley and Alter 2000). This is thought to be due primarily to injecting drug use, suggesting that the burden of liver disease attributable to hepatitis C has yet to reach its peak.

Countries such as Italy and Japan display a low prevalence among children and young adults but a sharp increase among older people. Here the risk of transmission was highest in the more distant past (30–50 years ago). It is assumed that the resulting burden of liver disease has already peaked in these populations.

The third pattern is characterized by a steady but high prevalence among all age groups. The risk of infection has remained high for many decades and is expected to continue to do so, leading to a persisting high level of liver disease.

Unfortunately, in many parts of eastern Europe and central Asia, data on the prevalence of infection remain extremely limited, making predictions of the future burden of disease difficult (Amato-Gauci and Ammon 2007).

Giardiasis

Giardiasis is a parasitic, cyst-producing protozoan known to settle in the human and animal bowel. Following infection, individuals are either asymptomatic or develop acute or chronic diarrhoea. Children and infants appear to be at higher risk of infection. Although contaminated surface waters are primary reservoirs of the parasite, transmission is most commonly through personal contact with infected persons, or through exposure to contaminated food or water. It is for this reason that outbreaks may be more common in nursing homes, day-care centres and orphanages (Amato-Gauci and Ammon 2007; Ekdahl and Andersson 2005).

Data from 11 EEA countries suggest a relatively stable trend since the mid-1990s (Amato-Gauci and Ammon 2007) but reported variations among countries are, at least in part, thought to reflect differences in the quality of surveillance. For this reason, authorities have sought to assess the burden of disease by monitoring travellers returning from endemic regions. Thus, a study among Swedish travellers found most cases originated in the Russian Federation, followed by Romania, Turkey, the former Yugoslavia and Bulgaria (Amato-Gauci and Ammon 2007). This may reflect a situation in which construction of housing and tourist resorts has expanded more rapidly than the supporting infrastructure, leading to weaknesses in the supply of clean water.

Infections have also been linked to migration, with a study from Sweden identifying an especially high prevalence among immigrants and refugees from Afghanistan (Ekdahl and Andersson 2005). Children adopted from eastern European countries were also identified as having a high prevalence of the disease, especially those adopted from Ukraine, Belarus, Latvia, Bulgaria and Romania (Ekdahl and Andersson 2005). A recent study of 30 GeoSentinal sites monitoring the frequency and cause of common illnesses among travellers returning from various regions also confirmed the disproportionately high prevalence of Giardiasis among travellers returning from south-central Asia (Freedman et al. 2006).

Influenza

Influenza is a viral disease of the respiratory tract, transmitted through large airborne droplets or fomites (Amato-Gauci and Ammon 2007). Three recognizable variations of the influenza virus are known to infect humans. These are influenza A, B and C. Seasonal influenza epidemics are known to occur during winter months. The intensity and variation of the winter epidemics and annual incidence is due to constant changes in the genetic make-up of the human influenza virus. The morbidity and mortality rates associated with the seasonal epidemic are 0.2% and 0.1% respectively, affecting mostly the elderly and the very young, as well as individuals with severe chronic conditions (Amato-Gauci and Ammon 2007).

Influenza is the classic example of a disease whose epidemiology reflects changes in the nature of the infectious agent. The pandemics that have occurred throughout history have emerged as a consequence of either antigenic shift within a subtype or recombination of genetic material between different subtypes. The speed with which the virus can traverse the globe has been increased greatly by the advent of intercontinental flights.

The constant threat of a pandemic and our inability to predict with precision when this threat might manifest, as well as the high level of resulting mortality, morbidity, and economic losses, has given influenza preparedness a very high political profile.

Immunization is effective (although recent research has questioned whether it is equally so in the very elderly) but must be repeated annually to provide coverage against newly emerging subtypes. Planning is essential. WHO has noted that ". . . once a pandemic begins it will be too late to accomplish the many activities required to minimize its impact" (Mounier-Jack and Coker 2006).

Legionnaires' disease

The Legionellae bacteria is important because of its ability to survive in high-temperature environments (Amato-Gauci and Ammon 2007). As a consequence, modern architecture has provided it with an evolutionary advantage as it can thrive in cooling towers, evaporative condensers, humidifiers, decorative fountains, and hot water systems. Infection is by airborne transmission. As a consequence, many outbreaks have been linked to large modern building complexes, such as tourist resorts. Treatment with antibiotics is generally effective but case fatality rates are disproportionately high among elderly and immuno-compromised individuals.

The overall reported incidence of Legionnaires' disease in the EU increased between 1996 and 2002, after which it plateaued at a rate of 1 per 100 000 (Amato-Gauci and Ammon 2007). Individuals over the age of 65 contribute approximately 81% of reported cases, with the age group 45–65 following close behind. The incidence is significantly higher in men than in women (Ricketts, McNaught and Joseph 2006).

While there are many localized outbreaks affecting individuals within a single country, the risk posed by cooling systems in tourist resorts, where individuals from many countries may come together briefly (and in large numbers as a result of low air fares), has posed a particular challenge for those engaged in surveillance. This has led to the creation of EWGLINET, a surveillance network monitoring travel-associated cases, linking, where possible, cases occurring in different countries back to a common source (Hutchinson, Joseph and Bartlett 1996).

In 2003–2004 the highest number of cases reported was from Spain, followed by Croatia and Switzerland. That same year, Bulgaria, Latvia, Lithuania, Poland and Slovakia reported the lowest incidence, but again, underrecognition of cases must be considered (Ricketts and Joseph 2005).

Leptospirosis

Leptospirosis is a zoonotic disease with symptoms such as fever, headache, chills, myalgia and conjuctival suffusion. Serious complications can result, including liver, kidney, lung, heart and cerebral involvement and haemorrhagic symptoms, albeit rarely. It infects humans mainly through contact with urine of infected animals or with contaminated soil or water. Since the mid-1980s there has been a shift from occupational to recreational exposure in some South-eastern European countries such as Bulgaria, reflecting changing patterns of human activity (Christova, Tasseva and Manev 2003).

Measles

Measles is a highly infectious disease of childhood. Although most cases are relatively mild, it can have very serious, and on occasions fatal, manifestations. It is, however, easily prevented by immunization. The WHO European Region has set a target of eliminating measles by 2010 but progress has been patchy in many countries. Since 2000 France, Germany and Italy have reported incidence rates between 5 and 42 per 100 000, whereas in some other countries these are 1 per 100 000 or lower (Amato-Gauci and Ammon 2007). In central and eastern Europe, there have been considerable reductions in incidence since the mid-1990s, reflecting increased financial support for immunization (Spika et al. 2003). In contrast, weak health and social infrastructures in some central Asian republics have made it difficult to extend immunization coverage (Veenema 2000).

Malaria

Carried by the *Anopheles* mosquito, four species of protozoans belonging to the genus Plasmodium (falciparum, vivax, ovale and malariae) are responsible for causing malaria in humans.

Once endemic in many parts of Europe (including areas such as southern England as recently as the 17th century) (Hutchinson and Lindsay 2006), malaria was eradicated from western Europe during the 20th century (de Zulueta 1998), with the exception of small numbers of imported cases and, exceptionally, transmission in the vicinity of international airports during warm weather (Van den Ende et al. 1998). It is, however, important to note that the conditions for transmission of malaria, in particular the presence of *Anopheles* mosquitoes, persist and there is an ever-present risk of re-establishment of the disease as a consequence of climate change. Malaria was also eradicated in the Soviet Union in the 1960s and 1970s, but in some places, such as Tajikistan, it has reappeared (Pitt et al. 1998). An epidemic in Afghanistan in 1998, resulting in an estimated 2–3 million cases, was critical in spreading malaria to other parts of central Asia, particularly along the border of Tajikistan (Kiszewski and Teklehaimanot 2004).

A deterioration in the agricultural infrastructure of the former Soviet Union in Azerbaijan has left large, dismantled irrigation canals (Temel 2004), built to support collective farms producing cotton. These are inappropriate for the new model of small, fragmented, private farms growing fruit and vegetables and have created ideal mosquito-breeding habitats. The situation is exacerbated by the dismantling of former state-organized antimalarial measures.

In Uzbekistan, eradication was achieved by 1961, only to reappear recently (Severini et al. 2004). This resurgence has been attributed to four factors:

- natural and climatic conditions favourable for malaria transmission;
- marked deterioration of malaria control in the neighbouring states Tajikistan, Afghanistan and Kyrgyzstan;
- migration between countries, particularly through people displaced from Tajikistan;
- shortage of trained staff, basic laboratory equipment and insecticides.

It is reasonable to assume that these factors are similarly important in Uzbekistan's neighbours.

Syphilis

Syphilis is an infection that is manifest as both an STI and through mother–child transmission, as congenital syphilis. Consequently, as with other STIs, its epidemiology reflects changes in human behaviour. Humans are the only reservoir for *Treponema pallidum*, the bacterium responsible for the disease (Amato-Gauci and Ammon 2007). Following an incubation period of 10–90 days, clinical presentation of syphilis initially includes a primary lesion, followed by a series of eruptions of mucocutaneous lesions, otherwise known as secondary syphilis. This stage is followed by long periods of latency, called latent or tertiary syphilis which may lead to tertiary syphilis lesions if left untreated. Serious vascular and neurological damage, as well as visceral and multi-organ involvement can occur in the absence of adequate treatment. The association of syphilis with HIV infection is of growing concern (Zeltzer and Kurban 2004).

The majority of cases occur in men, and within the age group of 25–44 years (Amato-Gauci and Ammon 2007). In western Europe, incidence decreased overall from 1996 to 2000 but, since then, there has been a steady rise in some places, especially in large cities among MSM and people using elicit drugs (Hook and Peeling 2004).

In eastern Europe and central Asia, syphilis has exhibited a pattern similar to that of HIV/AIDS and hepatitis C, reaching epidemic proportions in the early 1990s following the collapse of the former USSR (Amato-Gauci and Ammon 2007). Dramatic and alarming increases were seen in many countries until about 1997 (Table 5.2), following which they began to decline, albeit to levels still far above those before independence. Care is, however, required in interpreting the recent decline, which is thought to result, in part, from a reduced intensity of case finding, and a shift in utilization from public to private/informal sectors, which were less likely to engage in formal case reporting (Riedner, Dehne and Gromyko 2000).

Widespread availability of treatment, coupled with a high level of awareness among health professionals, meant that, prior to the 1990s congenital syphilis was very rare in eastern Europe and the former Soviet Union, but there has been a slight resurgence in some countries in recent years (Walker and Walker 2007).

Tick-borne encephalitis

The distribution of TBE in Europe has changed markedly since the early 1990s. The disease is endemic in central Europe (especially Austria, Croatia and Slovenia) and northern Europe (the Baltic states, Sweden and Finland) (Gritsun, Lashkevich and Gould 2003) but has been declining in the former and increasing in the latter (Charrel et al. 2004).

The most common hosts of the virus are small rodents, with ticks serving as vectors and reservoirs of the virus. Infections occur most frequently between April and November, with the transmission of infection arising when a very complex set of conditions come together, including temperature, humidity, patterns of land use, and human activity. The prevalence of ticks infected with the TBE virus in Europe has been found to vary, on average, from 0.5% to 5%, with the Russian Federation having recorded a prevalence of 40% in some regions.

The reasons for the changing distribution are increasingly well understood. Initial work suggested that climate change was the driving force but a detailed study of TBE in the Baltic states around the time of the collapse of the Soviet

Table 5.2 Trends in the incidence of syphilis in central Asia

Country	Baseline to peak year	Percentage increase	Rate in 2003
Kazakhstan	1991–1997	100+ fold increase	50 times rate in 1991
Kyrgyzstan	1990–1997	90-fold increase	30 times rate in 1991
Tajikistan	1990–1998	90-fold increase	6 times rate in 1991
Uzbekistan	1990–1997	30-fold increase	15 times rate in 1991

Source: Renton et al. 2006.

Union indicates that changing human activity may have played a major role (Sumilo et al. 2007). Between 1992 and 1993, the incidence of TBE in Estonia increased by 64%, while in Latvia the figure was 175% and Lithuania 1065%. These changes have been linked to a number of phenomena taking place at that time. One was the collapse of collective farming, with a shift in land cover from agriculture and pasture to wooded land leading to increases in the rodent populations, the reservoirs for the TBE virus. Another was changing behaviour, with more people visiting forests. The decline in central Europe seems, at least in part, to reflect the expansion of immunization coverage (Zenz et al. 2005).

Tularaemia

Tularaemia is caused by the bacterium *Francisella tularensis*. It is a zoonosis involving animals such as rabbits, hares, squirrels, foxes and ticks, which serve as both reservoirs and transmitters of the infection (Amato-Gauci and Ammon 2007). It can be spread by a variety of routes, including tick bites, ingestion, inhalation, or contact with the conjunctiva, each leading to different clinical manifestations. Tularaemia attracted attention from researchers in the United States and the USSR in the 1980s because of its potential as a biological warfare agent, but since then interest waned before being rekindled in recent years as outbreaks have occurred in areas where the disease was thought to have been controlled. These include northern Scandinavia, Turkey and Slovakia (Tarnvik and Berglund 2003).

Its method of transmission means that outbreaks often occur in response to situations where contact between humans and wild animals is changing. An example is the emergence of disease following the conflict in Kosovo in 1999–2000 (Tarnvik and Berglund 2003). Elsewhere, hunting of hares and crayfish fishing have been implicated in outbreaks in Spain, whereas two outbreaks reported in Bulgaria are thought to result from increases in rodent populations leading to contamination of water or food (Christova et al. 2004).

Tuberculosis

Caused by *Mycobacterium tuberculosis*, TB is a disease affecting many human organs but most often the lungs (Amato-Gauci and Ammon 2007). It is most commonly acquired through the inhalation of bacteria-rich droplets from another person with pulmonary disease, but alimentary infection can arise from ingestion of contaminated milk. Only 5–10% of those infected go on to develop active disease but this is much higher in individuals who are immuno-compromised, for example as a result of infection with HIV.

TB is a disease of poverty. A total of 86% of cases reported in 2005 within the WHO European Region were from outside the EU, and mostly from countries of the former Soviet Union (Amato-Gauci and Ammon 2007). Within the EU, the highest incidences are found in the three Baltic states and, in all countries, TB disproportionately affects migrants, homeless people, prisoners and drug users. In the context of an overall decline in incidence, a few EU countries, such as

Sweden and the United Kingdom, have experienced recent increases, largely attributed to cases among migrants from high-incidence countries (Amato-Gauci and Ammon 2007).

In all the countries of the former Soviet Union, the incidence of TB remains higher than in the early 1990s, although some countries are experiencing recent declines, most notably the three Baltic states. Rates are, however, continuing to increase in central Asia (Dye 2006).

Factors driving the epidemic in this region include economic decline, a growth in marginalized populations and weaknesses in TB control programmes (many of which continue to use ineffective forms of treatment from the Soviet era (Dye 2006). Those in prison have a greatly elevated risk of infection, although the incidence in Russian prisons at least has reduced substantially in recent years (Bobrik et al. 2005). A case-control study undertaken in the Russian Federation confirmed the importance of being in prison as a risk factor, although affecting a small number of people. In terms of the population-attributable risk the most important factors were unemployment and drinking unpasteurized milk (Coker, McKee and Atun 2006).

Effective pharmaceuticals to treat TB have been available since the 1940s. Yet, reflecting the perennial ability of microorganisms to adapt to changing circumstances, resistance is becoming a major problem in some countries. The former Soviet Union has been described as "one large hot spot for MDR-TB" (Cox et al. 2004). This reflects several factors, in particular disrupted courses of treatment, especially when individuals are discharged from prison and are unable to access care rapidly in the outside world, but also, in some places, the use of counterfeit and thus inactive drugs. Thus, rates of MDR-TB can be considered a marker of health system failure.

TB infection is now inextricably linked with HIV, an issue that is explored in detail in several subsequent chapters of this book. Consequently, effective control measures must take a holistic approach, addressing the causes of both diseases, many of which overlap, while providing integrated and sustainable treatment models (Atun et al. 2007).

Variant Creutzfeldt-Jakob Disease

The disease known as vCJD is another disease whose emergence is a direct result of changes in human behaviour. It is caused by prions (a form of infectious protein) and its clinical manifestation is characterized by progressive neurological deterioration and death (Amato-Gauci and Ammon 2007).

It is now clear that the spread of this disease to humans (there are other inherited forms of CJD) was a direct consequence of changes in the production of animal feed in the 1990s. So far, 199 fatal cases have been documented worldwide, out of which 162 have been in the United Kingdom and three of which were due to infected blood transfusions. Other European countries to have reported the disease include France, Ireland, Italy, Portugal, Spain and the Netherlands (Amato-Gauci and Ammon 2007). Although initial concerns about the potential extent of infection with this agent do not seem to have been realized, the political and economic implications of this disease, and in particular the failings that allowed it to emerge, have been substantial (Amato-Gauci and Ammon 2007).

West Nile virus

This is another infection that has spread rapidly from its origin. First isolated in Uganda in 1937, West Nile virus has subsequently been reported in other parts of Africa, parts of Europe, west and central Asia, Australia and the Middle East, finally reaching North America in the 1990s (Mukhopadhyay et al. 2003). West Nile virus is a Flaviviridae, belonging to the genus *Flavivirus*. Wild birds and mosquitoes serve as reservoirs, with most infections in humans resulting from mosquito bites (Amato-Gauci and Ammon 2007).

Following an incubation period of 1–6 days after an infectious bite, symptoms of West Nile virus reflect the age of the infected individual, ranging from a mild fever and Dengue-like clinical presentation in young children to meningo-encephalitis in the elderly. There are no effective treatments or preventive measures beyond avoiding mosquito bites (Amato-Gauci and Ammon 2007).

Outbreaks have been reported from Romania (1996), the Russian Federation (1999) and more recently France and Portugal. In addition, novel virus strains closely related to West Nile virus are circulating in central Europe and southern parts of the Russian Federation (Vorou, Papavassiliou and Tsiodras 2007). The reasons for the changing pattern of West Nile virus remain poorly understood but seem likely to include a combination of climate change and changes in land use. However, migration patterns of birds are also important and two isolates in birds in the same part of Hungary were found to have genetic structures consistent with separate origins, in central Africa and in Israel (Bakonyi et al. 2006). The strain of virus detected in the United States is similar to a strain that had previously been circulating in Israel (Lanciotti et al. 1999).

Antimicrobial resistance

Antimicrobial resistance is considered separately in this chapter. It is of critical importance in a book about the health system response to communicable disease, as its emergence is entirely a consequence of health systems. In the constant evolutionary struggle between humans and microorganisms, in which the latter can multiply at a vastly quicker pace than the former, the emergence of strains of microorganisms that are resistant to antibiotics and, increasingly, anti-viral agents (especially in the case of HIV), is virtually inevitable. However, the widespread variation in the rate at which resistance emerges in different populations provides clear evidence that much can be done to slow this process. It is now quite clear that antibiotic misuse is the "main selective pressure driving resistance" (Goossens et al. 2005).

The use of antibiotics varies markedly within and between countries. Often they are prescribed unnecessarily for viral infections, or broad-spectrum antibiotics are used to counter infections caused by unknown microorganisms in the hope that they will have an effect (Amato-Gauci and Ammon 2007;

Goossens et al. 2005). There is a strong association, at an ecological level, between antibiotic use (or misuse) and the development of antimicrobial resistance (Goossens et al. 2005; Jacobs 2003).

Clearly, the solution lies in more careful and judicious use of antibiotics, yet this requires the existence of a range of governance and quality-assurance mechanisms, locally, nationally and internationally, that often do not exist (Goossens et al. 2005).

Within the EU antibiotic resistance tends to increase as one moves from northern Europe to South-eastern Europe (Amato-Gauci and Ammon 2007). This correlates with other evidence on the type of antibiotics used in ambulatory care. In Nordic countries the most common products are older, narrow-spectrum antibiotics, while newer, broad-spectrum antibiotics are used more often in other parts of Europe.

It must, however, be noted that the available data provide an incomplete picture. In many parts of central and eastern Europe and the former Soviet Union, surveillance systems have failed to keep pace with developments elsewhere (Coker, Atun and McKee 2004).

Conclusions

This brief overview highlights the ways in which the pattern of communicable disease in a population is shaped by many different factors, many of which are constantly changing. This region has been characterized by major political and economic transition, beginning in the 1980s and continuing to the present day. The opening of borders has facilitated movement of people and goods, bringing with them many benefits but also many risks. This is exemplified by the spread of HIV, often following the route taken by heroin, from central Asia to western Europe. The political changes have been accompanied by profound changes in human activity. Thus, a move away from traditional patterns of agriculture (such as the monoculture of cotton) to small-scale privatized farms, coupled with greater mobility among a population who can now use their cars to go into forests, has led to marked changes in the pattern of many zoonotic and arthropod-borne infections. The accompanying social change, characterized by winners (the new middle classes and the oligarchs) and losers (those in prison or without homes) has left the latter exposed to infections that had once been brought under control.

Clearly, transitions in western Europe have been much less extensive but even here changes in human activity and land use have impacted on patterns of disease. The emergence of vCJD in the United Kingdom illustrates how a country with an advanced economy and well-developed surveillance system can be vulnerable and suffer when economic and technological forces combine perversely.

Changes in the health system have also played a role, both positive and negative. Initially, in some countries, a breakdown in established immunization programmes allowed some diseases, such as measles and diphtheria that had almost disappeared, to re-emerge. Elsewhere, expanded coverage allowed these diseases to be virtually eliminated, while expansion of immunization against

TBE is a factor in the decline of this disease in central Europe. On the other hand, increased ease of access to antibiotics, without accompanying improvements in the way that they are used, has created the enormous problem of resistance.

Although the effects are only slowly becoming apparent, it is impossible to ignore the consequences of climate change. A warmer world allows insect vectors to extend their range. When this is coupled with rapidly increasing international travel, allowing infectious agents to move far beyond their traditional homes, the consequences are potentially alarming. It is important not to lose sight of the fact that the economic development of many parts of Europe, such as southern Italy, only became possible with the eradication of malaria in the 1950s. The occurrence in Europe of West Nile virus and, more recently, of Chikungunya fever, a disease normally found around the Indian Ocean, are portents of dangers to come (Angelini et al. 2007).

No analysis of the factors influencing the pattern of communicable disease would be complete without considering the political context. In recent years, some communicable diseases have been discussed at the highest political levels, such as successive G8 summits. Influenza, a disease posing a threat to everyone, regardless of their social position, is an example. Yet others, especially those affecting predominantly the poor and marginalized, have received much less attention. At the level of the EU, a robust response to the threat posed by communicable disease has been mounted, as described by Reintjes in Chapter 8 of this book. This endeavour has not been matched by a similar response in the rest of this region. Worse, in a few countries, political authorities have failed to disclose the scale of communicable disease, most obviously in Turkmenistan.

The key message of this chapter is that a changing world provides opportunities and challenges, for both humans and microorganisms, in their ongoing evolutionary struggle. As discussed in subsequent chapters, health systems have a key role to play in this struggle on the part of humans.

References

Amato-Gauci, A. and Ammon, A. (2007). *The first communicable disease epidemiological report*. Stockholm: European Centre for Disease Prevention and Control.

Angelini, R., Finarelli, A. C., Angelini, P., et al. (2007). An outbreak of Chikungunya fever in the province of Ravenna, Italy, *Euro Surveill*, 12(9): E070906 1.

Ashbolt, N. (2004). Microbial contamination of drinking water and disease outcomes in developing countries. *Toxicology*, 198(1–3): 229–238.

Atun, R. A., Lebcir, R. M., Drobniewski, F., McKee, M. and Coker, R. J. (2007). High coverage with HAART is required to substantially reduce the number of deaths from tuberculosis: system dynamics simulation, *International Journal of STD & AIDS*, 18: 267–273.

Bakonyi, T., Ivanics, E., Erdelyi, K., et al. (2006). Lineage 1 and 2 strains of encephalitic West Nile virus, central Europe, *Emerging Infectious Diseases*, 12(4): 618–623.

Bobrik, A., Danishevski, K., Eroshina, K. and McKee, M. (2005). Prison health in Russia: the larger picture, *Journal of Public Health Policy*, 26(1): 30–59.

Charrel, R., Attui, H., Butenko, A., et al. (2004). Tick-borne diseases of human interest in Europe, *European Society of Clinical Microbiology and Infectious Disease*, 10: 1040–1055.

Christova, I., Tasseva, E. and Manev, H. (2003). Human leptospirosis in Bulgaria, 1989–2001: epidemiological, clinical, and serological features, *Scandinavian Journal of Infectious Diseases*, 35(11–12): 869–872.

Christova, I., Velinov, T., Kantardjev, T. and Galev, A. (2004). Tularaemia outbreak in Bulgaria, *Scandinavian Journal of Infectious Diseases*, 36(11): 785–789.

Coker, R. J., Atun, R. A. and McKee, M. (2004). Health-care system frailties and public health control of communicable disease on the European Union's new eastern border, *Lancet*, 363(9418): 1389–1392.

Coker, R., McKee, M., Atun, R., et al. (2006). Risk factors for pulmonary tuberculosis in Russia: case-control study, *British Medical Journal*, 332: 85–87.

Cox, H., Orozco, J., Male, R., et al. (2004). Multidrug-resistant tuberculosis in central Asia, *Emerging Infectious Diseases*, 10(5): 865–872.

Custer, B., Sullivan, S., Hazlet, T., et al. (2004). Global epidemiology of hepatitis B virus, *Journal of Clinical Gastroentorology*, 38(10 Supplement): 158–168.

de Zulueta, J. (1998). The end of malaria in Europe: an eradication of the disease by control measures, *Parassitologia*, 40(1–2): 245–246.

Dittman, S., Wharton, M., Vitek, C., et al. (2000). Successful control of epidemic Diphtheria in the states of the Former Union of Soviet Socialist Republics: lessons learnt, *Journal of Infectious Diseases*, 181(Supplement 1): 10–22.

Dye, C. (2006). Global epidemiology of tuberculosis, *Lancet*, 367: 938–940.

Ekdahl, K. and Andersson, Y. (2005). Imported Giardiasis: impact of international travel, immigration and adoption, *American Journal of Tropical Medicine and Hygiene*, 72(6): 825–830.

Freedman, D., Weld, L., Kozarsky, P., et al. (2006). Spectrum of disease and relation to place of exposure among ill returned travellers, *New England Journal of Medicine*, 354(2): 119–130.

Friedman, S., Kottiri, B., Neaiqus, A., et al. (2000). Network-related mechanisms may help explain long-term HIV-1 seroprevalence levels that remain high but do not approach population-group saturation, *American Journal of Epidemiology*, 152(10): 913–922.

Godinho, J., Renton, A., Vinogradov, V., et al. (2005). *Reversing the Tide: priorities for HIV/AIDS prevention in central Asia*. Washington, D.C.: World Bank.

Goossens, G., Ferech, M., Vander-Stichele, R. and Elseviers, M. (2005). Outpatient antibiotic use in Europe and association with resistance: a cross-national database study, *Lancet*, 365: 579–587.

Gritsun, T., Lashkevich, V. and Gould, E. (2003). Tick-borne encephalitis, *Antiviral Research*, 57: 129–146.

Hook, E. and Peeling, R. (2004). Syphilis control – a continuing challenge, *New England Journal of Medicine*, 351(2): 122–124.

Hutchinson, E. J., Joseph, C. and Bartlett, C. L. (1996). EWGLI: a European surveillance scheme for travel-associated Legionnaires' disease, *EuroSurveillance*, 1(5): 37–39.

Hutchinson, R. A. and Lindsay, S. W. (2006). Malaria and deaths in the English marshes, *Lancet*, 367(9526): 1947–1951.

Jacobs, M. (2003). Worldwide trends in antimicrobial resistance among common respiratory tract pathogens in children, *Pediatric Infectious Disease*, 22: 109–119.

Kiszewski, A. and Teklehaimanot, A. (2004). A review of the clinical and epidemiological burdens of epidemic malaria, *American Journal of Tropical Medicine and Hygiene*, 71(2 Supplement): 128–135.

Kozukeev, T., Ageilat, S., Maes, E. and Favorov, M. (2006). Risk factors for brucellosis – Leylek and Kadamjay districts, Batkan *Oblast*, Kyrgyzstan, January–November 2003, *Morbidity and Mortality Weekly Report*, 55(Supplement 1): 31–34.

Lanciotti, R. S., Roehrig, J. T., Deubel, V., et al. (1999). Origin of the West Nile virus responsible for an outbreak of encephalitis in the north-eastern United States, *Science*, 286(5448): 2333–2337.

Memish, Z. A. and Balkhy, H. (2004). Brucellosis and international travel, *Journal of Travel Medicine*, 11: 49–55.

Mounier-Jack, S. and Coker, R. (2006). How prepared is Europe for pandemic influenza? Analysis of national plans, *The Lancet*, 367: 1405–1411.

Mounier, S., McKee, M., Atun, R. and Coker, R. (2007). HIV/AIDS in central Asia. In: *HIV/AIDS in Russia and Eurasia*. New York: Palgrave, pp. 67–100.

Mukhopadhyay, S., Kim, B., Chipman, P., Rossmann, M. and Kuhn, R. (2003). Structure of West Nile virus, *Science*, 302(5643): 248.

Nylen, G., Dunstan, F., Palmer, S., et al. (2002). The seasonal distribution of campylobacter infection in nine European countries and New Zealand, *Epidemiology and Infection*, 128: 383–390.

Pappas, G., Papadimitriou, P., Akritidis, N., Christou, L. and Tsianos, E. V. (2006). The new global map of human brucellosis, *Lancet Infectious Diseases*, 6(2): 91–99.

Pitt, S., Pearcy, B. E., Stevens, R. H., et al. (1998). War in Tajikistan and re-emergence of Plasmodium falciparum, *Lancet*, 352(9136): 1279.

Poovorawan, Y., Chatchatee, P. and Chongsrisawat, V. (2002). Epidemiology and prophylaxis of viral hepatitis: A global perspective, *Journal of Gastroenterology and Hepatology*, 17(Supplement): 155–166.

Rechel, B. and McKee, M. (2007). The effects of dictatorship on health: the case of Turkmenistan, *BioMed Central*, 5(21): 1–10.

Renton, A., Gzirishvilli, D., Gotsadze, G. and Godinho, J. (2006). Epidemics of HIV and sexually transmitted infections in central Asia: Trends, drivers and priorities for control, *International Journal of Drug Policy*, 17: 494–503.

Ricketts, K. and Joseph, C. (2005). Legionnaires' disease in Europe 2003–2005, *EuroSurveillance*, 10(10–12).

Ricketts, K., McNaught, B. and Joseph, C. (2006). Travel-associated Legionnaires' disease in Europe: 2004, *EuroSurveillance*, 11: 4–6.

Riedner, G., Dehne, K. and Gromyko, A. (2000). Recent declines in reported syphilis rates in eastern Europe and central Asia: are the epidemics over, *British Medical Journal*, 76: 363–365.

Severini, C., Menegon, M., Luca, M. D., et al. (2004). Risk of Plasmodium vivax malaria reintroduction in Uzbekistan: genetic characterization of parasites and status of potential malaria vectors in the Surkhandarya region, *Tropical Medicine and Hygiene*, 98: 585–592.

Spika, J., Wassilak, S., Pebody, R., et al. (2003). Measles and rubella in the World Health Organization European region diversity creates challenges, *Journal of Infectious Diseases*, 187(Supplement 1): 191–197.

Sumilo, D., Asokliene, L., Bormane, A., et al. (2007). Climate change cannot explain the upsurge of tick-borne encephalitis in the Baltics, *Public Library of Science ONE*, 2(6): e500.

Tarnvik, A. and Berglund, L. (2003). Tularaemia, *European Respiratory Journal*, 21: 361–373.

Temel, T. (2004). Malaria from the gap: need for cross-sector co-operation in Azerbaijan, *Acta Tropica*, 89: 249–259.

UNAIDS (2006). *Report on the global AIDS epidemic*. Geneva: UNAIDS.

Van den Ende, J., Lynen, L., Elsen, P., et al. (1998). A cluster of airport malaria in Belgium in 1995, *Acta Clinica Belgica*, 53(4): 259–263.

Veenema, T. (2000). Health systems and maternal and child survival in central Asian Republics, *Journal of Nursing Scholarship*, 32(3): 301–306.

Vorou, R., Papavassiliou, V. and Tsiodras, S. (2007). Emerging zoonoses and vector-borne infections affecting humans in Europe, *Epidemiology and Infection*, 1–17.

Walker, G. J. and Walker, D. G. (2007). Congenital syphilis: a continuing but neglected problem, *Seminars in Fetal and Neonatal Medicine*, 12(3): 198–206.

Wasley, A. and Alter, M. (2000). Epidemiology of hepatitis C: geographic differences and temporal trends, *Seminars in Liver Disease*, 20(1): 1–16.

Zeltzer, R. and Kurban, A. (2004). Syphilis, *Clinical Dermatology*, 22: 461–468.

Zenz, W., Pansi, H., Zoehrer, B., et al. (2005). Tick-borne encephalitis in children in Styria and Slovenia between 1980 and 2003, *Pediatric Infectious Diseases*, 24(10): 892–896.

chapter *six*

Communicable disease in Latin America and the Caribbean

Oscar Echeverri, Patricio Marquez, Enis Baris

Introduction

Since colonial times, outbreaks of disease have been common in the countries of Latin America and the Caribbean, largely as a result of maritime trade and export of agricultural products and minerals that helped integrate them into the world economy, as well as the development of indigenous commercial interests (Marquez and Joly 1986). The history of public health in Latin America and the Caribbean is replete with efforts in sanitation, hygiene and disease control, especially directed at old scourges such as yellow fever and malaria.

The latter years of the 19th century and the early 20th century saw various attempts by the Latin American countries and the United States to adopt uniform quarantine regulations at different international conferences, under the aegis of the newly established Pan American Sanitary Bureau (1902). These sought to remove barriers to steam navigation, and to codify new preventive measures into specific health legislation and programmes based on the great microbiological discoveries of Pasteur, Koch and Klebs that had revolutionized public health practice in Europe.

The creation of national health departments, beginning in the late 19th century, responded directly to the need for sanitation campaigns against yellow fever in major port cities, resting on the acceptance and application of the germ theory in disease causation that were supported by leading Latin American scientists such as the Brazilians Oswaldo Cruz and Carlos Chagas, and the Cuban Carlos J. Finlay. As a result of these efforts, great inroads were made in the conquest of many of the diseases that had warranted quarantine, particularly yellow fever, commonly known as "Yellow Jack". This represented the principal scourge of international trade throughout the colonial period, up to the beginning of the 20th century. The completion of the Panama Canal in 1914 was only possible because of the success of major public health efforts against yellow fever and malaria, diseases that took a heavy toll in terms of lives lost among construction workers. In turn, the activities undertaken to help build the canal added further impetus to the development of sanitation programmes in the countries of the region by supporting research on the aetiology and transmission of yellow fever and malaria which led to the design of more effective control measures.

In subsequent periods, the activities of the national health departments expanded with the support of the International Health Commission of the Rockefeller Foundation to undertake land sanitation programmes centred on the control of hookworm infection and malaria, with the aim of improving the productivity of workers in exporting regions, such as those growing bananas and coffee. By the 1950s, most of the national health departments had evolved into the current ministries or secretariats of health.

In the last three decades of the 20th century and in the early 21st century, as discussed in the following sections of this chapter, the most important public health achievements in the Latin American and Caribbean region have continued to be in the areas of communicable disease control and basic sanitation, although these efforts have remained a secondary priority of the governments. Mortality rates have declined in virtually every country of the Americas, mainly at the expense of important declines in communicable diseases (with mortality falling from 95 per 100 000 people in 1980 to 57 per 100 000 in 2000) (PAHO 2002a). However, rapid population growth, especially in urban areas, along with migration, climatic changes (e.g. the El Niño phenomenon), stubborn inequality and social conflicts are bringing communicable diseases, new and old, back to the forefront of public health priorities in Latin America and the Caribbean.

The current burden of communicable diseases in Latin America and the Caribbean

Communicable diseases in Latin America and the Caribbean fall into two main groups: "tropical diseases" (for example malaria, dengue, cholera, leishmaniasis and yellow fever that are discussed in this chapter) and the "non-tropical diseases" group of diseases (such as TB and HIV also discussed in the context of Latin America and the Caribbean) that can be found worldwide. Most of the diseases in the first group are vector-borne, active between the tropics of Cancer and Capricorn.

Communicable tropical diseases

Among vector-borne diseases, malaria and dengue are important in Latin America and the Caribbean due to their social, economic and political implications. Although both require a mosquito – the vector – climate changes may facilitate the growth, in the medium and long term, of breeding places that will take these diseases into areas once free from them.

Malaria

Four types of malaria parasites of the genus plasmodium can infect humans: P. falciparum, P. vivax, P. ovale, and *P. malariAedes*. The most important ones in Latin America and the Caribbean are *P. vivax*, due to its high prevalence, and *P. falciparum*, due to its high lethality. Mosquitoes of the genus anopheles are the main vectors transmitting the disease (Nájera, Liese and Hammer 1993).

Malaria exists in 21 out of the 34 countries of Latin America and the Caribbean. The most affected countries are those that form part of the Amazon Basin: Bolivia, Brazil, Colombia, Ecuador, Guyana, French Guiana, Peru, Surinam and Venezuela. In 1995, 1.3 million cases were recorded – the highest number of cases ever recorded since reporting was established. Thereafter, the reported number of cases has been decreasing, with periodic reversals, until 2000, when the rate stabilized at approximately 1.14 million cases. Brazil, with a population of 180 million people, contributed 54% of all cases, followed by Colombia (44 million) with 9.5%; Ecuador (13 million) with 9%; Peru (26 million) with 6%; Venezuela (25 million) and Bolivia (9 million) with 3%; Guyana (0.8 million) with 2%; and Suriname (0.4 million) with 1% (PAHO 2002a). The only two Caribbean countries with malaria are Dominican Republic and Haiti, where almost all cases are due to *P. falciparum*, compared to only 18% in the rest of Latin America and the Caribbean, where *P. vivax* predominates. The *P. falciparum* in the Amazon region is resistant to drugs, while in the Caribbean it is not.

The burden of malaria in the general population is accounted for mainly by morbidity rather than mortality (Figure 6.1 and Figure 6.2). In 2000, the worldwide malaria death rate was 2 per 1000. In Latin America and the Caribbean, this rate was 0.02, compared to 9 in Africa and 0 in Europe. The mortality rate ranged from 12 per 100 000 in Bolivia, to 5 per 100 000 in Guyana, 2 per 100 000 in Haiti, and 1 per 100 000 in Colombia, Ecuador and Guatemala. By contrast, in 2000 the incidence of cases was 143 per 100 000 population, although in

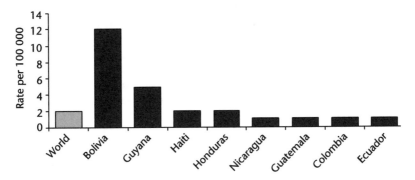

Figure 6.1 Malaria mortality rate in the world and in Latin America and the Caribbean, 2000

Source: (Adapted from) PAHO 2002b.

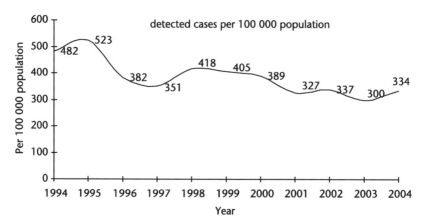

Figure 6.2 Malaria morbidity in Latin America and the Caribbean, 1994–2004

Sources: (Adapted from) PAHO 2002b and from PAHO 2005b.

high- and medium-risk areas, the incidence increased to 403.5 per 100 000 population (PAHO 2002a). Malaria deaths are concentrated in children, pregnant women and people with concomitant morbidity, such as diarrhoea, TB and HIV/AIDS. Figure 6.2 shows a disappointing morbidity trend with a small reduction over 1994–2004, due mainly to irregular support for vector control activities and inconsistent supply of antimalarial treatment.

The Roll Back Malaria initiative launched by WHO in 1998 proposed four main interventions aimed at halving the prevalence of the disease by 2010: (1) early diagnosis and treatment; (2) planning and implementation of selected preventive measures; (3) detection, control and prevention of outbreaks; and (4) strengthening of local health teams to deal with malaria. In response, nine countries sharing the tropical Amazon rainforest (where the disease endemicity is the highest in the region), the Central American countries, Dominican Republic, Haiti, and Mexico are all implementing national programmes and cooperating together. Other Caribbean countries are strengthening their surveillance systems to prevent reintroduction of malaria. Although all Latin American and Caribbean countries endorsed the initiative and have implemented programmes, the incidence has remained practically unchanged, and in some countries, drug-resistant malaria continues to rise due to environmental, social, and political factors. However, early diagnosis and treatment seems to have achieved some mortality reduction. In 1994, the total number of malaria deaths was 816, when 24% of all malaria infections were with *P. falciparum*, compared to only 277 reported malaria deaths in 2000, except 10 cases occurring in the Amazon Basin, when 26% of all malaria infections were with *P. falciparum* (PAHO 2002a).

Health sector reform in Latin America and the Caribbean has done little to strengthen the capacity of local and national health facilities to carry out early diagnosis and treatment of malaria and in some countries systems have actually weakened. Budgetary allocations for malaria control remained almost unchanged between 1997 and 1999, at approximately US$ 88 million; only in

2000 was there an increase to US$ 97 million, mainly from external sources such as loans and international aid. Success and sustainability in malaria control, however, require interventions that go beyond the confines of the health sector to involve environmental management practices that will permanently reduce the number and size of breeding sites for the anopheles vector (Lindsay et al. 2004).

The experience of Europe is not a good premonition for Latin America and the Caribbean, although transmission of malaria in Europe has been interrupted the prospect of eradication seems to be receding. For example, in Italy, local transmission of *P. vivax* malaria was recently reported (Baldari et al. 1998; Simini 1997). Debatable efficacy of existing vector control and treatment strategies (Baird 2005) and the growing parasite resistance to antimalarial drugs raise the threat of resurgence of malaria in Latin America and the Caribbean. The dream of eradicating malaria or "disappearing malaria" envisaged by Fred L. Soper, ex-Director of the Pan American Health Organization (PAHO) (Soper 1959), could remain just that, a dream.

Dengue

Dengue affects 2.5 billion people in the world, making it the most important viral mosquito-borne disease affecting humans. Its global distribution is comparable to that of malaria. Before 1970, only nine countries reported fatal dengue haemorrhagic fever, compared to at least 60 countries in 2005 (CDC 2005).

Dengue and dengue haemorrhagic fever are caused by one of four closely related, but antigenically distinct, virus serotypes (DEN-2, DEN-3, and DEN-4, DEN-1). DEN-3 is the virus responsible for dengue haemorrhagic fever. Infection with one of these serotypes does not provide cross-protective immunity to the others, so persons living in a dengue-endemic area can have four dengue infections during their lifetimes. Dengue is primarily a disease of the tropics, and dengue viruses are maintained in a cycle that involves humans and *Aedes aegypti*,[1] a domestic, day-time biting mosquito that prefers to feed on humans.

Dengue has been present in Latin America and the Caribbean for more than two centuries but was well controlled until the first half of the 20th century. Low endemicity remained throughout many parts of the region until 1981, when a major epidemic of dengue haemorrhagic fever occurred in Cuba, resulting in 344 203 cases, of which 116 143 needed hospitalization and 158 died. Since then, the situation has worsened with epidemic outbreaks in Mexico, Central America, most countries in South America and the Caribbean. In 1998, the number of new cases recorded reached 741 794, of which, 12 396 were dengue haemorrhagic fever, and a new epidemic outbreak occurred in 2002 with 1 015 420 cases, of which 14 374 were dengue haemorrhagic fever (Figure 6.3). However, following major efforts involving the Government and civil society since the mid-1980s, the number of reported cases in Cuba was reduced from 344 203 cases in 1981 to 14 443 in 2002 (De La Torre et al. 2004).

DEN-3 (causing dengue haemorrhagic fever) had not been reported for more

[1] http://www.cdc.gov/ncidod/dvbid/dengue/ae-aegypti-feeding.htm, accessed 29 November 2007.

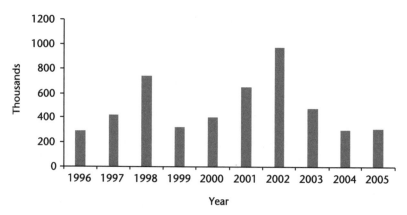

Figure 6.3   Notified cases of dengue in Latin America and the Caribbean, 1996–2005

Sources: Data from PAHO EID Updates (1996–2003) (http://www.paho.org/english/AD/DPC/
CD/eid-eer-ew.htm) and various PAHO reports on Basic Health Indicators (PAHO 2002–2005).

Note: 2005 data are from January–November.

than 20 years in Latin America and the Caribbean. In 1994, however, it was
detected in Central America (Panama, Nicaragua and Costa Rica) and in 1995
in El Salvador, Honduras, Guatemala and Mexico. Then, in 1997, cases were
reported from Belize and Guyana, and in 1998 it had spread to several Caribbean
islands (CDC 2005). If it spreads to South America, it is expected give rise to
major outbreaks among the large susceptible populations. It should be noted
that there is a higher risk of dengue haemorrhagic fever in locations where two
or more serotypes circulate simultaneously. The re-emergence of dengue or
dengue haemorrhagic fever as a major public health problem has been most
dramatic in the American region. The campaign to eradicate *Aedes aegypti* in
Central and South America in the 1950s and 1960s, which was aimed at preventing urban yellow fever, concentrated the outbreaks of dengue to the Caribbean
islands. However, in 1970, the United States discontinued efforts to eradicate
Aedes aegypti and the campaign dwindled throughout Latin America and the
Caribbean, leading to infestation of countries previously free of the vector. As
a result, the geographic distribution of *Aedes aegypti* in Latin America and the
Caribbean is now more extensive than before 1970. By 1997, 18 countries in the
American region had reported confirmed dengue cases and dengue haemorrhagic fever is now endemic in many of these countries (CDC 2005). After epi-
demic outbreaks in the Central American and the Andean regions during the
1990s, a major outbreak began in the Southern Cone in 2001, peaking in 2002
(Figure 6.4).

After very high levels of dengue haemorrhagic fever seen in the Andean
Region in 2001, the frequency has subsequently declined, although this region
still has the highest frequency in Latin America and the Caribbean.

In his 1998 presidential address to the American Society of Tropical Medicine,
Guerrant affirmed ". . . dengue hemorrhagic fever was practically eradicated
before 1981 in the Americas. However, it has returned throughout much of

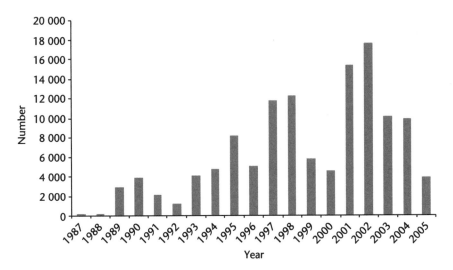

Figure 6.4 Dengue haemorrhagic fever trends in Latin America and the Caribbean, 1987–2005

Sources: Reports to PAHO from ministries of health of the respective countries: CDC, Caribbean Epidemiology Center (CAREC) and CIRE Antilles Guyana, French Guiana (1987–2006).

Central and South America ..." (Guerrant 1998). Weakening public health infrastructure following health reforms has contributed to this resurgence. Other reasons for the expansion of dengue in Latin America and the Caribbean are widespread mosquito infestations due to poor or absent vector control; inadequate waste disposal, with non-biodegradable containers increasing breeding places; increased travel and migration; and expanding urban populations, with growth concentrated in slums and in peri-urban settings.

As an effective vaccine to protect against the various viral strains is still several years away (Halstead et al. 2005; Gubler 1998), prevention by elimination of breeding places remains the most important intervention, followed by use of mosquito repellents, long sleeve shirts and screened doors. Firm and sustained commitment by governments, with civil society involvement, particularly to disseminate knowledge and change attitudes and practices among the population, are key factors in vector control.

Yellow fever

The widespread dissemination of the *Aedes aegypti* throughout the Americas makes the return of yellow fever to urban areas a permanent threat. Although urban yellow fever has not been reported in the region since 1942, more than 1900 cases of sylvatic (jungle) yellow fever have been notified from Bolivia, Brazil, Colombia, Ecuador, Peru, French Guiana, and Venezuela since the mid-1990s. The steady increase of reported cases between 1996 and 1998 prompted a vaccination campaign in the region, covering 77 million people between 1998 and 2002,[2] leading to reduced incidence in 2001 and 2002, but in 2003 Colombia reported an outbreak with 112 cases, followed by Peru which reported 67 cases in 2004. The outbreak in Colombia was associated with poor vaccination efforts and displacement of peasants to urban areas as a result of the armed conflict in the northern part of the country.

In spite of obvious risks, programmes for yellow fever are given little priority in public health and health insurance programmes and they remain underfunded.

Communicable non-tropical diseases

Cholera

Cholera had disappeared from the Americas in the 20th century, until 1991 when it reappeared in Peru, spreading to Ecuador and Colombia, and then through South and Central America, affecting all countries of Latin America except Uruguay and the Caribbean in the following three years. In 1991, approximately 82% of all cases reported in Latin America and the Caribbean were in Peru, where the incidence reached 27 per 100 000 population. Nearly a million cases were reported in the region and almost 9000 people died between January 1991 and December 1993. The mortality rate was less than 1%, due in large part to the provision of oral rehydration therapy.

Between 1991 and 1995 cumulative cholera incidence ranged from 0.06 per 100 000 in Paraguay up to 2738 per 100 000 in Peru. The Andean countries, and Nicaragua and Guatemala in Central America experienced the largest number of cases in the region. Public health measures kept the case fatality rate low (0.92%). It has since declined (Figure 6.5).

Little is known about how cholera disappeared from the Americas at the end of the 19th century and how it will behave after having reappeared in 1991 (Blake 1993). The association between cholera and development is increasingly recognized and some studies have found that the infant mortality rate and the Human Development Index (HDI) are better predictors of cholera incidence than access to potable water. In Latin America and the Caribbean, infant mortality of 40 per 1000 live births and HDI above 0.72 are the thresholds below which the risk of cholera increases (Ackers et al. 1998). The 1991 epidemic was widely publicized in the mass media, creating public apprehension. Cholera became synonymous with underdevelopment, increasing the pressure on governments to respond rapidly (Panisset 2000).

Tuberculosis

TB continues to be a public health threat in every Latin American and Caribbean country in spite of the availability of measures to control the disease. In 1999 almost a quarter of a million cases of TB were reported in the Americas. Of these,

---

[2] Yellow fever vaccine is highly effective and inexpensive. A single dose will confer immunity to at least 95% of individuals vaccinated for at least 10 years.

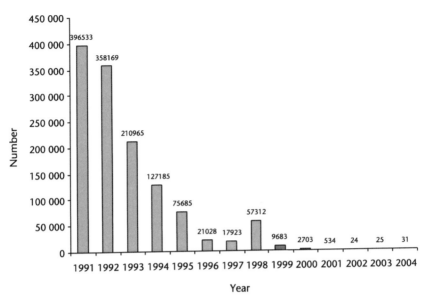

Figure 6.5 Notified cholera cases in Latin American countries, 1991–2004

Source: PAHO 2005b.

nearly 140 000 were new cases, predominantly affecting people between the ages of 15 and 55 (PAHO 2002a). Since 1980, rates of TB in the Americas have fluctuated, affecting countries to different degrees. In the second half of the 1980s, five countries experienced major increases in the number of notified cases: two in Central America, two in South America and the United States. In the 1990s, the number of countries with significant increases in reported cases rose to 17 and in 1998 the region as a whole reported the largest number of cases in a year since 1980 (262 809). Between 2000 and 2003, four countries reported a major increase in the number of cases: Colombia, Guyana, Haiti and Panama (WHO 2005).

In spite of PAHO efforts urging governments to assign high priority to TB control measures and the launch of the new "Stop Tuberculosis" strategy in 1998, Latin America and the Caribbean faces difficulties in achieving the target of reducing TB prevalence by 50% by the year 2010 and implementing effective strategies to control drug resistance and TB–HIV co-infections. Since 2000 the decline in incidence has been disappointing (Figure 6.6).

Figure 6.6 hides an important fact: the population of the United States and Canada comprise more than one third (38%) of the total population of the Americas, but together these countries account for only approximately 7% of all TB cases. In 2000, there were 217 037 new reported TB cases or 46 per 100 000 population in Latin America and the Caribbean (with 12 129 smear-positive cases or 23 per 100 000 population) (PAHO 2004c), an incidence at least 15 percentage points above the Americas as a whole. In Latin America and the Caribbean, the five social factors mentioned above, in addition to increased numbers of people with HIV/AIDS, have increased the risks of contagion and at

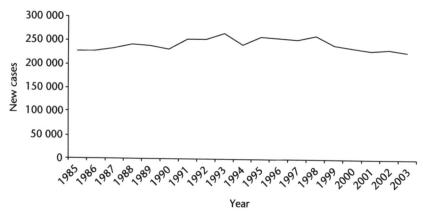

Figure 6.6   Trends in tuberculosis incidence in the Americas, 1985–2003

Source: WHO 2005.

the same time have created pressure on health care and TB control programmes (Arbelaez et al. 2004).

PAHO's estimates of TB incidence were used to cluster the Latin American and Caribbean countries into four groups. Using data from two years (2000 and 2003), four countries have changed for the worse and only one has improved. With the exception of Ecuador and Dominican Republic, the countries in the first group (> 85) have the worst socioeconomic indicators in Latin America and the Caribbean, highlighting the importance of the five social factors already mentioned.

In the 1990s, Brazil alone – with 34% of the total population in Latin America and the Caribbean – reported 33% of all cases of TB in the region, and Peru – with 5% of the total population in Latin America and the Caribbean – reported 17%. The slight decrease of 5.4% in reported cases in 1998–1999 was concomitant, with a 9% increase of smear-positive cases. A plausible explanation is that some countries with high rates (Bolivia, Peru, Ecuador, Dominican Republic, Brazil, Guatemala, Mexico and Panama) have improved the performance of TB control programmes.

Progress in reducing cases of TB has been unsatisfactory over the period 1990–2003. According to WHO data (WHO 2005), in 1990 the number of new cases (including those with HIV+) in the 22 continental countries ranged from 9 per 100 000 population in Canada to 397 per 100 000 in Peru, while in 2003 the range was from 5 per 100 000 in the United States to 225 per 100 000 in Bolivia (Figure 6.7). Although there has been a reduction from nine to four in the number of countries with 85 per 100 000 or more new cases, the number with rates between 50 and 84 has remained almost the same. Bolivia, Ecuador and Peru, despite some progress, continue to experience the highest incidence rates, with 225, 188 and 138 per 100 000 people, respectively. Only one third of all continental countries have an incidence below the average for the whole region of the Americas and just four countries have achieved substantial reductions in more than a decade: Chile 73%; Nicaragua 59%; Peru 53%; and El Salvador 47%.

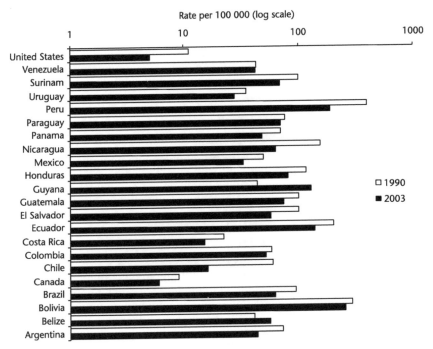

Figure 6.7 Estimated tuberculosis incidence in continental Latin American countries, 1990–2003*

Source: WHO 2005.

Note: * PAHO estimates 26 new cases per 100 000 people for the region, based on annual reports from national TB control programmes in the region.

Among the Caribbean countries, Haiti and Dominican Republic are the hardest hit by TB. Although both have achieved a 32% reduction in incidence between 1990 and 2003, they continued to have the highest rates in the Caribbean in 2003, with 232 and 96 cases per 100 000 population, respectively. The remaining Caribbean countries have incidence rates below 25 per 100 000, with the Bahamas with 40 per 100 000 and Anguilla with 25 per 100 000 as exceptions (Figure 6.8).

In 1990, overall TB prevalence in the Americas was 100 per 100 000, falling to 58 per 100 000 in 2003. The usual ratio of prevalence to incidence of 2:1 has been slightly reduced, mainly due to some reduction in the number of new cases, while old cases continue to accumulate.

In the same period (1990–2003 and using WHO data), progress in mortality reduction has been modest (Figure 6.9). In 1990, mortality rates in the 22 continental countries ranged from 1 per 100 000 in Canada to 58 per 100 000 in Peru, while in 2003 the range was from 0 in the United States to 34 in Bolivia. Three more continental countries had less than 10 deaths per 100 000. However, four countries have achieved substantial reductions: Chile from 9 to 1 per 100 000, Nicaragua from 23 to 8 per 100 000, Peru from 58 to 23 per 100 000 and El Salvador from 15 to 9 per 100 000. Bolivia, Ecuador and Peru continue to

Rate per 100 000 (log scale)

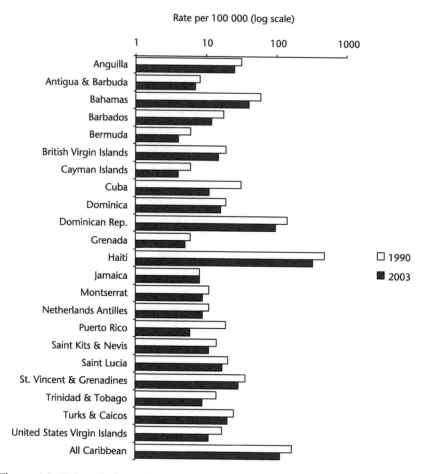

Figure 6.8 Tuberculosis incidence in the Caribbean countries, 1990–2003
Source: WHO 2005.

experience the highest mortality rates, with 34, 28 and 23 deaths per 100 000 people, respectively. Two countries increased death rates: Guyana from 8 to 24 and Paraguay from 11 to 13.

Haiti and Dominican Republic have the highest death rates from TB among the Caribbean countries. Although both have achieved 20% reductions in deaths between 1990 and 2003, in 2003 rates are still high at 71 and 17 deaths per 100 000, respectively. The remaining Caribbean countries have mortality rates between 1 and 5 per 100 000, except the Bahamas, where it is 7 per 100 000 (Figure 6.10).

Resistance to anti-tuberculosis drugs

In Latin America and the Caribbean, initial MDR-TB (in patients treated for the first time) was high in four countries all with very high TB incidence rates,

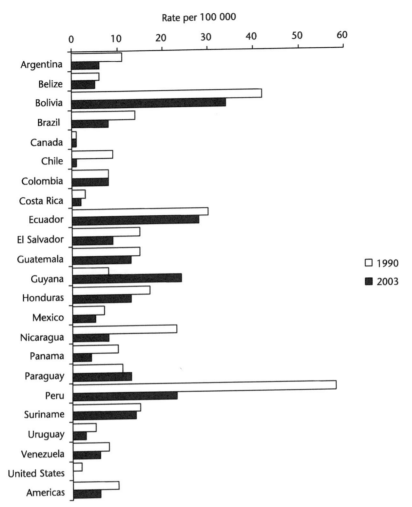

Figure 6.9 Tuberculosis mortality in continental American countries, 1990–2003

Source: WHO 2005.

namely, Dominican Republic, Ecuador, Peru and Guatemala. The most serious problem, however, was found in those with acquired MDR-TB in patients already treated. Again, countries with high incidence of TB had a high percentage of acquired MDR-TB: Ecuador 24.8%, Dominican Republic 19.7%, Guatemala 22.4% and Peru 12.3%. Mexico and Argentina also had high rates at 22.4% and 9.4%, respectively.

The rapid spread of MDR-TB drew attention to the consequences of poor control, with low coverage and inappropriate therapy. Another serious consequence was a possible negative impact on the expansion of the DOTS strategy for non-resistant TB patients. The alternative of scaling up DOTS-plus to tackle

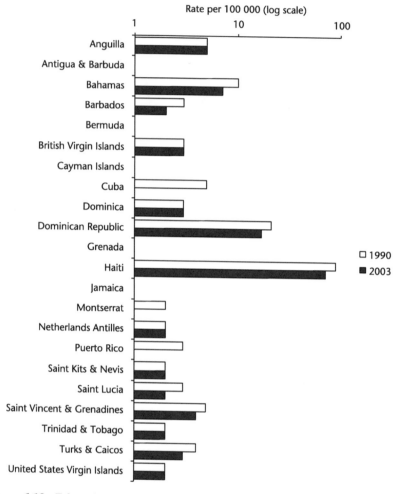

Figure 6.10   Tuberculosis mortality in the Caribbean countries, 1990–2003
Source: WHO 2005.

MDR-tuberculosis in Latin America and the Caribbean is a costly undertaking since it is 100 times more expensive than standard DOTS. (DOTS-plus is a TB treatment based on drug susceptibility testing and individualized or standardized treatment regimes involving four to eight pharmaceuticals, monthly smear microscopy and culture until six to eight months of negative cultures have been obtained.)

WHO/PAHO have set a target of detecting with smear tests 70% of estimated new TB cases and curing at least 85% of them by 2005, reducing the global burden of TB by 50% from its 2000 level, by means of the DOTS strategy. Table 6.1 summarizes the coverage achieved in Latin America and the Caribbean.

By 2000, DOTS had reached 65% of the population in Latin America and

Table 6.1 Coverage of the DOTS Strategy by country, the Americas, 2002

> 90%	> 50–89%	10–49%	<10%	No DOTS
Argentina***	Bolivia**	Brazil*		English-speaking
Belize*	Costa Rica*	Colombia*		Caribbean*
Chile*	Mexico***	Dominican		Suriname*
Cuba*	Panama*	Republic***		
El Salvador***	Venezuela*	Ecuador**		
Guatemala*		Guyana*		
Honduras*		Haiti***		
Peru*		Paraguay*		
Puerto Rico*				
Nicaragua*				
Uruguay*				
USA*				

Source: (Adapted from) PAHO 2004d.

Notes: * Countries with no changes; ** Countries with improved actual coverage but within the same range category; *** Countries with improved actual coverage beyond the range category.

the Caribbean. However, by 2002, countries with high TB incidence rates such as Brazil, Guyana and Paraguay had achieved few further advances in DOTS coverage. Although Dominican Republic and Haiti have made important strides, they still have low coverage, as has Colombia, with less than 50% coverage. Soon Mexico will reach 90% or more coverage, together with Bolivia. Significant progress has been made in Argentina and El Salvador, which together with Guatemala, Honduras, Peru and Nicaragua have reached coverage levels above 90%, the same as in Chile, Cuba, Uruguay and the United States.

By 2000, the WHO goal of 85% treatment success rate among sputum smear-positive patients in nine priority countries had only been achieved in Honduras and Peru. Bolivia, Mexico and Nicaragua were close to the goal, while Brazil, Haiti, Ecuador and Dominican Republic had low rates of treatment success, necessitating a review of their strategies and greater efforts to reach the desired goal.

The unsatisfactory advances in controlling TB in Latin America and the Caribbean during more than a decade coincided with important changes in the organization and financing of health services. Health sector reforms were introduced in some countries beginning in the mid-1980s, many of which assigned a low priority to public health problems, concentrating efforts on personal health care. Current rates of TB are a serious threat to public health in Latin America and the Caribbean; political commitment and allocation of resources to tackle TB through strengthened DOTS and sound DOTS-plus programmes have been less than satisfactory. Basic TB research has been insignificant. Health sector reforms, therefore, should be reappraised to ensure that they deliver effective public health programmes that go beyond medical care.

Tuberculosis co-infection with HIV

The pattern of TB in Latin America and the Caribbean has increasingly been complicated by the epidemic of HIV/AIDS, as many people infected with HIV develop TB and many TB patients are co-infected with HIV, which is now driving the TB epidemic in many countries; TB is the leading killer of HIV-positive people. On average across the region, 5% of the new cases of TB are attributable to HIV infection. Only Cuba and Uruguay maintain systematic surveillance of co-infection rates and have estimated prevalence rates of 1.4% and 1.3%, respectively; TB–HIV co-infection prevalence rates range from 2.5% in Honduras up to 34% in Peru and 64% in Haiti (Table 6.2). TB and HIV/AIDS programmes share common challenges: HIV control should be a priority for TB prevention, and TB control should be a priority of HIV/AIDS prevention and care programmes. Preventing and treating TB–HIV co-infection offers a unique opportunity to combine the principles and logistics of both DOTS and ARV delivery. However, some countries have reduced their support for TB control programmes.

TB can be controlled in Latin America and the Caribbean because it is well known what needs to be done, how to do it and how much it will cost. Failure to take forceful action now will have disastrous consequences for the region and for the world.

HIV/AIDS

In the Americas, the primary mode of HIV transmission among adults is unprotected heterosexual intercourse. In women, there is growing evidence that the main risk factor for being infected is risky behaviour by their male partners.

In Latin America in 2004 approximately 240 000 people (estimated between 170 000 and 430 000) were infected with HIV, between 1.3 to 2.2 million people were living with HIV, with approximately 0.5% of all youngsters aged 15–24

Table 6.2 Prevalence of co-infection tuberculosis/AIDS in some Latin American countries, 1999–2002

Country	Year	% tuberculosis cases among PLWHA	Type of HIV/AIDS epidemic
El Salvador	2002	11.5	Concentrated
Guyana	2000	13.7	Generalized
Haiti	1999	63.8	Generalized
Honduras	2002	9.0	Generalized
Nicaragua	2002	2.5	Concentrated
Panama	2002	24.8	Generalized
Peru	2001	34.0	Concentrated

Source: (Adapted from) PAHO 2005a.

Note: PLWHA: People living with HIV/AIDS.

years and 0.8% of all women living with HIV. Approximately 95 000 people have died of AIDS.

In Central America, HIV infections have been rising in El Salvador, Nicaragua and Panama since the late 1990s, but HIV prevalence remains highest in Guatemala and Honduras (over 1% of adults). Infected men outnumber infected women by a ratio of 3:1 and the epidemic is largely concentrated in urban areas.

In the Andean area, HIV is spreading increasingly to the partners of men who buy sex and to MSM.

In Brazil, with one third of the total population of Latin America and the Caribbean, the epidemic initially affected mostly MSM and then injecting drug users. Now, heterosexual transmission is responsible for a growing share of HIV infections, with women increasingly affected. As in other countries in the region, sex workers and poor women have high infection rates, fluctuating between 7% and 23% in Santos and São Paulo.

National prevalence of HIV among pregnant women has remained stable at below 1% since the early 2000s, but in some areas, as in Rio Grande do Sul, prevalence fluctuates between 3% and 6%. Injecting drug users constitute at least half of AIDS cases. In Porto Alegre the prevalence of infection in this group was 64% in 2003, while in Itajai it was 31%. Harm-reduction programmes in some cities have been very successful, notably in Salvador where prevalence fell from 50% in 1996 to 7% in 2001.

Spending priorities do not adequately address the main features of the epidemic in Latin America and the Caribbean. For instance, sex between men is a driving force in the epidemic throughout the region, with Peru the notable exception; however, prevention efforts aimed at this group are not a priority, while expenditure on prevention among sex workers is more prominent. In the case of injecting drug users, only Argentina and Brazil appear to have prioritized prevention spending on this group.

Brazil remains the best example of provision of treatment. Its health system offers all people living with HIV (PLHIV) access to ARV drugs, achieving substantial increases in survival time for AIDS patients from 18 months for those diagnosed in 1995 up to 5 years for those diagnosed in 1996. Also, Argentina, Cuba, Costa Rica and Panama have achieved significant mortality reductions after expanding ARV treatment.

The Caribbean is the second most affected region in the world, with an average adult HIV prevalence of 2.3%, with the highest frequency of HIV infected women in the Americas and with AIDS as the leading cause of death among adults aged 15–44 years (Marquez 2001). Prevalence exceeds 2% in five countries: the Bahamas, Belize, Guyana, Haiti, and Trinidad and Tobago. In 2004, more than 440 000 people were living with HIV, including 53 000 new cases (Caribbean Epidemiology Center 2005). Almost two thirds of the epidemic is occurring through heterosexual intercourse, while intravenous drug use is insignificant except in the Bahamas and Puerto Rico. However, a powerful prejudice against MSM and gender, social and economic inequalities are powerful forces maintaining the epidemic amid stigma, misconceptions and denial.

Women are hardest hit in Dominican Republic and Jamaica, where some girls have sexual relationships with older men ("sugar daddies") who are more likely to be HIV-positive (Caribbean Epidemiology Center 2005).

Haiti continues to be the most affected country in the region, although some studies are showing a decline in HIV prevalence. Pregnant women with HIV attending antenatal clinics have shown a reduction from 4.5% in 1996 to 2.8% in 2003–2004 (Caribbean Epidemiology Center 2005).

In the Bahamas between 2000 and 2003, the number of reported AIDS cases and deaths declined from 320 to 164 and from 272 to 185, respectively. This hopeful new trend coincides with stronger prevention efforts and the expansion of ARV treatment since 2000 (Caribbean Epidemiology Center 2005).

The World Bank has included the fight against HIV/AIDS as part of its agenda for reducing poverty in Latin America and the Caribbean. An example of this commitment is the US$ 155 million Multi-Country HIV/AIDS Prevention and Control Program in the Caribbean (World Bank 2001) that started in 2001 and now funds projects for 9 countries and another for regional institutions. Under this programme, in 2001 Barbados became the first country to receive World Bank funding for scaling up treatment with ARV drugs as part of a comprehensive approach that includes prevention, treatment and care, and institutional development. The success in Barbados is encouraging: new HIV diagnoses among pregnant women dropped from 0.7% to 0.3% between 1999 and 2002, and mother-to-child transmission has been reduced by 69% between September 2000 and December 2002. In addition, the introduction in 2001 of ARV treatment for PLHIV has reversed the upward trend in AIDS mortality, with a decline from 114 in 1998 to 50 in 2003, while hospital admissions for treatment of opportunistic infections fell by 42% in the same period (Marquez 2004).

In the capital of Dominican Republic, HIV prevalence among pregnant women aged 15–24 years has declined from approximately 3% in 1995 to below 1% in 2003, but nationally HIV prevalence among pregnant women remains over 2%. A focus of great concern is the 4.9% HIV prevalence among sugar cane plantation workers, where there are many immigrants from neighbouring Haiti.

Cuba, at 0.05%, has the lowest HIV prevalence in the Caribbean, reflecting strong preventive measures and universal free access to ARV therapy. However, there is great concern about the 5-fold increase in prevalence between 1995 and 2000 (Caribbean Epidemiology Center 2005). Most new HIV transmission is occurring during sex between men.

The year 1992 was a turning point for trends in AIDS in the region. While North America shows a sustained downturn, the Caribbean region has been experiencing a relentless increase and continental Latin America has seen a slowdown in the rate of increase (Figure 6.11). These patterns can be explained by two main factors: introduction of ARVs with different degrees of access, and a rapid increase of conversions from HIV infections into AIDS cases, reflecting the age and intensity of the epidemic in the region.

Governments have undertaken similar efforts in prevention, albeit with different emphases, but have employed different approaches in delivering ARVs. Cuba and Barbados have led the way with free ARVs while others are considering it, or still reluctant to commit themselves to this important component of HIV/AIDS control, largely on grounds of cost.

The health sectors in Latin America and the Caribbean have responded to the HIV/AIDS epidemic in two main ways. Insurance schemes include individual medical care for HIV/AIDS as a catastrophic condition with various adverse

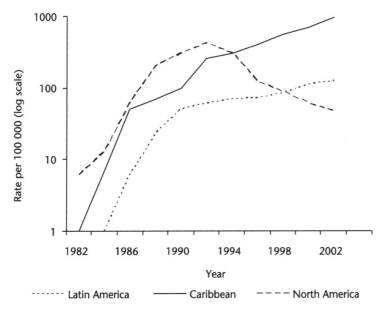

Figure 6.11   AIDS incidence rates in the Americas, 1982–2002

Source: Several data sources combined by authors.

manifestations; while health promotion, disease prevention, and now scale-up treatment programmes under the domain of public sector institutions and NGOs are funded largely with international donations from the Global Fund, and in some cases with loans, credit or grants from the World Bank. In spite of recent efforts and increasing funding, infected individuals have great difficulty in gaining access to proper treatment, except in those countries where governments have decided to provide ARV and care free of charge (i.e. Brazil, Barbados and Cuba). At the same time, health promotion and disease prevention activities receive little attention both in terms of financing and societal effort to control the epidemic. The consequence of this situation is that, despite public commitment by governments, the HIV/AIDS epidemic continues its relentless advance as the most serious threat to health and economic development (with very few exceptions) in the region.

Vaccine-preventable diseases

The countries in Latin America and the Caribbean, with support from PAHO and other international partners such as UNICEF, have achieved success in reducing vaccine-preventable diseases, most notably the eradication of smallpox in 1971 followed by poliomyelitis in 1991. The Americas was the first region in the world to accomplish these achievements. Interruption of indigenous measles transmission is now advanced. Currently, the countries in Latin

America and the Caribbean are striving to attain the goal of 95% coverage of all antigens included in national immunization programmes, particularly targeting hard-to-reach rural areas and marginal urban settlements. The vaccines in use in the Americas include: Bacille Calmette-Guerin (BCG, for TB); DPT, DT, and TT (for diphtheria, pertussis, tetanus); Hep A and Hep B (for hepatitis); Influenza; OPV and IPV (for poliomyelitis); Polysaccharide and conjugate pneumococcal (for pneumococcal disease); MMR, MR, M (for measles, mumps, rubella); yellow fever; Varicella (for chickenpox); and Hib conjugate (for haemophilus influenza type b).

Seven vaccine-preventable diseases present a very different trend compared with that of tropical infectious diseases in Latin America and the Caribbean. Poliomyelitis, measles, rubella, diphtheria, tetanus, and whooping cough have largely been controlled. This is the outcome of the excellent immunization programmes throughout the Americas supported by the Expanded Program on Immunization (EPI), launched in 1977 by PAHO, building upon smallpox eradication efforts.

A critical contribution to the vaccination achievements in Latin America and the Caribbean has been PAHO's Revolving Fund for Vaccine Procurement, established in 1979 to purchase vaccines, syringes, needles and cold-chain equipment. This has assured the supply of high-quality vaccines for national immunization activities (Box 6.1).

The whole region is now free of indigenous wild poliovirus transmission, and endemic transmission of the indigenous measles virus. Great progress has been achieved toward the goal of eliminating rubella and Congenital Rubella Syndrome (CRS) by 2010, and controlling neonatal tetanus as a public health concern. Vaccine coverage in children aged 1 year in Latin America and the

---

Box 6.1 Contributions of the PAHO Revolving Fund for Vaccine Procurement

- Makes vaccines affordable as the result of competitive procurement of bulk purchases, with the attendant economies of scale, which both keeps prices low and helps manufacturers make long-term production plans and capital investments.
- Enables delivery of technical cooperation directly to health authorities responsible for immunization programmes.
- Requires a specific line item in countries' budgets to cover recurrent costs, 5-year work plans, and the appointment of a national immunization programme manager.
- Introduces new and additional vaccines rapidly and at affordable prices. Two examples are the Haemophilus influenza type B vaccine, used in only two countries in 1996 and now widely used in most countries in the Americas; and the hepatitis B vaccine, used only for risk groups in 1997 and today part of routine immunization.

Source: PAHO 2002c.

Caribbean has been above 80% since 1999 (Figure 6.12). A cautionary note is that in 12 countries over 50% of the municipalities have coverage below 95%; among them Colombia, Venezuela and Peru (PAHO 2004a). This makes the region vulnerable to outbreaks of some vaccine-preventable diseases. However, vaccination has contributed to a decrease in childhood mortality from 51 per 1000 live births (1990–1995) to 31 per 1000 by 2003 and has spared thousands from birth defects and millions from serious illness.

Poliomyelitis

The number of polio cases was reduced from 6653 in 1970 to 0 in 1992 (Figure 6.13), and the region was certified as free of circulation of the indigenous wild poliovirus in 1994 (Robbins and de Quadros 1997). Latin America and the Caribbean will continue vaccination until the world is certified as polio free (PAHO 2002c).

Measles

In 1994, the Americas established the goal of interrupting indigenous measles transmission by the year 2000. Intensified vaccination and surveillance, coupled with the active search for cases in health centres and high-risk communities, has brought about a sharp reduction in the incidence of measles. In 2002, all cases in Canada (6), Brazil (1) and the United States (37) were imported, while Colombia and Venezuela, with vaccine coverage below 80%, were the only

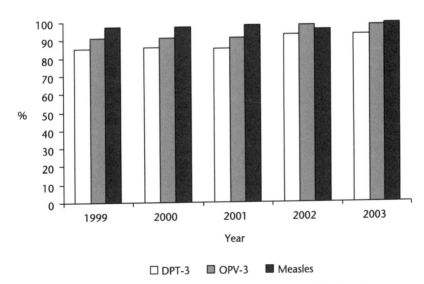

Figure 6.12   Immunization coverage in children aged 1 year in the Americas, 1999–2004

Source: (Adapted from) PAHO 2004a.

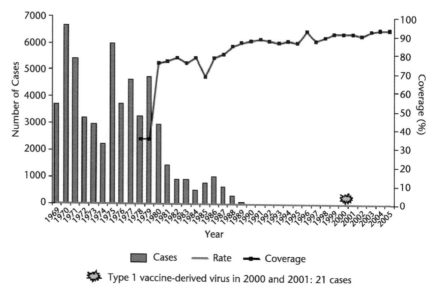

Cases ▬ Rate ■ Coverage

🌟 Type 1 vaccine-derived virus in 2000 and 2001: 21 cases

Figure 6.13 OPV3 vaccination coverage and incidence of paralytic poliomyelitis, the Americas, 1969–2001

Source: PAHO 2007.

countries reporting 140 and 2392 indigenous cases, respectively. The outbreak in Venezuela occurred following imported cases from Europe in 2001. After major vaccination campaigns in both countries, the last reported case occurred in Venezuela in September 2002. In 2003, Mexico reported 44 cases (26 confirmed indigenous) and the United States 45 (19 imported). No confirmed indigenous measles circulation has occurred anywhere in the region since then. However, the risk remains, due to insufficient coverage during routine and campaign vaccination and inadequate investigation of some cases (de Quadros et al. 2004). To reduce this risk, PAHO has recommended a 3-pronged vaccination strategy that has been highly successful in other countries applying it: first, a one-time nationwide campaign ("catch-up"), targeted at children aged 9 months to 14 years; second, a routine vaccination of children aged >1 year ("keep-up"); and third, periodic mass vaccination campaigns every 3–4 years ("follow-up") targeting children aged 1–4 years, regardless of their previous vaccination status. The interruption of measles virus transmission is maintained by keeping high population immunity through this 3-pronged strategy.

Neonatal tetanus

Elimination of neonatal tetanus is near to being achieved in the Americas. The incidence dropped by 95% from 1988 to 2003, with only 116 cases in 2003 (PAHO 2005b). However, between 2001 and 2003, Haiti, with a population of only 8 million inhabitants, reported almost 50% of the total number of cases in the region of the Americas. Neonatal tetanus is a very good indicator of the quality of prenatal care and of how health reforms may affect public health priorities. A single neonatal tetanus case should be considered a failure of the health care system.

Rubella

Cuba was the first country to eliminate rubella and congenital rubella syndrome in the Americas. The last reported case in Cuba occurred in 1989. In 2003 the ministries of health adopted the goal of eliminating rubella and congenital rubella syndrome in the Americas by 2010. By September 2004, all countries and territories in the region, except Haiti, had introduced vaccines containing the rubella antigen (MR or MMR) in their national child vaccination programmes (Castillo-Solorzano and Andrus 2004).

The success of Cuba and the English-speaking Caribbean countries (cost–effectiveness per prevented case of congenital rubella syndrome was US$ 2900 in the English-speaking Caribbean) facilitated strengthening the commitment to rubella elimination in Latin America. For instance, the Presidents of Costa Rica and Ecuador launched campaigns with executive decrees, facilitating inter-sectoral coordination of public and private institutions. In Brazil, social mobilization was the key to the success of a vaccination campaign aimed at adults. In El Salvador, vaccination focused initially on institutional populations (schools, factories, etc.) and high transit-density areas.

Diphtheria

The highest reported number of diphtheria cases ever recorded in the region was 6857 in 1978. Cases have declined continuously to 113 cases in 2000 and 68 in 2001, but rose slightly again to 164 in 2002.

Colombia (2000) and Paraguay (2002) reported outbreaks with 11 and 15 cases, respectively (PAHO 2005b). Haiti and Dominican Republic continue to have endemic diphtheria; in 2004, each country reported an outbreak of 51 and 65 suspected cases, respectively. A total of 24% were confirmed in Dominican Republic and 37% in Haiti, and the case fatality rate was 43% and 46%, respectively (PAHO 2004b). Coverage of children under 1 year with DPT3 was 48% in Haiti and 75% in 2003. Most cases in these four countries have occurred among poor people with limited access to health care services and low vaccination coverage.

Pertussis

Pertussis incidence has declined drastically in the last few years, from 22 093 cases in 1999 to 863 in 2003. Chile, Peru, Paraguay, Panama and Ecuador have reported relatively large numbers of cases until 2002. Thereafter, the reduction has been generalized in Latin America and the Caribbean (PAHO 2005b).

Immunization programmes are now positioned to complete eradication of vaccine-preventable disease from Latin America and the Caribbean, thanks to the effective performance of the EPI and the creation of a culture of vaccination among the population. However, pockets of poverty must be tackled vigorously to end the transmission of these diseases. A good measure of the success of the health system as a whole is the attainment of immunization goals. Immunization programmes are among the priorities that must be included in basic health packages of health insurance.

Vaccine-preventable diseases have become the paradigm of success (and sometimes failure) of public health interventions, involving massive coverage with effective vaccines of susceptible populations, using efficient logistics systems, strong surveillance systems and clear programme policy and guidelines. However, the success, above all, comes from the fact that in most countries there is an unambiguous political commitment to achieve the proposed goals of eradication and control.

Conclusion

Communicable diseases prevalent in Latin America and the Caribbean have different epidemiological patterns intimately related to the presence of vectors, population growth and distribution, climatic changes, persistent inequality and social conflicts. Vector-borne diseases have recurrent patterns of outbreak and control or silent occurrence due to ecologic variables that are difficult to manage, mainly because of social, political and economic limitations on the application of effective technological measures for controlling vectors and treating sick people. The other group of "non-tropical" communicable diseases that exists in the region and around the world has a more predictable pattern. Control measures are more amenable to elicit sustained reductions in occurrence through public health measures, behavioural changes and the use of therapeutic and immunologic technologies. Furthermore, the creation of advocate groups in different countries to constantly oversee effective health action, such as the expanded programme of immunizations supported by PAHO, has rendered satisfactory results in the control of vaccine-preventable infections. However, recent changes in the health systems of the region including decentralization of health services, along with "horizontalization" and integration of vertical health programmes, have brought unconvincing results (see Chapter 8). A more objective and thorough analysis of alternative health system reforms may bring the changes needed to achieve efficiency, effectiveness and equity in controlling communicable diseases in Latin America and the Caribbean, although keeping the region free of communicable diseases remains a long-held aspiration.

References

Ackers, M. L., Quick, R. E., Drasbek, C. J., Hutwagner, L. and Tauxe, R. V. (1998). Are there national risk factors for epidemic cholera? The correlation between socioeconomic and demographic indices and cholera incidence in Latin America, *International Journal of Epidemiology*, 27(2): 330–334.

Arbelaez, M. P., Gaviria, M. B., Franco, A., et al. (2004). Tuberculosis control and managed competition in Colombia, *International Journal of Health Planning and Management*, 19(Suppl 1): 25–43.

Baird, J. K. (2005). Effectiveness of antimalarial drugs, *New England Journal of Medicine*, 352(15): 1565–1577.

Baldari, M., Tamburro, A., Sabatinelli, G., et al. (1998). Malaria in Maremma, Italy, *Lancet*, 351(9111): 1246–1247.

Blake, P. A. (1993). Epidemiology of cholera in the Americas, *Gastroenterol Clinics of North America*, 22(3): 639–660.

Caribbean Epidemiology Center (2005). *Annual Report 2004*. Port of Spain: CAREC/Pan American Health Organization.

Castillo-Solorzano, C. and Andrus, J. K. (2004). Rubella elimination and improving health care for women, *Emerging Infectious Diseases*, 10(11): 2017–2021 (http://www.cdc.gov/ncidod/EID/vol10no11/04-0428.htm, accessed 27 November 2007).

CDC (2005). *Fact Sheet: Dengue and dengue fever*. Atlanta, G.A.: United States Centers for Disease Control (http://www.cdc.gov/ncidod/dvbid/dengue/index.htm, accessed 27 November 2007).

De La Torre, E., Lopez, C., Marquez, M., Gutierrez Muniz, J. A. and Rojas, F. (2004). *Salud Para Todos Si es Posible [Health for all is possible]*. Havana: Cuban Public Health Society.

de Quadros, C. A., Izurieta, H., Venczel, L. and Carrasco, P. (2004). Measles eradication in the Americas: progress to date, *Journal of Infectious Diseases*, 189(Suppl 1): 227–235.

Gubler, D. J. (1998). Dengue and dengue hemorrhagic fever, *Clinical Microbiology Reviews*, 11(3): 480–496.

Guerrant, R. L. (1998). Why America must care about tropical medicine: threats to global health and security from tropical infectious diseases, *American Journal of Tropical Medicine and Hygiene*, 59(1): 3–16.

Halstead, S. B., Heinz, F. X., Barrett, A. D. and Roehrig, J. T. (2005). Dengue virus: molecular basis of cell entry and pathogenesis, 25–27 June 2003, Vienna, Austria, *Vaccine*, 23(7): 849–856.

Lindsay, S., Kirby, M., Baris, E. and Bos, R. (2004). *Environmental management for Malaria control in the East Asia and Pacific (EAP) Region. Discussion Paper. April*. International Bank for Development and Reconstruction.

Marquez, P. (2001). *HIV/AIDS in the Caribbean. Issues and Options. A World Bank Country Study*. Washington, D.C.: World Bank.

Marquez, P. (2004). Scaling up the Struggle: Barbados HIV/AIDS Prevention and Control, *Development Outreach*, 6(2): 12–14.

Marquez, P. V. and Joly, D. J. (1986). A historical overview of the ministries of public health and the medical programs of the social security systems in Latin America, *Journal of Public Health Policy*, 7: 378–394.

Nájera, J. A., Liese, B. and Hammer, J. (1993). Malaria, in D. T. Jamison (ed.) *Disease control priorities in developing countries*. New York; Oxford: Oxford University Press for the World Bank.

PAHO (2002a). *Health in the Americas. Scientific and Technical Publication No.587*. Washington, D.C.: Pan American Health Organization.

PAHO (2002b). *La Salud en las Américas. volumen I*. Washington, D.C.: Pan American Health Organization.

PAHO (2002c). *Charting a Future for Health in the Americas*. Washington, D.C.: Pan American Health Organization.

PAHO (2004a) A Culture of Prevention: A model for control of vaccine-preventable diseases. XVI meeting of the Technical Advisory Group on Vaccine-preventable Diseases. Mexico city, November 3–5.

PAHO (2004b). EPI Newsletter, 26(3). Washington, D.C.: Pan American Health Organization (http://www.paho.org/english/ad/fch/im/sne2603.pdf, accessed 27 November 2007).

PAHO (2004c). *Tuberculosis Fact Sheet.* Washington, D.C.: Pan American Health Organization.

PAHO (2004d). *Status of TB operations (Region of the Americas, 2004).* PowerPoint presentation, 19 March 2004. Washington, D.C.: Pan American Health Organization.

PAHO (2005a). *Epidemiological status of TB (Region of the Americas, 2004).* PowerPoint presentation, 30 March 2004. Washington, D.C.: Pan American Health Organization (http://www.paho.org/common/Display.asp?Lang=E&RecID=6433, accessed 27 November 2007).

PAHO (2005b). *Health Analysis and Information Systems Area. Regional Core Health Data Initiative; Technical Health Information System.* Washington, D.C.: Pan American Health Organization (http://www.paho.org/Project.asp?SEL=TP&LNG=ENG&ID=44&PRGRP=docs_gen, accessed 27 November 2007).

PAHO (2007). *Protecting the Health of the Americas: Moving from Child to Family Immunization.* Final Report. XVII Meeting of the Technical Advisory Group on Vaccine-Preventable Diseases July 2006, Guatemala.

Panisset, U. B. (2000). *International Health Statecraft. Foreign Policy and Public Health in Peru's Cholera Epidemic.* Lanham, Maryland: University Press of America, Inc.

Robbins, F. C. and de Quadros, C. A. (1997). Certification of the eradication of indigenous transmission of wild poliovirus in the Americas, *Journal of Infectious Diseases,* 175(Suppl 1): 281–285.

Simini, B. (1997). First case of indigenous malaria reported in Italy for 40 years, *Lancet,* 350: 717.

Soper, F. L. (1959). *Some 1959 Impressions of World-Wide Malaria Eradication. Paper delivered as the 24th Annual Charles Franklin Craig Lecture before the American Society of Tropical Medicine and Hygiene, Indianapolis, Indiana, October 28, 1959.*

WHO (2005). *Global Tuberculosis Control: surveillance, planning, financing.* Geneva: World Health Organization.

World Bank (2001). *Project Appraisal Document for Proposed Loans in the Amount of US$25 million to the Dominican Republic and US$15.15 million to Barbados in support of the First Phase of the US$155 million Multi-Country HIV/AIDS Prevention and Control Adaptable Program Lending (APL) for the Caribbean Region. Report No. 22184-LAC.* Washington, D.C.: World Bank.

chapter seven

Health systems and systems thinking

Rifat Atun, Nata Menabde

Introduction

In 1979 Theodore W. Schultz, Nobel Laureate for economics, argued that population quality was the "decisive factor" of production. He emphasized the merits of investing in education and health, while identifying the main channels through which health could boost economic productivity.

Improved health, as measured by life expectancy and adult survival rates, exercises a positive impact on human capital formation and hence on economic growth. In turn, sustained growth rates allow for better health conditions. Improved health boosts economic productivity and growth (Schultz 1980; Schultz 1979). Hitherto, the relationship between economic growth and health had emphasized the impact of economic growth on improved health. There is now strong empirical evidence demonstrating a two-way relationship, indicating that improved health significantly enhances economic productivity and growth (Atun and Gurol-Urganci 2005; Suhrcke et al. 2005).

Health systems play an important role in improving health. WHO estimates that, between 1952 and 1992, half the gains in global health resulted from application of new knowledge and technology in health systems, with the remaining gains due to income improvements and better education (WHO 1999).

Yet, in spite of increasingly large proportions of national incomes invested in health care, the performance of many health systems remains suboptimal in terms of the desired outcomes of higher and more equitable population health, protection from financial risk, and user satisfaction. For example, the United States, which spends 16% of its GDP on its health system, has some of the worst health outcomes of all developed countries, over 40 million people uninsured – and hence without adequate financial risk protection when ill – and an increasingly dissatisfied population. Similarly, in the United Kingdom, with health systems which to date have emphasized equity of access and outcomes, substantial new investment in the health system in recent years has yet to deliver desired results in terms of improved health outcomes, increased efficiency and enhanced user satisfaction. The health systems in most countries of central and eastern Europe have failed to respond adequately to changing patterns of demand. In particular, in many of the countries of the former Soviet Union, health systems with roots in the Semashko model have found it difficult to meet the substantial challenges brought about by the changing context. They have been confronted by a rapid transition from command to market economies accompanied by financial instability, widening of socioeconomic inequalities, decline in funding for social sectors (including health), dramatic falls in life expectancy and re-emergence of communicable diseases (Atun 2005; Atun, Ibragimov and Ross 2005; Coker, Atun and McKee 2004a; Shkolnikov, McKee and Leon 2001).

Failure by health systems to respond to emerging challenges also affects the delivery of communicable disease programmes. Many constraints faced by communicable disease programmes are due less to the technical content of the programme but rather the shortcomings of health systems (Raviglione and Pio 2002). Conversely, where they succeed, their success is often determined by the performance of health systems (Walt 2004; WHO 2003). Hence, addressing health systems issues more broadly, rather than the communicable disease programme alone, increases the chances of sustainability for these programmes. Indeed, WHO has identified comprehensive engagement with and strengthening of health systems as necessary starting points for the successful scale-up of communicable disease programmes (Jong-wook 2003; WHO 2006).

Unfortunately, with the exception of a small number of studies, our understanding of the interaction between health systems and communicable disease programmes remains limited (Atun et al. 2004; Atun et al. 2005b; Atun et al. 2005c). This understanding is further constrained by our inadequate understanding of health systems. This chapter explores the approaches and frameworks used for health system analysis. Building on these approaches and drawing on systems, complexity and organizational theories, it offers a novel analytical framework for analysing health systems.

The introductory section of this chapter is followed by a brief review of health system definitions, key approaches and analytical frameworks used to measure health system performance, and those used for analysing health reforms, including more recent definitions of health systems and analytical concepts developed to explain better the causal relations between health system elements and health system goals. The third section describes a novel framework developed for analysis of health systems: one that draws on systems thinking. This section also briefly describes what systems are, how they behave and why understanding of systems behaviour is important, in particular what an understanding of complex systems can contribute.

Health systems: definitions, measuring performance and analysis of health systems performance

Early definitions conceptualized health systems in terms of actors within them, economic relationships or flows of funds (Box 7.1). More recent definitions, such as that by WHO, describe health systems as all the activities whose primary purpose is to promote, restore or maintain health (WHO 2000).

Measuring health systems performance

Several frameworks have been developed to explore or measure the performance of health systems (Hsiao 1992; Jee and Or 1999; Murray and Frenk 2000; OECD

Box 7.1 Early definitions of health systems

Drawing on earlier work by Evans (1981), who identified four main sets of actors in health care systems (the population to be served; health care providers; third-party payers; and government as regulator) and described several alternative sets of market and non-market relationships between them, Hurst and colleagues at the Organisation for Economic Co-operation and Development (OECD) define health systems in terms of fund flows and payment methods between population groups and institutions. They identify seven major subsystems of financing and delivery of health care, namely three voluntary insurance systems (comprising the private reimbursement model, the private contract model and the private integrated model), three compulsory insurance- or tax-funded models (comprising the public reimbursement model, the public contract model and the public integrated model) and the direct, voluntary out-of-pocket payment model (Hurst 1991; OECD 2001).

Others have described health systems in terms of the economic relationship between demand, supply and intermediary agencies which influence the supply–demand relationship (Cassels 1995; Janovsky and Cassels 1996). The demand side comprises individuals, households and populations whose actions (individually or as households) influence health outcomes (for example through risk behaviour and health-seeking patterns). The supply side includes the institutions that produce human and material resources for health care, the service providers (public, private or non-profit-making organizations), individuals and informal unpaid carers. The agencies include the State, government institutions responsible for the financing, regulation and purchasing of health care, and other institutional purchasers (such as private insurers, public insurance funds, district health authorities or health maintenance organizations) that identify health needs for defined populations and purchase clinical and support services from providers using a variety of contractual mechanisms.

1992). Of these, perhaps the most well known is the WHO Performance Assessment Framework (PAF), which was used to compare the performance of WHO member countries and formed the basis of the WHO *World Health Report 2000* (WHO 2000).

The WHO PAF assessed health systems performance in terms of attainment of a number of goals: average level of health, distribution of health, average responsiveness, distribution of responsiveness and fairness of financial contribution (Box 7.2). Both the *World Health Report 2000* and the WHO PAF generated significant debate (Williams 2001) on measuring health system performance at national level and spurred WHO to refine the PAF framework.

Analysing health systems reform

There are several frameworks that have focused on analysis of health system reforms. That developed by Kutzin enables exploration of health systems reform through a financing lens (Kutzin 2001; Kutzin 1995), although in earlier studies he and McPake suggest a 3-step approach to evaluating health reforms to describe (Kutzin and McPake 1997):

• key contextual factors driving reform
• the reform itself and its objectives, and
• the process by which the reform was (is being) implemented.

The approach developed by Frenk focuses on the dimensions of health system

---

Box 7.2 World Health Organization Performance Assessment Framework

WHO identifies key health system goals as the level and distribution of health and responsiveness, and fairness in financial contribution. The indicator used to summarize the overall health of different populations is disability-adjusted life expectancy (DALE). Responsiveness measures how people view their experience when they come into contact with the health system in clearly specified domains: dignity, autonomy, confidentiality (together comprising respect for persons), prompt attention, quality of basic amenities, access to social support networks during care, and choice of provider (comprising client orientation), while Fairness in Financial Contribution measures the distribution of financial contributions of households to the health system.

The health system functions that are discharged to attain these goals include delivering personal and non-personal health services; raising, pooling and allocating the revenue to purchase those services; investing in people, buildings and equipment; and acting as the overall stewards of the resources, powers and expectations entrusted to them.

reform and interrelationships among health system components (Box 7.3) (Frenk 1994).

In contrast to earlier definitions of health systems, Hsiao conceptualizes a health system as "a set of relationships where the structural components (means) [sic] and their interactions are associated and connected to the goals the system desires to achieve (ends) [sic]" (Hsaio 2003). Hsiao expands the analytical framework for health system reform by linking what he calls the "macro-level", namely "the total size, shape and functioning" of the health sector with aggregate outcomes (Hsiao 2003). In doing so, he develops a causal model, whereby the major components of the health system which he calls the "control knobs" (i.e. explanatory variables) can largely account for observed outcomes of the health system (i.e. dependent variables) (Box 7.4).

Hsiao conceptualizes a health system as a "means to an end" – a system which "exists and evolves to serve societal needs". He then goes on to define a health system ". . . by those principal casual components that can explain the system's outcomes." In his definition of a health system, Hsiao limits the boundaries of a health system to the "components" which ". . . can be utilized as policy instruments to alter the outcomes." In doing so, when developing his causal model he includes ". . . structural variables" (which he calls control knobs) "that can be altered by policy to influence outcomes within several years" while excluding from this causal relationship variables such as culture ". . . that cannot be changed, except in the long term." A control knob is used by policy-makers to achieve a desired goal or an intermediate goal, but achieving these also depends on the interactions among all the control knobs (Box 7.4).

Although the frameworks described above enable us to measure health system

---

Box 7.3   Frenk's dimensions of health reform

Frenk conceptualizes the health system as a set of relationships among five major groups of actors: the health care providers, the population, the State as a collective mediator, the organizations that generate resources, and the other sectors that produce services that have health effects.

He uses the relationships among providers, population, and the State to form the basis for a typology of health care modalities. The type and number of modalities present in a country make it possible to characterize its health system. He identifies four policy levels at which health system reform operates: systemic, which deals with the institutional arrangements for regulation, financing and delivery of services; programmatic, which specifies the priorities of the system, by defining a universal package of health care interventions; organizational, which is concerned with the actual production of services by focusing on issues of quality assurance and technical efficiency; and instrumental, which generates the institutional intelligence for improving system performance through information, research, technological innovation and human resource development.

Box 7.4 Analysis of health reform: Hsiao's control knobs

Hsiao describes the goals ("ends") of a health system as "good health for all, financial risk protection for all, and satisfaction of the people, while maintaining an affordable health system." Health systems are concerned with improving both the level and distribution of these goals: hence, ensuring equity dimension is also taken into account. In achieving these goals, health systems also aim to improve access, quality and/or efficiency of services (which Hsiao calls intermediate goals) as achieving these ultimately affects the goals of system.

Hsiao identifies five major "control knobs" of a health system (each with a set of instruments) which policy-makers can use to achieve health system goals. These include: (i) financing and its organizational organization (which has four instruments comprising financing modalities, funds allocation, rationing and institutional arrangement for financing); (ii) macro-organization of provision (for which there are three fundamental decisions, namely, choice of public monopoly versus competition, the *degree* of vertical integration, and ownership of health facilities (whether public, private non-profit-making or profit-making); (iii) payments (to individuals and organizations) which form the basis of incentive structure – the payments are concerned with the method of payment and the amount of payment per unit and the incentives, in the form of "financial reward and risk bearing", that these create for patients, institutional providers, health professionals employed by institutions or practising independently, and pharmaceutical suppliers; (iv) regulations, which Hsiao refers to as the "coercive power to impose constraints on organizations and individuals"; and (v) persuasion – use of a number of means to influence people's beliefs, expectations, lifestyles, and preferences.

performance or enable policy-makers better to conceptualize health systems and their elements and how the control knobs can be used to achieve health system goals, they are not designed specifically to analyse health systems and they are therefore less useful in analysing health system behaviour. Indeed, few studies have explored the behaviour of health systems or how elements of health systems interact to produce outcomes.

Further, there is also limited analysis of why many well-intentioned policies and managerial decisions aimed at improving the performance of health systems have not led to the intended outcomes and in many cases have led to unexpected or even undesired outcomes.

One explanation for this phenomenon is that too often, the tools and methods used for analysis, policies aimed at redesigning or changing health systems, and the heuristics used to generate managerial decisions are too simplistic for health systems that are complex. The behaviour of complex systems is generally difficult to predict. Often in such systems isolated interventions lead to perturbations whose magnitude and direction may not be readily predictable. Isolated interventions to parts of a complex system often upset the equilibrium of the whole system and influence the elements or subsystems to resist this intervention – so as to prevent system change – leading to "policy resistance".

Hence, better understanding of health systems and how health system elements interact to produce results requires a more nuanced understanding of systems behaviour. This is discussed in more detail below.

Systems and dynamic complexity

A system is a set of elements, connected together, which form a whole, thereby possessing properties of the whole rather than of its component parts (Checkland 1981). A system's activity is the result of the influence of one element on another. This influence is called feedback, which can either be positive (amplifying) or negative (balancing) in nature (Senge 1990).

Systems can be closed or open. Closed systems are completely autonomous and independent of the activity around them, in contrast to open systems which interact with their environment.

Systems are dynamic and complex, made up of many interconnected and interdependent elements which form extensive networks of feedback loops with time delays and non-linear relationships: it is these characteristics that are the sources of dynamic complexity in systems.

Given this interconnectedness and complexity, a system response occurs as a result of the interactions among the system's elements, rather than the result of change in a single component. This is the essence of systems thinking: ". . . the ability to see the world as a complex system", comprising many interconnected and interdependent parts (Sterman 2001). Systems thinking, which has its roots in a range of disciplines such as engineering, computing, cybernetics and cognitive psychology, views the system as a whole rather than its individual component parts. It takes into account behaviour of systems over time rather than static "snapshots" (Senge 1990).

Systems thinking postulates that disturbances in systems arise due to a particular kind of complexity, namely "dynamic complexity". Hence, an understanding of "dynamic complexity" is a necessary step in understanding the underlying causes of complexity and systems thinking.

There are three drivers of dynamic complexity in systems:

- presence of feedback loops
- variable time lags between the cause and effect of an action, and
- existence of non-linear relationships among the system's elements.

Dynamic complexity arises when:

- the short- and long-term consequences of the same action are dramatically different;
- the consequence of an action in one part of the system is completely different from its consequences in another part of the system; and
- obviously well-intentioned actions lead to non-obvious counter-intuitive

results (Forrester 1961; Richardson 1995; Sterman 1994; Sterman 1989a; Sterman 1989b).

Understanding dynamic complexity is a means to identifying the leverage points in a system to improve its performance and avoid policy resistance (Box 7.5).

Box 7.5 Dynamic complexity

Feedback loops

Most human thinking is based on the event-oriented, linear and open-loop (without feedback loops) view of the world. Such thinking encourages interpretation of successive events as being linked by linear cause–effect relationships. However, in reality, such linear cause and effects links rarely exist. Actions taken by an agent in a system upset the system's equilibrium and trigger reactions from other agents to restore the system's balance. These reactions generally affect the initial action, establishing a circular loop of cause and effect. This circular relationship, known as "feedback", lies at the heart of systems thinking as systems consist of many inter-related feedback loops. The reaction of multiple feedback loops to an action is the principal cause for "policy resistance" observed in the real world as the system attempts to restore its initial equilibrium. Similarly, inadequate understanding of the structure of the feedback loops in a system can also lead to counter-intuitive results or "side-effects" for many actions, as incomplete conceptualization of the feedback loops in a system leads to poor prediction of results by the decision-makers (Sterman 2001).

There are two types of feedback loops. With reinforcing (positive) loops, any disturbance within the loop variables is reinforced and amplified causing an exponential growth (or decline) in the system. With self-correcting (negative) loops, any disturbance is resisted as the system moves towards a state of equilibrium. Although one can infer the behaviour of each of these loops in isolation, in a system which includes many interacting feedback loops it becomes impossible to predict how the system will behave (Ford 1999).

Time delays

It is commonly assumed that a trigger or intervention is followed by an action. However, in real life, causes and effects are often not close in time and space (Sengupta, Abdelhamid and Bosley 1999; Sterman 2000). These delays create more dynamically complex systems as they slow the learning process by reducing the ability to accumulate experience, test hypotheses, and apply findings to improve a particular situation. Further, if the results are not immediately apparent, agents will continue to pursue their goals

---

without allowing sufficient time for the system to adapt. In these situations, systems either overshoot or lag behind their equilibrium: especially when delays are "unobservable".

Non-linear relationships

The response (effect) of the system to an action (cause) is not always linearly proportional. The presence of such relationships in a system increases dynamic complexity because the response of the system to a disturbance will be different, as it will depend on its current state. The same action may trigger completely unpredictable consequences, as the response of the system is contingent upon the existing balance of power among the feedback loops.

One reason for poor decision-making in complex systems is that managers often focus on "detail complexity", reducing the amount of information used, simplifying mental cause–effect maps and limiting themselves to a number of static options when making decisions, instead of focusing on "dynamic complexity" characterized by networks of relations, feedback loops and non-linearity (Sengupta and Abdelhamid 1993). This reductionist linear approach fails to provide an accurate representation of the real world and ignores possible wider impacts of the decisions. This "bounded rationality" (Simon 1982) is further reinforced in situations of dynamic complexity due to the limits on the cognitive skills and information-processing capability of the human mind. The human mind often ignores feedback structures, non-linearities in the system and the time delays between actions and consequences. This leads to "misperception of feedback", so that even when information is available, consequences of interactions cannot rapidly and correctly be deduced (Diehl and Sterman 1995).

Health systems as complex dynamic systems

Health systems exhibit all the key characteristics of complex dynamic systems. For example:

- health systems involve many interacting feedback loops and the results of these interactions cannot be readily deduced using linear representations;
- the effects of decisions are often separated in time and space and the consequences of actions are not immediately visible;
- health systems involve many non-linear relationships, hence it is difficult to accurately predict outcomes given a particular intervention involving a system element.

These relationships extend beyond the system elements, as health systems are intricately linked to the context within which they exist. This complexity in health care has been noted by others as an example of complex adaptive systems (Plsek and Greenhalgh 2001).

The contexts within which health care organizations and health systems exist are also dynamic and complex. Furthermore, there is a bidirectional interaction between health systems and their context. This bidirectional interaction further increases the dynamic complexity of health systems.

The tools and procedures traditionally applied by policy-makers and managers are inadequate for understanding these complexities, solving emerging problems and capitalizing on opportunities. Effective management of this complex web of interdependence and the interactions between system elements and the context requires acquisition, absorption and interpretation of vast quantities of information, often beyond the capability of decision-makers (Senge 1990). This leads to a simplistic analysis of situations, so that the most important sources of the problem are either missed or overlooked and the interventions aimed at eliminating these problems lead to unforeseen consequences and "policy resistance" (Sterman 1994).

As noted by Figueras, McKee and Lessof (2004): "In practice, policy-makers tend to focus their attention on individual initiatives that all too often are perceived as 'magic bullets' that will cure all of the health sector's ills . . . need is for a better understanding of the intricacies and complexities of health systems as a whole, and the nature of the interrelationships between their different elements."

Managing dynamic complexity in health systems

To date, in health systems analysis, analytical approaches have not adequately taken into account the context or understood the context to be separate from the system. In reality the context and the health system are not separate but intricately linked, with a bidirectional relationship between them: changes in the context influence system elements and in turn interventions to system elements effect the context (Atun et al. 2007c).

So, what can be done to manage better within this environment of dynamic complexity? The first step is to adopt systems thinking, instead of the linear and reductionist approaches which prevail in health systems. Second, the relationship between health systems and the context within which they exist needs to be better understood: hence, analytical approaches used to explain changes and outputs should not focus on the health system alone but also include the context within which the health systems exist. In addition, as a continuation of the above analysis, the interaction of system elements and programmes (such as communicable disease control programmes which are embedded within these) need to be studied in order to learn how changes in programmes and system elements influence each other. Yet, to understand better how health systems interact with their context and with the programmes embedded within them, one needs to adopt inductive approaches and multi-method research programmes that draw on both quantitative and qualitative methods of inquiry. These two points are discussed in more detail in the next section.

Towards systems thinking in health systems

Systems thinking originated in the 1920s within several disciplines, including biology and engineering, as a response to growing technological complexities that confronted engineering and science. It evolved further with system dynamics developed in 1956 by Jay Forrester at the Massachusetts Institute of Technology, who recognized the need for better methods of testing new ideas in social systems (in the same way as ideas are tested in engineering) (Forrester 1961). Systems thinking helps in understanding social systems, as engineering principles help understanding the mechanical system. In systems thinking an organization or system and its respective environment (context) is viewed as a complex whole of interrelated and interdependent parts, rather than separate entities (Cummings 1980).

Systems thinking takes into account structures, patterns of interaction and events as components of larger structures. It is a discipline for seeing the whole: a framework for seeing interrelationships and repeated events rather than things, for seeing and patterns of change rather than static "snapshots". Systems thinking encourages looking at organizational dynamics, instead of getting over-involved in the details of a situation, and the interrelationships in the system. It helps anticipate, rather than react to events and thus to better prepare for emerging challenges.

Systems thinking is commonly divided into "hard" and "soft" types: with the former referring to approaches used to resolve problems occurring in the natural sciences, and the latter referring to approaches used to solve managerial problems (Checkland and Scholes 1990).

In practice, shifting to systems thinking means placing a greater emphasis on the more careful thinking through of possible consequences of actions, generating scenarios through group working and joint thinking: taking into account the interlinkages between system elements, the linkages between the systems and the context within which the system sits.

These "soft systems" approaches can be combined with formal modelling methods (such as systems dynamics modelling (Lane and Oliva 1998)) to represent system dynamics and simulate system behaviour according to explicit assumptions (Sterman 1989a). System dynamics modelling enables hypothesis testing and generation of scenarios, as well as enhanced joint thinking, group learning and shared understanding of problems (Box 7.6).

Box 7.6 Systems dynamics modelling

Systems dynamics modelling uses both qualitative and quantitative analysis to develop models that represent complex systems. The approach enables involvement of different key stakeholders in the modelling process, as well as in the generation of policy options or scenarios which can be tested using the model developed. This interaction of varied stakeholders (such as policy-makers, managers, clinicians and service users) leads to more rapid use and integration of available knowledge and aids organizational learning, but also generates views on the impact of health system interventions on outcomes (Royston et al. 1999; Sterman 2000). Although systems dynamics is used increasingly to aid decision-making in health care services (Dangerfield, Fong and Roberts 2001; Wolstenholme 1993) and to inform control of communicable diseases (Atun et al. 2007b; Atun et al. 2005a; Atun et al. 2007a), it has yet to be applied to health systems.

Analysis of the context, the health system and health programmes

Multimethod analytical approaches offer a means to understand better the relationship between the health system and the context within which the system exists (Atun et al. 2006).

A health system is made up of elements that interact together to form a complex system whose sum is greater than its parts. The interactions of these elements affect the achievement of health system goals. Although these goals may differ in emphasis between different countries, essentially many are similar (see below). As identified earlier, the health system interacts with the wider context within which it is situated. Therefore, a framework which analyses health system functions also needs to analyse simultaneously the context with which it interacts. Figure 7.1 describes below a framework which enables simultaneous analyses of the health system and the context.

As with the WHO PAF and the analytical frameworks developed by Hsiao and Frenk, this framework uses health, financial risk protection and consumer satisfaction as the ultimate health systems goals, but further expands them to take into account the context within which the health system functions, namely, the demographic, economic, political, legal and regulatory, epidemiological, sociodemographic and technological contexts (DEPLESET). As each country and health system has a distinct history which influences the trajectory of system development, the analysis of the context also captures the political economy of the health system. Collectively, analysis of these contextual elements enables us to determine the opportunities and the threats faced by the health system in the short and the long term.

The framework identifies four levers available to policy-makers when managing the health system. Modification of these levers enables policy-makers to achieve different intermediate objectives and goals. These levers include:

- "stewardship and organizational arrangements", which describe the policy environment and the regulatory environment, stewardship function and structural arrangements for purchasers, providers and market regulators;
- "financing" (how the funds are collected and pooled);
- "resource allocation and provider payment systems" (how the pooled funds and other available resources, such as human resources, capital investment or equipment, are allocated and the mechanisms and methods used for paying health service providers); and

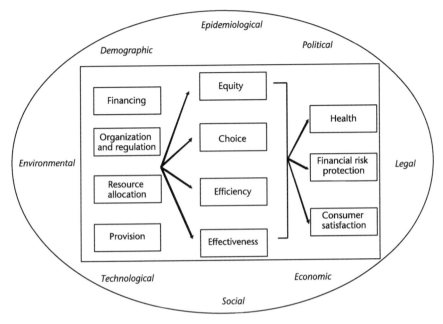

Figure 7.1   A framework for analysing health systems and the context

Source: Atun et al. 2007c.

- "service provision", which refers to the "content", that is, the services that the health sector provides rather than the structures within which this "content" is delivered.

The intermediate goals identified in the framework (equity, efficiency (technical and allocative efficiency), effectiveness and choice) are frequently cited by others as end goals in themselves.

The framework is extended and used to develop a Systemic Rapid Assessment (SYSRA) toolkit which allows simultaneous and systematic examination of the broad context, the health care system and the features of health programmes (such as communicable disease control programmes). The SYSRA toolkit is modular in structure and has two linked elements that are applied simultaneously: a "horizontal" element to analyse the health system within which the communicable disease control programme is embedded and a vertical element to analyse the programme itself (Box 7.7). The SYSRA toolkit employs a multimethods approach to research and analysis, undertaken by a multidisciplinary team (Atun et al. 2004). The empirical evidence arising from the analysis is used iteratively for cross-referencing and triangulation, hypothesis generation and testing, to inform organization learning and decision-making and to further systems thinking (Coker, Atun and McKee 2004b).

Using the framework and the approach described, we have been able to demonstrate in a number of settings (Box 7.8 and Box 7.9) that the context, the interaction between health system elements and context–health system

Box 7.7 Systemic Rapid Assessment toolkit

The toolkit is based loosely on a "T" model and has two elements which are explored both individually and in terms of their linkages to each other. The "horizontal element" has modules to assess the macro context and the health system within which the infectious disease programme is embedded from a variety of perspectives: political, legal, social, demographic, economic, technological, financing, organizational arrangements, resource allocation, provider payment systems and provision. The "vertical element" has modules which allow assessment of key elements relating to the infectious disease programme, such as epidemiology, service delivery, diagnostics laboratory networks and treatment.

The modular structure allows flexibility according to the area in question, context and resource availability. Each module addresses a specific area (e.g. legal, political, financing and epidemiology) and uses a predefined set of key questions to obtain the necessary information rapidly. A multimethods approach by a multidisciplinary team enables cross-referencing and triangulation of data. Where possible, the toolkit utilizes routine datasets.

The toolkit has three stages of analysis. The first stage ("screening"), involves reviews of documents and analysis of data to address predefined questions for each module that are applied to provide qualitative and quantitative information on the context, past patterns and other historical information, trends, responses to emerging challenges, processes and mechanism for the programme in question.

The second stage involves a field visit and interviews with key informants, purposively identified to capture a representative group, to rapidly elicit more detail on the health system and vertical programme in order to fill gaps identified by the screening questions, and to elucidate information obtained during stage one. Qualitative data predominate, but routine quantitative data, especially in the areas of financing and epidemiology, are also collated for analysis to identify areas for further in-depth longitudinal analysis at stage three. Through an iterative process of information gathering and discussions, the team triangulates the findings for scenario building. The second stage typically takes 3–5 working days for a team to complete.

The aim of stage three is to provide detailed qualitative and quantitative information on areas identified as being critical to the success of the programme and not easily collated during the rapid assessment stages (stages one and two). This new information is collected over a longer period of time and used to inform programme implementation.

interactions affect the way rules, norms and enforcement mechanisms are interpreted to generate system responses that may not be easy to predict and may indeed be counter-intuitive (Atun et al. 2005b; Atun et al. 2005c).

Box 7.8   Health system barriers to sustainable tuberculosis control

The Russian Federation has the 11th highest TB burden in the world in terms of the total estimated number of new cases that occur each year. But in spite of an extensive TB control system, the country has one of the lowest case-detection rates for new smear-positive cases and the lowest rates for treatment success of DOTS.

Although economic evaluations have shown cost–effectiveness of the WHO approved methods that favour minimizing hospital stays, TB patients in the Russian Federation continue to undergo long hospital stays. Lengthy hospital stays have been attributed to the traditional Russian clinical and pathophysiological concepts of TB that encourage hospitalization and differ from those of WHO and the international community, but research using a systems approach has demonstrated a complex health systems and sociopolitical and cultural context which has led to policy resistance and hindered broad adoption and diffusion of DOTS. First, hospital funding, based on the existing number of beds and bed occupancy (while numbers of staff and other inputs are based on bed numbers), has created perverse incentives for health service providers to maintain existing beds and hospitalize TB patients. Second, federal guidelines and tariffs for payment stipulate long periods of hospitalization, which need to be observed for providers to be paid. Third, large numbers of staff are employed in TB control facilities, and downsizing or redistributing these resources would be politically difficult to achieve. Fourth, hospitals play a dual role for clinical and social care as social support networks in the community are poorly developed. As financing regulations in the Russian Federation prevent a shift of funds from health to social sectors, or pooling of health and social sector budgets, development of multisectoral policies that might address the social problems of TB patients is hindered. Fifth, the "not-invented-here" syndrome prevails. As DOTS has been seen as a "foreign" product, not befitting Russian constructs of clinical medicine and "evidence", its adoption requires behavioural change amongst providers.

Barriers to adoption and diffusion relate less to the understanding of the "technology" associated with DOTS but more to inherent disincentives created by health system factors (financing, organizational structure and provider payment systems) and to the sociocultural norms which need to be addressed if the DOTS strategy can be successfully and sustainably scaled up in the Russian Federation.

A key lesson emerging from the case studies described above and below is that when attempting to address HIV and TB epidemics, technical solutions alone are not adequate to mount effective and sustainable scaled-up responses, as these responses are influenced by complex health systems and the sociopolitical

Box 7.9 How the health system context influences HIV control

Drawing on methodologies used for rapid situational assessments of vertical programmes for tackling communicable disease, we analysed HIV control programmes in Pskov, Samara and Tatarstan, three regions of the Russian Federation with centrally directed programmes (Atun et al. 2005b).

The analysis shows that although many similarities exist between the three regions studied, there are differences as regards stages of the epidemic, organizational arrangements, the political environment, social attitudes to HIV (seen by some as a problem of risk groups and unlikely to affect the "normal" population), finances allocated to HIV, monitoring and clinical management of HIV/AIDS patients, civil society involvement, interorganizational links and multisectorality of responses to the HIV epidemic.

Each region displays some commonalities arising from the Soviet traditions of public health control. Yet, despite an apparently clearly set out federal policy, accompanied by funding, there is considerable diversity in the priorities identified, policies pursued and translation of policies into action.

Although each region draws on a common legislative framework, the interpretation of the law differs. In Tatarstan, policy-makers have seized the opportunity to galvanize their community to mount a multisectoral response to HIV prevention and control, while in the other two regions the gaps in the legal basis for combating HIV has prevented an appropriate public health response to the emerging epidemics.

There is a complex political economy within which efforts to control HIV sit, an intricate legal environment and a high degree of decentralization of financing and operational responsibility. This complex environment and the interaction between the system elements have affected the way the rules, norms and enforcement mechanisms are interpreted to generate system responses that are counter-intuitive. For instance, we observed the following elements: in Pskov, despite limited multisectoral response and little political commitment, an excellent harm-reduction programme; in Samara, a leading reformist region with an internationally supported STI–HIV control programme, along with a fragmented response and no harm-reduction programmes; and in Tatarstan, not a leading reformist region as regards health, a sophisticated multisectoral response.

environment within which the communicable disease programmes are embedded. An effective scaled-up response to communicable disease challenges must take these into account.

Conclusions

Contextual and health system factors influence the translation of policies to action. Therefore, a broader and more sophisticated analysis of the context and health system elements than that usually undertaken by specific programmes will enable better prediction of the effects of a specific policy and promotion of sustainability. A simplistic situational analysis may result in the most important causes of the problem being overlooked and a risk that decisions made to eliminate a problem could have unforeseen consequences and result in "policy resistance". One way to reduce this policy resistance is to adopt "systems thinking", which requires a detailed analysis of the context and drawing on lessons learnt to devise effective responses.

When managing communicable disease programmes to control TB or HIV, technical solutions alone are not adequate to mount effective scaled-up responses. This is because the responses are influenced by the health system organization, design and financing and the context within which these programmes are embedded. An effective scaled-up response to prevention and control of these conditions must take these factors into account.

Understanding the health systems contexts and embedding communicable disease programmes within them is a necessary prerequisite to scaling up new programmes and achieving sustained success.

References

Atun, R. A. (2005). The health crisis in Russia, *British Medical Journal*, 331(7530): 1418–1419.

Atun, R. A. and Gurol-Urganci, I. (2005). *Health expenditure: an 'investment' rather than a cost? Working Paper 05/01*. Chatham House, London: Royal Institute of International Affairs, International Economics Programme.

Atun, R. A., Ibragimov, A. and Ross, G. (2005). *The World Bank Report No. 32354-ECA. Review of experience of family medicine in Europe and central Asia: Executive Summary. (In Five Volumes) Volume I. Human Development Sector Unit, Europe and central Asia Region.* Washington, D.C.: The World Bank.

Atun, R. A., Lennox-Chhugani, N., Drobniewski, F., Samyshkin, Y. and Coker, R. (2004). A framework and toolkit for capturing the communicable disease programmes within health systems: Tuberculosis control as an illustrative example, *European Journal of Public Health*, 14: 267–273.

Atun, R. A., Lebcir, R., Drobniewski, F. and Coker, R. (2005a). Impact of an effective multi-drug-resistant tuberculosis control programmes in the setting of an immature HIV epidemic: system dynamics simulation model, *International Journal of STD & AIDS*, 16 (8): 560–570.

Atun, R. A., McKee, M., Drobniewski, F. and Coker, R. (2005b). Analysis of how health system context influences HIV control: case studies from the Russian Federation, *Bulletin of the World Health Organization*, 83(10): 730–738.

Atun, R. A., Samyshkin, Y. A., Drobniewski, F., et al. (2005c). Barriers to sustainable tuberculosis control in the Russian Federation health system, *Bulletin of the World Health Organization*, 83(3): 217–223.

Atun, R. A., Menabde, N., Saluvere, K., et al. (2006). Introducing a complex health innovation – primary health care reforms in Estonia (multimethods evaluation), *Health Policy*, 79(1): 79–91.

Atun, R. A., Lebcir, R. M., Drobniewski, F., McKee, M. and Coker, R. J. (2007a). High coverage with HAART is required to substantially reduce the number of deaths from tuberculosis: system dynamics simulation in the setting of explosive HIV epidemic and tuberculosis, *International Journal of STD & AIDS*, 18: 267–273.

Atun, R. A., Lebcir, M. R., McKee, M., Habicht, J. and Coker, R. J. (2007b). Impact of joined-up HIV harm-reduction and multidrug-resistant tuberculosis control programmes in Estonia: system dynamics simulation model, *Health Policy*, 81: 207–217.

Atun, R. A., Kyratsis, I., Gurol, I., Rados-Malicbegovic, R. and Jelic, G. (2007c). Diffusion of complex health innovations-implementation of primary care reforms in Bosnia and Herzegovina: a qualitative study, *Health Policy and Planning*, 22(1): 28–39.

Cassels, A. (1995). Health Sector reform: Some key issues in less developed countries, *Journal of International Development*, 7(3): 329–348.

Checkland, P. (1981). *Systems thinking, systems practice*. Chichester: Wiley.

Checkland, P. and Scholes, J. (1990). *Soft systems methodology in action*. Chichester: Wiley.

Coker, R. J., Atun, R. and McKee, M. (2004a). Health care system frailties and public health control of communicable diseases on the European Union's new eastern border, *Lancet*, 363: 1389–1392.

Coker, R. J., Atun, R. A. and McKee, M. (2004b). Untangling Gordian knots: improving tuberculosis control through the development of 'programme theories', *International Journal of Health Planning and Management*, 19: 217–226.

Cummings, T. G. (1980). *Systems theory of organizational development*. New York: Wiley.

Dangerfield, B. C., Fong, F. and Roberts, C. A. (2001). Model-based scenarios for the epidemiology of HIV/AIDS: the consequences of highly antiretroviral therapy, *System Dynamics Review*, 17(2): 119–150.

Diehl, E. and Sterman, J. D. (1995). Effects of feedback complexity on dynamic decision-making, *Organizational Behavior and Human Decision Processes*, 62(2): 198–215.

Evans, R. G. (1981). Incomplete Vertical Integration: The Distinctive Structure of the Health-Care Industry, in J. J. van der Gaag and P. M (eds) *Health, economics, and health economics*. Amsterdam: North Holland.

Figueras, J., McKee, M. and Lessof, S. (2004). *Health systems in transition: learning from experience. First Edition*. Brussels: European Observatory on Health Systems and Policies.

Ford, D. N. (1999). A behavioural approach to feedback loop dominance analysis, *System Dynamics Review*, 15(1): 3–36.

Forrester, J. W. (1961). *Industrial dynamics*. Cambridge, MA: The MIT press.

Frenk, J. (1994). Dimensions of health system reform, *Health Policy*, 27: 19–34.

Hsiao, W. C. (1992). Comparing health care systems: what nations can learn from one another, *Journal of Health Politics, Policy and Law*, 17: 613–636.

Hsiao, W. C. (2003). *What Is A Health System? Why Should We Care?* Cambridge, Massachussetts: Harvard School of Public Health.

Hurst, J. W. (1991). Reforming health care in seven European nations, *Health Affairs (Millwood)*, 10(3): 7–21.

Janovsky, K. and Cassels, A. (1996). Health Policy and Systems Research: Issues, Methods and Priorities, in K. Janovsky (ed.) *Health policy and systems development: An agenda for research*. Geneva: World Health Organization.

Jee, M. and Or, Z. (1999). *Health outcome measurement in OECD countries: toward outcome-oriented policy-making (DEELSA/ELSA/WP1(98)6/ANN)*. Paris: Organisation for Economic Co-operation and Development.

Jong-wook, L. (2003). Global health improvement and WHO: shaping the future, *Lancet*, 362(9401): 2083–2088.

Kutzin, J. (1995). *Health financing reform: a framework for evaluation. Revised working document. WHO/SHS/NHP/96.2* Geneva: World Health Organization Health Systems Development Programme.

Kutzin, J. (2001). A descriptive framework for country-level analysis of health care financing arrangements, *Health Policy*, 56(3): 171–204.

Kutzin, J. and McPake, B. (1997). *Methods for Evaluating Effects of Health Reforms. Current Concerns. ARA Paper number 13, World Health Organization, WHO/ARA/CC/97.3.* Geneva: World Health Organization.

Lane, D. C. and Oliva, R. (1998). The greater whole: towards a synthesis of system dynamics and soft system methodology, *European Journal of Operational Research*, 107: 214–235.

Murray, C. and Frenk, J. (2000). A framework for assessing the performance of health systems, *Bulletin of the World Health Organization*, 78(6): 717–731.

OECD (1992). *The Reform of Health Care: A Comparative Analysis of Seven OECD Countries. Health Policy Studies No. 2.* Paris: Organisation for Economic Co-operation and Development.

OECD (2001). *The Reform of Health Care: A Comparative Analysis of Seven OECD Countries.* Paris: Organisation for Economic Co-operation and Development.

Plsek, P. E. and Greenhalgh, T. (2001). Complexity science: The challenge of complexity in health care, *British Medical Journal*, 323: 625–628.

Raviglione, M. C. and Pio, A. (2002). Evolution of WHO policies for tuberculosis control, 1948–2001, *Lancet*, 359(9308): 775–780.

Richardson, G. P. (1995). Loop polarity, loop dominance and the concept of dominant polarity, *System Dynamics Review*, 11(1): 67–88.

Royston, G., Dost, A., Townshend, J. P. and Turner, H. (1999). Using System Dynamics to help develop and implement policies and programmes in health care in England, *System Dynamics Review*, 15(3): 293–313.

Schultz, T. W. (1979) Nobel Prize Lecture. The Economics of Being Poor [electronic publication]. The Nobel Foundation (http://nobelprize.org/economics/laureates/1979/index.html, accessed 15 September 2006).

Schultz, T. W. (1980). Nobel Lecture: The Economics of Being Poor, *The Journal of Political Economy*, 88(4): 639–651.

Senge, P. M. (1990). *The fifth discipline: the art and practice of the learning organization.* New York: Doubleday.

Sengupta, K. and Abdelhamid, T. K. (1993). Alternative conceptions of feedback in dynamic decision environments: an experimental investigation, *Management Science*, 39(4): 411–428.

Sengupta, K., Abdelhamid, T. K. and Bosley, M. (1999). Coping with staffing delays in software project management: An experimental Investigation. IEEE Transactions on systems, *Management and Cybernetics*, 29(1): 77–91.

Shkolnikov, V., McKee, M. and Leon, D. A. (2001). Changes in life expectancy in Russia in the mid-1990s, *Lancet*, 357(9260): 917–921.

Simon, H. A. (1982). *Models of bounded rationality.* Cambridge, MA: The MIT press.

Sterman, J. D. (1989a). Misperceptions of feedback in dynamic decision-making, *Organizational Behavior and Human Decision Processes*, 43(3): 301–335.

Sterman, J. D. (1989b). Modeling management behavior: misperception of feedback in a dynamic decision-making experiment. *Management Science*, 35(3): 321–339.

Sterman, J. D. (1994). Learning in and about complex systems, *System Dynamics Review 1994*, 10(2–3): 291–330.

Sterman, J. D. (2000). *Business dynamics. Systems thinking and modeling for a complex world.* Buckingham: Mc-Graw Hill/Irwine, International Edition.

Sterman, J. D. (2001). Systems dynamic modelling: tools for learning in a complex world, *California Management Review*, 43: 8–25.

Suhrcke, M., McKee, M., Sauto Arce, R., Tsolova, S. and Mortensen, J. (2005). *The contribution of health to the economy in the European Union.* Brussels: European Commission.

Walt, G. (2004). WHO's World Health Report 2003, *British Medical Journal*, 328(7430): 6.

WHO (1999). *World Health Report 1999*. Geneva: World Health Organization.

WHO (2000). *World Health Report 2000 – Health systems: improving performance*. Geneva: World Health Organization.

WHO (2003). *World Health Report 2003: shaping the future*. Geneva: World Health Organization.

WHO (2006) *World Health Organization. The 3 by 5 initiative* [web site] (http://www.who.int/3by5/en, accessed 16 September 2006). Geneva: World Health Organization.

Williams, A. (2001). Science or marketing at WHO? A commentary on 'World Health 2000', *Health Economics*, 10(2): 93–100.

Wolstenholme, E. F. (1993). A case study in community care using system thinking, *Journal of the Operational Research Society*, 44: 925–934.

chapter eight

International and European responses to the threat of communicable disease

Ralph Reintjes[1]

Communicable diseases, a re-emerging threat to public health

Epidemics have significantly influenced the course of history (see Chapter 4): in the 5th century the downfall of the Roman Empire was accelerated by an outbreak of plague (McNeill 1976), while in the 14th century the enormous devastation caused by another plague epidemic undermined the authority of the church, contributing to the subsequent reformation (Davis 1996). The 20th century, with the advent of antibiotics and vaccines, saw tremendous scientific advancements in the control of infectious disease, leading, by the 1950s, to the widely held assumption that communicable diseases would in the future not cause significant harm. The re-emergence of old communicable diseases, such as TB and the emergence of new threats, such as SARS, influenza and HIV/AIDS since the mid-1980s, have shown that this optimism was unrealistic. Communicable diseases as well as threats of bioterrorism (e.g. anthrax) pose major challenges to health systems. Changes in lifestyle and behaviour, influenced by factors such as increasing urbanization and easier travel, contribute to the changing threats to human health caused by communicable diseases (Table 8.1) (MacLehose, McKee and Weinberg 2002). According to the *World Health Report 2001*, 14.4 million deaths, comprising 26% of global mortality during the year 2000, can be attributed to communicable diseases. The most frequent causes of death were lower respiratory tract infections, TB, diarrhoea, malaria and HIV/AIDS (WHO 2001).

[1] I would like to thank Amena Ahmad and Ralf Krumkamp for their valuable support and comments on earlier versions of this paper, as well as Nolene Sheppard for reviewing the language within it.

Table 8.1 A selection of evolving threats to human health from infectious diseases

Challenge	Examples
New technology	Modified cattle food resulted in prion transmission to cattle which led to nearly 200 000 cases of BSE in cattle and over 100 cases of human vCJD (Ministry of Agriculture Fisheries and Food 2000).
Travel and trade	The globalization of the food industry has led to the possibility of contaminated food being distributed internationally; e.g. consumption of chocolates contaminated with salmonella produced in one factory was related to cases notified in six European countries (Werber *et al.* 2005).
Climate change	Climatic changes are causing shifts in the distribution patterns of communicable diseases to geographical areas where they were not common in the past.
Microbial adaptation	Increasing poverty, lack of resources and inadequate treatment has led to dramatic increase in cases of MDRTB in countries of the former Soviet Union (Kimerling *et al.* 1999). Other drug resistant pathogens, e.g. MRSA, are spreading especially in hospitals and nursing homes worldwide (Mellmann *et al.* 2006).
Human behaviour	Relaxation of social norms and attitudes combined with a significant increase in intravenous drug use and commercial sex trade in eastern Europe has led to epidemics of syphilis (Riedner *et al.* 2000) and HIV infections (UNAIDS/WHO 2001).
Impaired immunology	The risk of contracting an opportunistic infection is rising on account of the immuno-compromised status of an increasing number of people (e.g. because of the spread of HIV infections or immunosuppressive drug therapy).

Source: (Adapted from) MacLehose, McKee and Weinberg 2002.

Notes: BSE: bovine spongiform encephalopathy; (v)CJD: (variant) Creutzfeldt-Jakob Disease; MDRTB: multidrug-resistant tuberculosis; MRSA: methicillin resistant *Staphylococcus aureus*; HIV: human immunodeficiency virus.

Rapid access to far-away destinations, with nearly 2 million international travellers each day, and increasing interconnectedness within Europe, where the widening and deepening of the EU has opened borders, has made the spread of communicable diseases easier than in previous decades. Historically, diseases travelled along sea routes taking long periods to spread globally, while now they can do the same within days using international air travel. This has led to intensive efforts both nationally and internationally to enhance communicable disease surveillance, prevention and control. Yet, there are significant disparities in the approaches used to tackle infectious diseases by public health authorities across Europe (MacLehose et al. 2001). Microorganisms pay no attention to borders; the surveillance and control of communicable diseases can only be successful if the systems in each individual country are well prepared, the available data are comparable and all systems are linked to allow effective cooperation (Ammon 2005). International cooperation is essential and international agencies, such as WHO and the European Commission (EC) with its newly established European Centre for Disease Prevention and Control (ECDC), play a major role in coordinating this process. This chapter reviews the existing structures that contribute to the international response to communicable disease.

International Health Regulations and response structures of WHO

Since its creation WHO has been responsible for collecting, analysing and interpreting data on communicable diseases worldwide and for administering the IHR, the mainstay of the international response to communicable disease. New patterns of collaboration between countries are constantly being developed to enable countries to respond appropriately to international threats to health. Several events in recent years, such as the threat of bioterrorism, SARS and avian influenza have exposed the shortcomings of the original IHR, first adopted in 1969. As a consequence, the WHA approved an innovative revision of the IHR as we know them (WHO 2005), as a means of enhancing the timely detection and control of events that may have a serious international health impact. They represent a clear shift from the traditional system by which WHO's member countries were required to notify a small number of communicable diseases, broadening this to create the means for a systematic analysis of health events of international concern (Rodier et al. 2006). The IHR (2005) represent a paradigm shift in several ways. First, the objects of surveillance are events, and no longer verified cases of certain diseases. This increases the sensitivity while it lowers the positive predictive value of the surveillance system. Second, member countries no longer have a monopoly as suppliers of epidemic information to WHO. Now WHO is allowed to use multiple sources of information, including the mass media and NGOs. Third, the power to define an event that invokes the use of the full power of the IHR (2005) has been moved from WHO's member countries. Even if a member country denies that an event is occurring in the country, WHO can recommend measures that affect the member country. Fourth, there are clear obligations for member countries to develop capacities for surveillance and response (Desenclos 2006).

Beyond the system arising from these regulations, there are several networks which support WHO in its quest to detect and respond rapidly to public health events of international concern.

For example, GOARN, established in 2000 with a secretariat based within WHO, is an electronically interconnected network of more than 120 institutions and experts worldwide, with specialized staff and technical resources. It constantly validates information about health-related events and acts as an international "strike force" which can be rapidly mobilized to pool resources and provide assistance in a broad range of areas concerned with the control of communicable disease outbreaks (Heymann 2006).

Information about communicable disease outbreaks today are mostly obtained through real-time electronic communications and the Internet, rather than from official Ministry of Health reports. A total of 61% of unverified reports to

WHO about a communicable disease outbreak, between January 2001 and October 2004, originated from unofficial electronic sources. A fear of economic repercussions, such as a decrease in trade and tourism that might result from measures taken to control outbreaks, explains why some countries have been reluctant to provide early information about a public health threat (Heymann 2006). The Global Public Health Intelligence Network (GPHIN), a GOARN partner, is a sensitive computer application which systematically scans the World Wide Web for keywords in different languages to identify reports of communicable disease outbreaks. The resulting information is then assessed by public health experts from, for example, WHO and action is then taken if required.

The role of Europe

European countries have participated in various WHO activities since the organization's earliest days. Nevertheless, information exchange was often slow and not very effective in initiating timely public health interventions. Even though the area of health was addressed in the original Treaty of Rome, which formed the legal basis for the establishment of the European Economic Community (EEC) in 1957, it was only limited to some aspects of occupational health for workers in the coal, steel and atomic energy sectors (McKee, Mossialos and Baeten 2002). The close causal link between trade and communicable disease spread was the driving force to establish a European competence in this field. In 1992, with the Treaty of Maastricht, this was achieved, providing a basis for cooperation between EU Member States in disease prevention and control. Its competency was further specified in the Treaty of Amsterdam in 1997. Today, the EC provides advice on measures to be taken in the event of a health crisis and coordinates the responses of the EU Member States. However, the EC does not have the mandate to implement these actions; this is the responsibility of the individual Member State.

Efficient and effective national surveillance and control systems is one of the basic requirements to ensure safety at national, European and international levels in the area of communicable disease. The progressive relaxation of borders within the EU necessitates a more coordinated approach. The free, unhindered movement of goods and people created a need for national surveillance organizations to communicate events to each other regularly and swiftly, and to use consistent surveillance systems and case definitions (Giesecke 1996). Common case definitions are important, in order to facilitate comparison of communicable disease incidence between countries. In 2002 the EC published guidelines on comparable case definitions to be used in the EU Member States (EC 2002).

However, the nature of disease surveillance in European countries as well as the public health approaches to controlling them still vary greatly (Desenclos, Bijkerk and Huisman 1993; Fenton and Lowndes 2004; MacLehose et al. 2001; Reintjes et al. 2006). A common international practice is to compare indicators such as disease notification rates across various countries. These indicators are generally obtained from each country's national surveillance data. Currently, there are 29 different national surveillance structures within the 27 EU Member

States, all of which differ in structure, design and quality (Desenclos, Bijkerk and Huisman 1993; Fenton and Lowndes 2004; Hawker 2005). As the surveillance systems within Europe vary considerably, so do the data collected within these systems. An example is the difference in sensitivity and timeliness of the various systems. To make the data comparable, to understand what they actually mean, and to assess how individual surveillance systems could be improved, studies benchmarking the national surveillance systems can be very helpful. Such a benchmarking study has been conducted to facilitate the integration of the Hungarian surveillance system into the EU. This study also highlighted areas for improvement in other national surveillance systems in Europe (Reintjes et al. 2006). Another example of important differences between European countries in the prevention and control of communicable diseases is the diversity in the organization and management of national vaccination programmes. Some countries (e.g. the United Kingdom, Finland, Hungary and the Netherlands) have a centrally organized national vaccination system, while in others (e.g. Germany) there is an expert commission that only recommends vaccination schedules. In the latter, the entire process of vaccine administration is a matter solely for the patients, their parents and the private physician consulted. These differences in health systems lead to obvious differences in vaccination status (e.g. approximately 80–85% of children under 24 months are immunized against MMR in Germany, while the figure is >95% in Hungary, Finland and the Netherlands) (Reintjes et al. 2006).

European networks

In recent years a number of international projects and networks have been developed in Europe. They have been financed partly by the EC, with additional contributions from national institutions (Sprenger, Bootsma and Reintjes 1998). They include disease-specific surveillance networks as well as infrastructure developments. Infrastructural developments aim to improve communication between national institutions, while at the same time supporting the development of comparable surveillance methods.

The European Programme for Intervention Epidemiology Training (EPIET)[2] has made a major contribution to training the next generation of Europe's communicable disease epidemiologists. During a 2-year period of "on the job" training, epidemiologists work on assignments at a national public health institute in an EU country other than their own. The objective of the programme is to foster a European network of trained epidemiologists who will be able and willing to cooperate (van Loock et al. 2001).

Eurosurveillance is an excellent example of infrastructure development.[3] This bulletin on disease surveillance and prevention is circulated rapidly within the European public health community.

In addition, there are a number of independent disease-specific networks. Table 8.2 lists these networks and demonstrates their diversity. The networks are

---

[2] www.epiet.org, accessed 29 November 2007.
[3] www.eurosurveillance.org, accessed 29 November 2007.

Table 8.2 Overview of a selection of European networks for the surveillance and control of communicable diseases

---

General surveillance network

BSN (Basic Surveillance Network)

Sexually transmitted / Blood-borne diseases

Euro-HIV (European Centre for the Epidemiological Monitoring of AIDS),

ESSTI (European Surveillance of Sexually Transmitted Infections)

Vaccine-preventable diseases

ESEN (European Seroepidemiology Network),

ELWGD (European Laboratory Working Group on Diphtheria),

EUVAC-NET (Surveillance Community Network for Vaccine Preventable Infectious Diseases),

EU IBIS (European Union Invasive Bacterial Infections Surveillance)

Zoonoses / Food-borne diseases

Enternet (International Surveillance Network for the Enteric Infections Salmonella and VTEC)

DIVINE-NET (Prevention of emerging (food-borne) enteric viral infections: diagnosis, viability testing, networking and epidemiology)

Respiratory diseases

Euro-TB (European Surveillance of Tuberculosis),

EISS (European Influenza Surveillance Scheme),

EWGLINet (European Working Group for Legionella Infections)

Antibiotic resistance / Nosocomial infections

EARSS (European Antimicrobial Resistance Surveillance Consumption),

ESAC (European Surveillance of Antimicrobial Consumption)

HELICS (Hospitals in Europe Link for Infection Control through Surveillance)

Others

ENIVD (European Network for Imported Viral Diseases)

EUNID (European Network of Infectious Diseases physicians)

Sources: Ammon 2005; Hawker 2005.

coordinated by institutions from different countries. The Basic Surveillance Network covers the most frequently notified communicable diseases (Ammon 2005). The tasks of disease-specific networks are briefly described using the following two examples of Enter-NET and the European Working Group for Legionella Infections (EWGLI).

Enter-NET (International Surveillance Network for the Enteric Infections Salmonella and verocytotoxin-producing Escherichia coli (VTEC)) is the international surveillance network for human gastrointestinal infections. Participants[4] in this network are the microbiologists in charge of the national reference laboratories for salmonella and *E. coli* infections and the epidemiologists responsible for the national surveillance of these diseases. Most countries of the EU, along with Australia, Canada, Japan, South Africa, Switzerland and Norway are members of this network. It conducts international surveillance of salmonellosis and verocytotoxin producing *Escherichia coli* (VTEC) O157, and monitors drug resistance.[5]

EWGLI[6] is a surveillance network for travel-associated Legionnaires' diseases, with 36 participating countries. The aim of the network is to detect outbreaks of Legionnaires' disease and thus identify potential sources. A total of 41% of all disease clusters detected by EWGLI in 1999 would have been missed by national systems operating alone (Lever and Joseph 2001).

In addition to the disease-specific networks, the Early Warning and Response System (EWRS) plays a key role in Europe. It consists of a web-based, password-secured notification system for important information that is transmitted to all EU Member States immediately. Decision 2119/98/EC requires each EU Member State to inform all other Member States and the EC (and since 2005, the ECDC) of outbreaks of notifiable diseases, as defined by the EU, as well as any intervention measures taken (EC 1998). The appearance of new diseases such as SARS or avian influenza must be reported immediately, following which an assessment of the risk takes place and intervention measures are decided. This procedure is especially important when an EU-wide approach is called for (Guglielmetti et al. 2006).

New structures within Europe

European Centre for Disease Control

An intensive debate about the best structure for the surveillance and control of communicable disease in Europe has been taking place for a long time. The central question is whether collaboration should be based on a network of disease-specific networks linking national centres across Europe or whether a single European centre, similar to the United States CDC would be more effective (Giesecke and Weinberg 1998; Tibayrenc 1997). In 1999 it was widely agreed that, given existing structures in Europe and the existing networks, a "network approach" would be the preferred approach for Europe (EC 2000). Nevertheless, in response to the threat of bioterrorism and the emergence of SARS, this decision was revised and the ECDC was created to strengthen Europe's defences against communicable disease. The necessary legislation was passed by the European Parliament and the Council of Ministers in the spring of 2004 and the ECDC was formally launched in September 2004 (EC 2004; Wigzell 2005). Based in Stockholm, this new EU agency provides

---

[4] http://www.hpa.org.uk/hpa/inter/enter-net_participants.htm, accessed 29 November 2007.
[5] http://www.hpa.org.uk/hpa/inter/enter-net_menu.htm, accessed 29 November 2007.
[6] www.ewgli.org, accessed 29 November 2007.

a structured and systematic approach to the control of communicable disease and other serious health threats to the citizens of the EU. The ECDC also reinforces the synergies between the existing national centres for disease control. At the core of its mandate, the ECDC is responsible for facilitating cooperation between national disease control agencies and other organizations, and coordinating European action to meet some of the key health challenges of the 21st century. The main tasks of the ECDC explained in more detail in the following subsections.

Epidemiological surveillance and networking of laboratories

The ECDC supports epidemiological surveillance activities at European level. To accomplish this, the Centre can either use its own staff, staff from the dedicated surveillance networks (Table 8.2), or in some instances, it can delegate tasks to a national centre of excellence. The Centre can also identify and maintain networks of reference laboratories and simultaneously enhance their quality and expertise.

Early Warning and Response System

This web-based, password-secured notification system requires "around the clock" availability of specialists in communicable diseases to disseminate critically important information in real time to EU Member States. The responsibility for action remains with EU Member States and the EC.

Scientific opinions

Public health decisions have to be based on scientific evidence. While dealing with communicable diseases, a wide variety of issues ranging from clinical medicine and epidemiology to standardization of laboratory procedures have to be considered. Creating one permanent scientific committee to cover all these issues would not therefore be appropriate. The ECDC instead pools together scientific expertise in the specific fields through its multiple EU-wide networks and via ad hoc scientific panels.

Technical assistance and communication

ECDC's rapid reaction capacity can also cover countries outside the EU, such as the EEA and European Free Trade Association (EFTA) countries. The Centre also has the ability to support, if necessary, the services of the EC which deals with humanitarian aid and other types of assistance in response to disease outbreaks in developing countries. In addition, the ECDC coordinates the evaluation of all EU Disease Surveillance Networks (ECDC 2006).

It is of the utmost importance that the EU and WHO work closely together. This is exemplified by the activities related to pandemic influenza preparedness planning. Since 2005, the EU and all its Member States have made considerable progress in strengthening their preparedness against pandemic influenza. The health systems in all countries have developed preparedness plans and, at national level, substantial efforts have been made to make these plans operational (Mounier-Jack and Coker 2006). To maintain the momentum and to further involve non-health care sectors, a working group comprising officials from the WHO Regional Office for Europe and independent experts was established.

A total of 27 countries participated in a preparedness review. These were the first 25 EU Member States, plus Iceland and Norway. By acting together, Member States and the EC, supported by EU agencies such as the ECDC, have made great progress in preparing Europe for a pandemic (ECDC 2007). The example discussed in the following subsection highlights how international response structures and cooperation among countries led to the containment of the SARS epidemic in 2003.

International response: the example of SARS

Reports of a major "flu outbreak" in mainland China were first picked up by the GPHIN and other partners of the GOARN in late November 2002, following which the "WHO Global Influenza Surveillance Network" was alerted. In response to requests for validation of these reports, the Chinese Ministry of Health confirmed that the cases were due to transmission of influenza type B virus (Heymann 2006). On 10 February 2003, the WHO office in Beijing received an email message describing a "strange contagious disease" outbreak in Guangdong, China, which had led to the death of more than 100 people, followed the next day by an official report from the Chinese Ministry of Health to WHO of approximately 300 cases and five deaths due to an atypical pneumonia of unknown cause, dating back to 16 November 2002, with reassurance that the outbreak was coming under control (Whaley and Mansoor 2006). Fear of a major influenza outbreak and the insufficient data from China led to heightened surveillance for respiratory diseases in Asia. Reports to WHO of two cases of avian influenza from Hong Kong on 19 February 2003 and a case of severe atypical pneumonia in Vietnam on 26 February, followed on 5 March by reports of infected health care workers in Hong Kong and Vietnam (Heymann 2006) led to WHO issuing a first global alert on 12 March 2003 regarding the appearance of a new contagious respiratory disease of unknown aetiology in Asia. The signs and symptoms were described and as a first measure WHO recommended the isolation of suspect cases, barrier nursing and the reporting of such cases to national authorities (WHO 2003c) and to WHO using electronic reporting formats (Heymann 2006). Subsequent reports of similar cases from Canada, Singapore, Taiwan and other Asian countries, along with the realization that SARS had spread to several countries in a short time via air travel resulted in WHO issuing a second stronger alert in the form of an emergency travel advisory on 15 March 2003. An initial case definition, based on clinical signs and symptoms, as well as a history of contact or travel to areas reporting these cases, was formulated (WHO 2003d).

During the 2002/2003 SARS epidemic over 8000 SARS cases were reported from 29 countries. Its transmission was successfully interrupted within less than four months of its first spread outside China. Science and communication systems of the 21st century, together with 19th century classical public health tools of case detection, contact tracing, quarantine and isolation, and infection control overcame the virus. Yet this was only possible due to the coordinated efforts of governments, international organizations, health care institutions and many dedicated people. The collaboration of countries and ready reporting of SARS cases (not covered by the IHR at that time) and the international response showed that countries were willing to forego their exclusive sovereign rights to solve a global threat (Heymann 2006; WHO 2003b; WHO 2003a).

WHO adopted a unique role in coordinating the global SARS containment efforts. Through its GOARN partners, it was able to mobilize expertise and resources rapidly to find answers to the key epidemiologic parameters, identify the causative agent and send teams to affected areas. The instant sharing of information among governments, epidemiologists, medical and public health experts and laboratory scientists enabled WHO to make evidence-based recommendations (Doberstyn 2006).

The EC formed a multidisciplinary SARS expert group to advise the Commission and national authorities on SARS-related issues. In June 2003 the Commission reported on the "Measures Undertaken by Member States and Accession Countries to Control the Outbreak of SARS" in Europe, and noted that ". . . on the whole, European countries have adopted rapid and consistent measures on early detection of cases, implementation of isolation measures and guidance to health professionals and the public on the identification of possible SARS cases." It was also evident that travel advice was inconsistent among European countries. SARS also exposed weakness in the health infrastructure in EU Member States and identified areas that needed increased European coherence. It reinforced the need for a European centre which would provide an operational platform for combining the expertise of EU Member States, organizing an EU-wide systematic approach to control communicable disease and strengthening cooperation with international partners such as the GOARN network. This culminated in the establishment of the ECDC in 2005 (EC 2003).

It also led to the initiation of several research projects by the EC to advise policy-makers on how to prepare for a potential new epidemic. A good example of a multidisciplinary concerted approach is the SARS Control Project. It seeks to identify effective and acceptable strategies for the control of SARS and other newly emerging infections in China and Europe. Within this study, a range of issues are studied, from surveillance to economics and from risk perception to policy evaluation (Krumkamp et al. [Submitted]).

Future prospects

SARS is a success story in the international struggle against communicable diseases. There is currently a high level of political commitment to strengthen pandemic influenza preparedness. The organizational and health system structures for the prevention and control of pandemics is under revision internationally. The rapid implementation of the decision to establish a new European agency, the ECDC, was exceptional.

Nevertheless, there are still a number of challenges ahead. In the field of pandemic preparedness there are several areas where further work is needed, including better integration across various government ministries. A pandemic would require cooperation from all elements of government and beyond. Most countries focus essentially on health sector plans and many report not yet having business continuity plans to ensure that essential public services outside the health sector will be able to cope with the sustained stress of a pandemic (e.g. transport, utilities, police, etc). Pandemic influenza is only one candidate disease that might test health systems in many unforeseen ways. The challenge for health systems will be to ensure they have the capacity to meet both the needs of today and the diseases of the future.

It is evident that coordinated national and international measures to ensure the sharing of robust information, knowledge and resources are necessary to prevent, detect and control communicable disease outbreaks. Yet these can only succeed if they are based on strong and effective national public health infrastructures. The strengthening of networks such as GOARN and institutions such as the ECDC is essential to tackle emerging threats. If the process of integration and improvement at international level seen since the mid-1990s can continue, the "network of networks and (international and national) institutions" could lead to where the world needs to be in order to protect public health most effectively.

References

Ammon, A. (2005). Strukturen der Überwachung und des Managements von Infektions-krankheiten in der EU. Die EU-Netzwerke für übertragbare Krankheiten und das Europäische Zentrum für die Prävention und die Kontrolle von Krankheiten (ECDC), *Gesundheitsblatt – Gesundheitsforschung – Gesundheitsschutz*, 48: 1038–1042.

Davis, N. (1996). *Europe: a history.* Oxford: Oxford University Press.

Desenclos, J. C. (2006). Are there "new" and "old" ways to track infectious disease hazards and outbreaks? *Euro Surveill*, 11(12): 206–207.

Desenclos, J. C., Bijkerk, H. and Huisman, J. (1993). Variations in national infectious diseases surveillance in Europe, *Lancet*, 341(8851): 1003–1006.

Doberstyn, B. (2006). *What did we learn from SARS?* In: SARS: How a global epidemic was stopped. Geneva: World Health Organization.

ECDC (2006) Evaluation of Networks. In: Minutes of the Sixth meeting of the Advisory Forum. European Centre for Disease Prevention and Control, Stockholm, 10–11 May 2006.

ECDC (2007). *Technical Report – Pandemic influenza preparedness in the EU.* Stockholm: European Centre for Disease Prevention and Control.

EC (1998). *Setting up a network for the epidemiological surveillance and control of communicable diseases in the community. OJ L 268, 03.10.1998.* Brussels: European Commission.

EC (2000). *Community Decision of 22 December 1999 on the communicable diseases to be progressively covered by the Community network under Decision No. 2119/98/EC of the European Parliament and of the Council (2000/96/EC), OJ L28. 3.2.2000.* Brussels: European Commission.

EC (2002). *Commission Decision 2002/253/EC laying down case definitions for reporting communicable diseases to the Community network under Decision No. 2119/98/EC of the European Parliament and of the Council. OJ L 86, 3.4.2002:44.* Brussels: European Commission.

EC (2003). *Measures undertaken by Member States and accession countries to control the outbreak of SARS. Report by the Commission.* Luxembourg: SANCO Public Health Directorate.

EC (2004). Regulation (EC) No. 851/2004 of the European Parliament and of the Council of 21.4.2004 establishing a European centre for disease prevention and control. OJ L 142, 30.04.2004:1. Brussels: European Commission.

Fenton, K. A. and Lowndes, C. M. (2004). The European Surveillance of Sexually Transmitted Infections (ESSTI) Network: Recent trends in the epidemiology of sexually transmitted infections in the European Union, *Sex Transm Infect* 80: 255–263.

Giesecke, J. (1996). Surveillance of infectious diseases in the European Union, *Lancet*, 348(9041): 1534.

Giesecke, J. and Weinberg, J. (1998). A European Centre for Infectious Disease? *Lancet*, 352(9136): 1308.

Guglielmetti, P., Coulombier, D., Thinus, G., Van Loock, F. and Schreck, S. (2006). The Early Warning and Response System for communicable diseases in the EU: an overview from 1999 to 2005, *EuroSurveillance*, 11(12): 215–220.

Hawker, J. (2005). *Communicable disease control handbook.* Oxford: Blackwell Science.

Heymann, D. L. (2006). SARS and emerging infectious diseases: a challenge to place global solidarity above national sovereignty, *Annals Academy of Medicing Singapore*, 35(5): 350–353.

Krumkamp, R., Duerr, H. P., Kassen, A., Eichner, M. and Reintjes, R. [Submitted]. Impact of public health interventions in controlling the spread of SARS – Modelling intervention scenarios. Augsberg: Kongress Medizin und Gesellschaft; Düsseldorf: Medical Science GMS Publishing House.

Lever, F. and Joseph, C. A. (2001). Travel-associated Legionnaires' disease in Europe in 1999, *EuroSurveillance*, 6(4): 53–61.

MacLehose, L., McKee, M. and Weinberg, J. (2002). Responding to the challenge of communicable disease in Europe, *Science*, 295(5562): 2047–2050.

MacLehose, L., Brand, H., Camaroni, I., et al. (2001). Communicable disease outbreaks involving more than one country: systems approach to evaluating the response, *British Medical Journal*, 323(7317): 861–863.

McKee, M., Mossialos, E. and Baeten, R. (2002). *The impact of EU law on health care systems.* Brussels: Peter Lang.

McNeill, W. H. (1976). *Plagues and Peoples.* Middlesex: Penguin.

Mounier-Jack, S. and Coker, R. J. (2006). How prepared is Europe for pandemic influenza? Analysis of national plans, *Lancet*, 367(9520): 1405–1411.

Reintjes, R., Thelen, M., Reiche, R. and Csohan, A. (2006). Benchmarking national surveillance systems: a new tool for the comparison of communicable disease surveillance and control in Europe, *European Journal of Public Health*.

Rodier, G., Hardiman, M., Plotkin, B. and Ganter, B. (2006). Implementing the International Health Regulations (2005) in Europe, *EuroSurveillance*, 11(12): 208–211.

Sprenger, M. J. W., Bootsma, P. A. and Reintjes, R. (1998). Infectious disease surveillance in Europe, *Nederlands Tijdschrift voor Geneeskunde*, 142(44): 2418–2423.

Tibayrenc, M. (1997). European centres for disease control, *Nature*, 389(6650): 433.

van Loock, F., Rowland, M., Grein, T. and Moren, A. (2001). Intervention epidemiology training: a European perspective, *Euro Surveill*, 6(3): 37–43.

Whaley, F. and Mansoor, O. D. (2006). *SARS Chronology. In SARS: How a global epidemic was stopped.* Geneva: World Health Organization/Western Pacific Region.

WHO (2001). *World Health Report 2001.* Geneva: World Health Organization.

WHO (2003a). *World Health Report 2003: shaping the future.* Geneva: World Health Organization.

WHO (2003b). *Severe acute respiratory syndrome (SARS): Status of the outbreak and lessons for the immediate future. 20 May* Geneva: World Health Organization, Communicable disease surveillance and response.

WHO (2003c). *WHO issues a global alert about cases of atypical pneumonia: cases of severe respiratory illness may spread to hospital staff. World Health Organization press release 12 March 2003.* Geneva: World Health Organization (http://www.who.int/csr/sars/archive/2003_03_12/en, date accessed 6 March 2008).

WHO (2003d). *World Health Organization situation update 15 March 2003.* Geneva: World Health Organization (http://www.who.int/csr/sars/archive/2003_03_15/en, accessed 27 November 2007).

WHO (2005). *IHR: International Health Regulations.* Geneva: World Health Organization (http://www.who.int/csr/ihr/en/, accessed 27 November 2007).

Wigzell, H. (2005). A European CDC? *Science*, 307(5716): 1691.

nine

HIV/AIDS and tuberculosis control in post-Soviet Union countries

Nina Schwalbe, Jeffrey Lazarus,
Olusoji Adeyi

Introduction

This chapter explores health system responses to communicable disease by looking at HIV/AIDS and TB in the 15 countries of the former Soviet Union, where health systems reform has been especially challenging to implement, in particular the national TB and HIV/AIDS control programmes which are separately organized in terms of financing, surveillance, management and service delivery. HIV and TB, both global public health emergencies, were chosen as illustrative cases as eastern Europe has one of the fastest growing HIV epidemics in the world.

History of the epidemics in the Europe and central Asia region

In the early 1990s, the former Soviet states saw the emergence of both HIV and TB epidemics. At that time, the two infections were not directly related and there were few cases of AIDS. In less than a decade, however, the region had the fastest growing HIV epidemic in the world. TB, which had been a low-incidence disease during the Soviet period, started to increase rapidly, beginning in the 1990s, due to worsening social conditions. By the year 2000, more than half of the former Soviet Union countries were categorized by WHO as high-incidence countries for TB. By 2004, 6.8% and 8.3% of diagnosed TB cases were estimated to be co-infected with HIV in the Russian Federation and Ukraine, respectively (WHO 2006a).

HIV/AIDS

Overall rates of newly diagnosed HIV infection continue to increase rapidly in the countries of the former Soviet Union. At the end of 2006, WHO/Joint United Nations Programme on HIV/AIDS (UNAIDS) estimated there to be 1.7 (between 1.2 and 2.6) million people with HIV (UNAIDS and WHO 2006) – of which 90% were in the Russian Federation and Ukraine alone – and the estimated prevalence among adults had surpassed 1% of the adult population in three countries: Estonia, the Russian Federation and Ukraine (WHO Regional Office for Europe 2006). Moreover, AIDS killed an estimated 84 000 (between 58 000 and 120 000) adults and children in 2005 – more than twice as many as in 2003.

In all of these countries, male injecting drug users comprise the majority of those infected (see Table 9.1) (Dehne et al. 1999; Hamers and Downs 2003). The next most affected populations are women who inject drugs, followed by partners of drug users of both sexes. Most new cases occur among those aged 20–39.

At the time of writing, all of the countries had only poor to moderate treatment coverage for HIV/AIDS, with coverage in the Russian Federation being under 10% of those in need (WHO Regional Office for Europe 2005). Data also show inequity with regard to access to treatment, especially for injecting drug users. In nine reporting countries of eastern Europe, for example, injecting drug users make up only 52% of those being treated, in spite of constituting 74% of reported cases. In real numbers, however, this meant 739 individuals being treated out of 65 313 people reported to be living with HIV (Donoghoe et al. 2007).

Table 9.1 Reported HIV/AIDS cases and tuberculosis incidence, selected countries, 2005

	Population (million)[a]	Adult HIV prevalence[a]	Proportion of persons aged <25 among PLWHIV (%)[a]	Proportion of injecting drugs users among PLWHIV (%)[a]	Proportion of males among PLWHIV (%)[a]	TB incidence per 100 000 population (2004)[b]
Estonia	1.33	> 1%	60	90	77	46
Georgia	4.47	< 0.1%	26	68	71	82
Kazakhstan	14.82	0.1–0.3%	38	84	76	155
Kyrgyzstan	5.26	0.1–0.3%	N/A	80	81	122
Latvia	2.30	0.8–1%	47	81	73	68
Lithuania	3.43	0.1–0.3%	55	83	89	63
Republic of Moldova	3.59	0.1–0.3%	44	74	73	138
Russian Federation	143.20	> 1%	61	87	75	115
Ukraine	46.48	>1.4%	n/a	71	66	101

Sources: [a] EuroHIV 2005; WHO Regional Office for Europe 2006; [b] WHO 2006a.

Notes: HIV: human immunodeficiency virus; PLWHIV: people living with HIV; TB: tuberculosis; n/a: not available.

Tuberculosis

Reported TB rates began to increase in 1992 in all of the countries, following the break-up of the Soviet Union and the resulting worsening of socioeconomic conditions, compounded by a faltering and underfunded health care system. Rates have remained high throughout the region, with 10 of the 15 countries now classified as high incidence (more than 70 per 100 000 population) (Institut de veille sanitaire, WHO Collaborating Centre for the Surveillance of Tuberculosis in Europe and Royal Netherlands Tuberculosis Association (KNCV) 2004). Furthermore, the countries of the region have some of the highest incidences of multi-drug resistant tuberculosis (MDR-TB). TB patients in the Baltic states and the Russian Federation are 10 times more likely to have MDR-TB than in the rest of the world (Aziz et al. 2004; WHO Regional Office for Europe 2002). Along with Kazakhstan and Uzbekistan, these countries constitute 6 out of the 10 global MDR-TB hotspots, with drug resistance in new patients as high as 14% (Aziz et al. 2004). TB has become endemic in the general population, with much higher prevalence rates in the prison setting, where close living quarters, poor air circulation and overcrowding promote the spread of the disease. The increased likelihood of TB transmission in prisons is well documented in the literature, but appears to have been exacerbated by inadequate treatment of the disease. Moreover, HIV infection, which fuels TB by facilitating progression to active disease, is further expected to contribute to continued high rates of TB.

Although by 2003 of all the 15 of the countries that had purportedly adopted the WHO recommended strategy for TB control (DOTS), none had reached the WHO-recommended target of both 70% case-detection and 85% cure rates. Further, the reported percentage of the population covered by DOTS was less than 50% in 7 of the 15 countries (WHO 2006a).

Data quality for HIV/AIDS and tuberculosis

Within the region, data on these diseases come from the following distinct sources: the national surveillance systems that report actual cases of TB and HIV/AIDS, WHO Headquarters, which reports estimates on TB, and UNAIDS/ WHO which report estimates on HIV/AIDS. The government figures, whether reported cases or estimates, often differ dramatically from those quoted by the multilateral agencies. And in the 2006 report on the global AIDS epidemic, UNAIDS states that due to more accurate data, estimates for 2005 are lower than those previously published, in spite of the inclusion of infected people over the age of 50 for the first time. They stress that the latest estimates cannot be compared directly with estimates published earlier and nor should they be compared directly to those to be published in the years to come.

HIV/AIDS

In most of the countries of the region, official government data come from actual case reporting (specific numbers of people who test positive for HIV or those who are diagnosed with AIDS). Such reporting, however, does not accurately reflect either the prevalence or the incidence of HIV or AIDS, as those people most at risk may not be getting tested nor presenting themselves to government health care facilities when sick (Nielsen and Lazarus 2006). For this reason, official government figures are considerably lower than those estimates reported by United Nations agencies. Table 9.1 presents an estimated prevalence for people aged 15–49 years, derived by UNAIDS/WHO using the Workbook method. The method estimates national adult HIV prevalence based on the HIV prevalence in high-risk populations, and their partners, together with estimations of the size of those groups. National prevalence estimates produced can then be imported into a software package called Spectrum to project the future trends in the number of people infected with HIV, as well as AIDS cases and AIDS deaths (Ghys, Walker and Gamett 2006; UNAIDS 2005). The concern with such modelling is that the size of the risk groups and their partners is very difficult to calculate with any degree of accuracy, as is the degree of HIV prevalence among the risk groups. Also, in many of the countries, at-risk groups such as injecting drug users, migrants, ethnic minorities and sex workers may overlap, complicating the accurate registration of new HIV cases, which in turn affects the accuracy of the estimates.

The only relatively complete and consistent dataset for post-Soviet countries is that collected from the countries themselves, e.g. from their national AIDS centres or other surveillance agencies, by the European Centre for the Epidemiological Monitoring of AIDS (EuroHIV). These data can serve to monitor trends over time, but are not an accurate portrayal of the magnitude of the problem, because, as described above, they present cases of newly diagnosed HIV infections and AIDS only and not the overall population prevalence. Box 9.1 discusses HIV estimates in Ukraine.

Tuberculosis

In the case of TB, governments in the region report actual cases. These are conveyed mid-year to the European Centre for the Epidemiological Monitoring of Tuberculosis (EuroTB) and the WHO Regional Office for Europe, which coordinates the efforts for the surveillance of TB in Europe. While EuroTB collects individual data based on case notification (and thus is consistent with government reporting), WHO calculates country estimates based on smear positivity and incidence, reflecting the fact that the number of reported cases is lower than the actual number of cases (WHO 2006a).

National efforts to control tuberculosis and HIV/AIDS in post-Soviet Union countries

Key issues and debates

The principal concern with regard to the control of both diseases in the countries of the former Soviet Union is the vertical isolation of the prevention and treatment efforts (where they exist) within the national disease control

Box 9.1   Improving national HIV estimates in Ukraine

In 2005, Ukraine initiated a process to review and improve the national HIV prevalence estimates following a lack of consensus among various stakeholders. A series of workshops and consultations were held to review the available data and estimates on HIV in the country, identify major gaps in the data, train national experts in the existing UNAIDS/WHO methods to produce estimates and to develop revised national HIV estimates for Ukraine. The process included a broad group of stakeholders on HIV in Ukraine, including epidemiologists and surveillance experts from both the regional and national levels, representatives from the Ministry of Health as well as United Nations organizations and both national and international NGOs such as the International HIV/AIDS Alliance in Ukraine, organizations representing PLHIV in Ukraine and the British Council.

Following the first consensus meeting held in April 2005, which highlighted the lack of information about the sizes of the most at-risk populations in Ukraine, the International HIV/AIDS Alliance in Ukraine, in partnership with UNAIDS, WHO and several Ukrainian sociological research institutions facilitated a series of special surveys in order to assess and develop estimates of the number of injecting drug users, female sex workers and MSM. These revised population size estimates were used together with data from the HIV prevalence studies carried out among selected populations in a number of regions in Ukraine to produce the revised national HIV prevalence estimates for Ukraine.

This process led to a decreased HIV prevalence estimate for Ukraine compared to earlier estimates. This decline does not represent an actual decline in the epidemic, but rather a more accurate estimate based on improved evidence. Ukraine is probably the country in the region which has undertaken the most serious efforts to improve their national HIV estimates. However, in spite of these efforts, serious issues persist. For example, there is a lack of behavioural surveillance to shed light on the frequency of the key risk behaviours facilitating HIV transmission in Ukraine, such as the extent of unprotected sex, unsafe injections (e.g. using shared or non-sterile injecting equipment), and the number of sexual partners and amount of sexual mixing between different risk groups. In particular, there is a lack of data on HIV among MSM and prisoners in Ukraine.

Source: Nielsen 2006; Ukraine Ministry of Health et al. 2006.

programmes. Each disease is managed in its own silo, originating at the central planning level and carrying down to the local level with its own distinct and separate medical specialists and service delivery mechanisms and structures. Although there have been attempts to integrate prevention and treatment of these infections in countries with newly reformed primary care systems, current protocols still refer patients to different facilities for all counselling, testing and treatment services.

A further obstacle to the integration of care is the fact that prison health services, which are particularly poor in all countries, are not linked to the civilian health care system. There is no recognition of the concept of equivalence, which calls for "providing prisoners with prevention, care, treatment and support for HIV/AIDS that is equivalent to that available to people in the community outside of prison" (UNODC, WHO and UNAIDS 2006). High rates of incarceration in the region, and the constant movement of people between the prison system and the civilian sector, add to the challenge of adequately addressing either infection.

History of HIV/AIDS services

The HIV/AIDS diagnosis and treatment system is similar in structure to that of TB. Although it does not have a long historical legacy per se, it has roots in the STI service, which also dates to pre-Soviet times and was established as a vertical system, with special centres, hospitals and professionals designated to deal with the diseases.

The Soviet Union registered its first official case of HIV in 1986. The case was described as a homosexual in the military who had had sexual relations with an African and then reportedly had sex with 15 other soldiers. However, because of the discrimination against homosexuality and the potential for scandal given its clear presence in the military, the case was minimized. The virus was only more widely reported in 1987, when found among 279 children in the city of Elista, resulting from the multiple use of syringes and other medical equipment without proper sterilization. In the late 1980s the disease also spread among the homosexual community in St Petersburg, but few of these cases were officially reported, given that homosexuality was at that time illegal.

The Government responded immediately to the Elista outbreak by instituting a vertical disease control programme, which provided for AIDS centres in each region. After the break-up of the Soviet Union all 15 countries adopted the same model, with an AIDS centre in each of the 89 *oblasts* (provinces/regions), controlled by the national Ministry of Health of the respective countries. By the mid-1990s, each country had also adopted national HIV/AIDS plans and in 2001 all countries became signatories to the United Nations General Assembly Special Session on AIDS (UNGASS) Declaration of Commitment on AIDS. This committed governments to execute extensive prevention and treatment efforts, which they again agreed to in the 2004 Dublin Declaration on Partnership to fight HIV/AIDS in Europe and Central Asia (Government of Ireland 2004).

Wide-scale HIV testing began at the end of the Soviet period (late 1980s), with contact tracing conducted as follow-up for individuals that test positive. Testing is mandatory for blood and organ donors and in some countries for professionals deemed to likely be in contact with PLHIV as well. In practice, many former Soviet Union countries also test pregnant women, homosexuals, patients undergoing operations, drug users, army conscripts, prisoners and foreigners requesting multi-entry visas. Approximately 17–20 million HIV tests have been performed each year since 1988 in the Russian Federation alone and testing rates are also among the highest in the world in the other countries (EuroHIV 2005). This sort of mass screening is not considered standard practice anywhere else in the world and, further, has not proved effective for controlling the epidemic in countries where the epidemic is concentrated among specific groups at risk, such as injecting drug users.

In all of the former Soviet Union countries, federal or national funds are allocated for technical support of HIV/AIDS services (e.g. supplies and testing kits), with local authorities responsible for all other costs related to maintaining services (staffing, facilities maintenance and prevention and outreach activities). As such, the quality of services differs greatly depending on the emphasis placed on the disease by local government authorities and the financial means they may or may not have to address it. Lack of quality control is further compounded by the fact that many of the countries have engaged in overall decentralization of government services.

History of tuberculosis services

The countries of the region have a long history of TB, as evidenced and recorded by such authors as Anton Chekhov and Fyodor Dostoyevsky, both of whom themselves suffered from the disease. The first TB programme was established in the Tsarist period and carried forward to the Soviet period. In the Soviet era, the programme functioned under the federal Ministry of Health and had its own set of hospitals, research institutes and a category of physician called "phtysiologists" for treating the disease. In addition to passive case finding, the TB control services carried out mass population screening. Criteria for screening included not just groups considered to be at a particular risk of TB (such as medical staff, school children or the military) but also the general population whenever they encountered the public system, such as to obtain a marriage certificate or to get a public sector job). Screening was performed by X-ray. Anyone found with active TB was either hospitalized or confined to sanatoria, with surgery as the most common treatment modality. At birth, children were (and still are) immunized with BCG and given booster doses in early childhood and adolescence.

Although diagnosis by X-ray, coupled with surgery and BCG have certainly been part of standard practice in many countries since the early 1900s, treatment began to change radically in the 1950s, with the introduction of anti-TB drugs, which were proven to be a much more effective form of treatment than surgery. Pharmaceuticals are also much cheaper and less labour intensive to administer. Similarly, both mass population screening and X-rays were replaced by active case finding, using sputum smear microscopy. As for BCG, the efficacy of this vaccine has been highly disputed, and is no longer used in much of the world, in part because it has not proven effective in adults and in part because once immunized, diagnosis for latent disease becomes more difficult. Lengthy hospitalizations and reliance on surgery for treatment made the Soviet TB programme quite labour intensive and not particularly cost efficient (Reichman 2002).

With all these caveats, the Soviet system was adequate in terms of controlling the spread of TB when it was a low-incidence disease. However, with political and economic turmoil in the early 1990s resulting in worsening socioeconomic conditions for the populations overall, an end to central planning in health and chronic pharmaceutical shortages (Garrett 2000), the incidence of TB began to rise rapidly throughout the region and by the late 1990s had reached high proportions, particularly in prisons (Veen and Godinho 2006) (see Figure 9.1).

The divide between prison and civilian health systems

In 2004, approximately 14% of the Russian Federation's known AIDS cases were in prison populations (AIDS Foundation East-West 2005). The two main modes of transmission were needle sharing among injecting drug users, within and

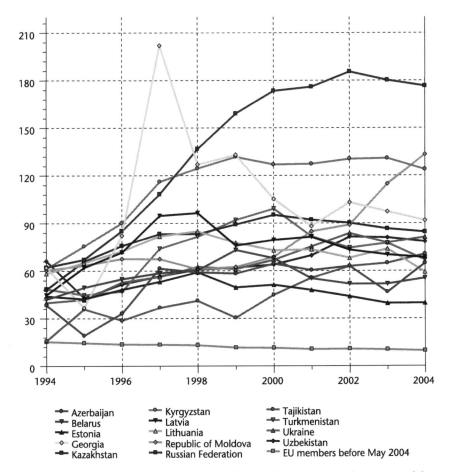

Figure 9.1 Tuberculosis incidence per 100 000 population in selected countries of the former Soviet Union, 1994–2004

Source: WHO Regional Office for Europe 2006a.

beyond penitentiary systems, and unsafe sex. At the same time, in some countries in the region, TB is reported to be 200 times more prevalent in prisons than in the general population (Aerts et al. 2000). Although many countries have been working to adopt pilot programmes for both condom promotion, needle and syringe exchange and the treatment of TB, the fact that prison health authorities in most former Soviet Union countries have no official relation to ministries of health has made it difficult for the integration of care or sharing of expertise between the two sectors.

Tensions as tuberculosis and HIV moved from low-incidence infections to epidemics

Although logical within the organizational framework of central planning, the Soviet health system suffered from many of the inefficient features of state-owned enterprises seen in the formerly socialist economies of eastern Europe and central Asia. Some of these features include a state monopoly over most health sector activities; lack of functioning labour markets, capital markets and insurance markets; a state monopoly over financing and ownership of most health services; rigid public bureaucracies with little management flexibility; and the pervasive lack of responsiveness to demand, along with little scope for dynamic evolution (Preker and Adeyi 2005). These factors have played out in the course of both the TB and HIV epidemics, as well as country responses to them.

For both diseases, a number of key problems emerged in the design and implementation of the programmes. First, the misplaced emphasis on mass screening versus active case finding among high-risk groups meant that although many tests were performed, they were not performed among the risk groups, thus those with the infection were often missed. Second, the vertical structure of services translated into significant problems with identification, referral and follow-up of patients. Third, the subspecialization within these infections by the medical establishment kept the necessary services from becoming part of the regular primary health care system. This approach is not appropriate for dealing with full-blown epidemics, where everyone entering the health system should be assessed for risk of disease, and referred appropriately. And, finally, the stigmatization and discrimination against people with TB or HIV – one associated with the destitute and with prisoners, the other with drug users, homosexuals and sex workers – meant slow implementation of national population-based education and information programmes and little mass media attention.

A secondary, but equally important, set of factors concerns history and "turf". In terms of history, the TB control establishment was over a century old, in fact, older than the Soviet Union itself. The HIV establishment, although relatively new, was rooted in the history of STI control, which was punitive in nature with intensive contact tracing and a lack of anonymity or confidentiality. The tie with the former system of STI services and lack of confidentiality set the stage for patient distrust of any promise of anonymity.

As for "turf", both systems have massive bureaucracies to protect. In the case of TB, this includes the network of TB doctors and surgeons, and hospitals and sanatoria that are reimbursed according to numbers of beds, rather than numbers of patients or types of treatment provided. In the case of HIV, the bureaucracy includes AIDS centres and staff in every region and major city of each country, as well as a massive laboratory infrastructure for testing.

International efforts and interventions

International agencies began to work in the countries of the former Soviet Union shortly after the political break-up in the early 1990s. These included bilateral donors, multilaterals, private foundations and international NGOs. Some worked with federal or national authorities, some worked directly with regional or local governments and some worked with the newly developing nongovernmental sector. The programmes ranged in size and scope from non-monetary exchanges to multimillion dollar infrastructure projects. In terms of HIV/AIDS, the first interventions began in the early 1990s and included information and education activities for the population as a whole via television, print, radio and the distribution of leaflets and condoms, as well as condom social marketing, support for NGOs for outreach activities among homosexuals and the training of medical personnel. The first harm-reduction programmes in the region were piloted in the mid- and late 1990s and by 2003 there were pilot programmes operating in all 15 countries of the region, although by the time of writing, services had not been brought to full scale in any of them.

In terms of TB, a number of international NGOs became engaged in the mid-1990s, including *Médecins Sans Frontières* (MSF), the Public Health Research Institute (PHRI), and the International Committee of the Red Cross (ICRC), focusing mostly on the prison sector as part of a humanitarian effort. WHO and bilateral donors followed soon after, working with the ministries of health and civil society and attempting to expand successful pilot programmes and introduce the DOTS strategy as the national protocol. In late 2006 WHO Regional Office for Europe launched a new set of HIV/AIDS treatment and care protocols, with the intent that the TB/HIV protocol will contribute to the better integration of these independent services (WHO Regional Office for Europe 2006).

With regard to both diseases, the pilot and scale-up phases of these efforts have met with varying degrees of success. This success has depended a great deal on the willingness of partners within/associated with countries to radically shift their attitudes and approaches to infectious disease control.

HIV/AIDS

Whereas local government has in many cases been quite receptive to implementing pilot programmes, political denial and stigma at national level have been major barriers to the countrywide scale-up of prevention projects (Donoghoe, Lazarus and Matic 2005). As the principal behavioural risk factor behind epidemics in this region is injecting drug use, followed by commercial sex, a lack of knowledge about the behavioural patterns of drug users and sex workers and the belief by governments that the epidemics could remain contained within these populations prevented early action in many of the countries. Even where successful pilot projects had been established, moving from pilot projects to countrywide programmes was not successful. This was in part because it required building coalitions across groups with disparate interests and constituencies (e.g. social conservatives, liberal activists, different government ministries, NGOs and religious groups) and in part because of the lack of willingness of governments to commit adequate resources to scale up. One of the more successful techniques used to shift the debate from a health issue to a central policy issue was presenting evidence that demonstrated the impact of HIV/AIDS on the labour force and consequently on the economy (Ruehl, Pokrovsky and Vinogradov 2002). Another was to create a strong local evidence base on the success of pilots engaging local experts and key decision-makers in their projects (Tkatchenko-Schmidt et al. 2007).

Tuberculosis

Despite the support of international organizations and the success of pilot projects in both the prison and civilian sectors, it has been very difficult for countries to develop and implement large-scale TB control programmes based on criteria recommended by WHO. In this case, institutional, policy, legal and social conditions for the large-scale implementation of evidence-based programmes proved even more challenging than the financial constraints. With such an extensive network of clinics, hospitals and specialists employed and invested in the Soviet system, inertia and interest groups have slowed the pace and depth of reforms (Adeyi et al. 2003).

HIV and tuberculosis programmes in prisons

As mentioned, international NGOs were involved in developing pilot projects in the prison system for both HIV and TB. In the area of HIV, prevention programmes included condom distribution, education campaigns and training for prison doctors. However, no country has to date agreed to pilot needle exchange programmes for prisoners, reflecting a denial of authorities to acknowledge active injecting drug use within prison walls.

As for TB projects, it was the prison authorities who were among the first to welcome international partners, both for treatment of drug-susceptible and drug-resistant TB. In most cases this was the result of morbidity and mortality among prison staff, coupled with a need for resources following the decrease in funding for prison services after the break-up of the Soviet Union.

What worked and what did not

There are a limited number of published studies evaluating HIV or TB programmes supported by international assistance, but a number of contextual and health system factors appear to have contributed to the success or failures of pilot programmes (Atun et al. 2005a; Atun et al. 2005b; Atun et al. 2005c; Coker et al. 2003; Tkatchenko-Schmidt et al. 2007).

Perhaps the biggest failure by international actors was the lack of understanding of the Soviet health care system and how it would need to be restructured to accommodate new thinking about prevention and treatment. For HIV, this meant a transition from the extensive system of testing to one that combines key public sector functions – of policy formulation, regulation, standard setting, financing, oversight, and support for service delivery – with those of NGOs, who are better able to reach high-risk groups. It also required changing fundamental beliefs that preventive and curative medicine should remain solely under a physician's control. For TB, changes aiming to simplify treatment protocols (short-course chemotherapy versus inpatient treatment) and replace X-ray diagnostics with sputum smear microscopy threatened the livelihood of thousands of health care professionals, who were completely invested in perpetuating the status quo.

Another barrier to rapid uptake of international prevention and treatment standards stemmed from a lack of public health training by medical professionals. Evidence "imported" from other countries was not acceptable, nor were materials or campaigns that had been designed specifically for the local market. It thus proved important to establish modern public health training, including social epidemiology and principals of evidenced-based medicine, for those involved in programme implementation and design. It was also critical to establish multiple pilots in varied settings (e.g. rural and urban *oblasts*, and prison and civilian populations) and to develop an evidence base, together with local decision-makers, regarding these programmes (Box 9.2).

Addressing the turf issues with regard to both diseases required an active process of stakeholder engagement. For harm-reduction programmes, a key to success in each country was the simultaneous engagement and education of three sectors in the start-up phase: departments of health, law enforcement officials and NGOs. For TB, it required engaging both civilian and prison authorities together.

Another turf issue which slowed progress was between multilateral agencies and international NGOs. In the mid-1990s, neither treatment of MDR-TB nor needle and syringe exchange programmes for the prevention of HIV were endorsed by WHO or the World Bank. There are no formal studies to establish what really happened, but anecdotes from people who worked in the region present a mixed picture. On the one hand, those working in the field at the time suggest that the tension and disagreement between these actors provided an excuse for resistance to change by local governments throughout the region.[1] On the other hand, there are perceptions that while pioneering NGO efforts helped to establish innovative programmes on a small scale, some central governments had strong reservations about what they regarded as overly abrasive approaches by some of those NGOs, which, in turn, made it more difficult for the World Bank to reach agreements with central governments to progress from small-scale experimentation to countrywide implementation of evidence-based approaches to HIV control, as well as DOTS for TB control.[2] A formal study of the political economy of change in TB and HIV policy in the region could clarify the complex factors and interactions that occurred during this period.

---

[1] Personal correspondence with representatives of the Open Society Institute, PHRI, the United Kingdom Department for International Development (DFID) and USAID.

[2] Personal correspondence with representatives of the World Bank.

Box 9.2 A case study of tuberculosis control in Latvia

In 1996, in Latvia, MDR-TB was reported in 14% of patients newly diagnosed with TB but without a history of treatment for this disease, and in 54% of those with a history of such treatment. In response, the Latvian National Tuberculosis Programme (NTP) began implementation of the WHO-recommended DOTS strategy. However, the short-course chemotherapy regimen of the DOTS strategy is generally ineffective in MDR-TB patients. Therefore, in addition to the DOTS strategy, special treatment strategies for MDR-TB are essential in settings where rates of MDR-TB are high.

After implementing the DOTS strategy and still documenting high rates of MDR-TB, in 1998 the Latvian NTP began implementing the DOTS-Plus strategy, using an individualized treatment approach. By 2000, full treatment for all patients with MDR-TB was available and was provided through a combination of hospital-based and ambulatory-based treatment with limited external support. A retrospective study showed that of the 204 patients assessed, 27% had been newly diagnosed with MDR-TB, and 73% had been previously treated with first-line or second-line drugs for this disease. Assessment of treatment outcomes showed that 66% were cured or completed therapy, 7% died, 13% defaulted and treatment failed in 14%. Of the 178 adherent patients, 76% were cured or completed treatment. The study suggests that when building an effective DOTS strategy, the DOTS-Plus strategy of identifying and treating patients with MDR-TB can be effectively implemented on a nationwide scale in a setting with limited resources.

Source: Lemaine et al. 2005.

Ultimately, however, responsibility for the failure of government stewardship to address important epidemics rests with the governments, not with external actors. Although both the treatment of MDR-TB and needle and syringe-exchange interventions have now been endorsed and are fully supported by the international community, success with regard to scaling-up pilots has only recently begun to take place and has required international financing as well as the development of partnerships between national health services, local and international NGOs, and multilateral agencies and governments.

The future: what will it take to achieve success?

The HIV/AIDS and TB epidemics continue to grow in most of the countries of the region and appear to be on a course to converge. In some countries that growth is nationwide, in others it primarily affects the most at-risk populations such as drug users, sex workers and migrants, and is geographically concentrated. A number of interventions and pilot projects in both the civilian and prison sectors have proven successful, but most only on an experimental basis.

With the exception of the Baltic states, now members of the EU, to date no country has implemented an adequate, fully comprehensive, nationwide programme for either disease. Two sources of financing, however, provide the opportunity for countries to scale up: the World Bank and the Global Fund to Fight AIDS, Tuberculosis and Malaria (GFATM).

At present, the World Bank is supporting loan, credit or grant agreements for TB- and HIV-specific projects in central Asia, the Republic of Moldova, the Russian Federation and Ukraine. GFATM has grants allocated for TB projects in 10 countries (Armenia, Azerbaijan, Belarus, Georgia, Kazakhstan, Kyrgyzstan, the Republic of Moldova, the Russian Federation, Tajikistan and Uzbekistan) and for HIV/AIDS in an additional six countries (Armenia, Azerbaijan, Belarus, Estonia, Kazakhstan and Ukraine). In addition, WHO coordinates three knowledge hubs in central and eastern Europe. These address second-generation surveillance (Croatia), harm reduction (Lithuania) and treatment (Ukraine).

These mechanisms have the potential to address the epidemic, only, however, if they prove to be a supplement to national government funding and commitment. In some instances, external financing has served as substitutes for, instead of additions to, local commitments and other sources of external finance. For example, in 2003, in Belarus, when the Government was notified that its GFATM grant application had been accepted, it cancelled its consultations with the World Bank for a loan to finance a TB control and primary health care development project.

In most former Soviet Union countries, governments continue to show a lack of commitment in a number of key areas. First, with regard to at-risk populations: stigma and discrimination remain a problem, and although testing is confidential, in most countries confidentiality is violated if someone who has tested positive seeks further treatment or information. Drug laws remain highly punitive, forcing users further underground and making them less likely to seek services. Needle and syringe exchange programmes have not yet been fully implemented on a national scale. Similarly, methadone, the most affordable of available opioid substitution therapies, has been piloted in a number of countries in the region, but without scale-up and thus remains largely inaccessible in most countries. Few NGOs are involved in government programmes, and there is inadequate representation of individuals affected by the diseases within the country coordinating mechanisms (CCMs)[3] for the GFATM grants.

Programmes also remain highly vertical and thus separated from other health care services. Despite the fact that TB is the largest killer of people with HIV, the disease programmes have yet to be integrated in any country past the pilot stage (WHO 2004). The diseases are diagnosed and treated through separate systems, and primary care doctors have not been brought into provision of care for either disease. Further, at national levels, prison and civilian health systems remain isolated from one another.

---

[3] CCMs are country-level partnerships, which submit grant proposals to the GFATM based on priority needs at national level. After grant approval, they oversee progress during implementation.

In conclusion, any attempts to control these epidemics must be placed into the overall context of the health system, political support for integrating care, the adoption of international standards of care and their adaptation to local contexts, with an emphasis on the achievement of sustained improvements in outcomes. International agencies working in these countries must understand the history of the health systems, including their cultural contexts, and design their interventions accordingly. Also, given that the affected populations of both diseases are predominately marginalized groups, both local and international efforts must address these diseases within the environmental context of the country (socioeconomic, political and cultural) and broaden the engagement of those outside the health care sector as well as those within it.

References

Adeyi, O., Fidler, A., Loginova, T. and Gracheva, M. (2003). Tuberculosis and AIDS control in Russia: closing the knowing-doing gap, *Eurohealth*, 9(4): 22–27.

Aerts, A., Habouzit, M., Mschiladze, L., et al. (2000). Pulmonary tuberculosis in prisons of the ex-USSR state Georgia: results of a nation-wide prevalence survey among sentenced inmates, *International Journal of Tuberculosis and Lung Disease*, 4(12): 1104–1110.

AIDS Foundation East-West (2005). Resource Centre [web site]. [electronic publication] AIDS Foundation East-West (www.afew.org, accessed 20 May 2005).

Atun, R. A., Baeza, J., Drobniewski, F., Levicheva, V. and Coker, R. (2005a). Implementing WHO DOTS strategy in the Russian Federation: stakeholder attitudes, *Health Policy*, 74(2): 122–132.

Atun, R. A., McKee, M., Drobniewski, F. and Coker, R. (2005b). Analysis of how health system context influences HIV control: case studies from the Russian Federation, *Bulletin of the World Health Organization*, 83(10): 730–738.

Atun, R. A., Samyshkin, Y. A., Drobniewski, F., et al. (2005c). Barriers to sustainable tuberculosis control in the Russian Federation health system, *Bulletin of the World Health Organization*, 83(3): 217–223.

Aziz, M. A., Wright, A., De Muynck, A. and Laszlo, A. (2004). *Anti-Tuberculosis Drug Resistance in the World – Third Global Report*. New York: Tuberculosis Alliance, World Health Organization (WHO); International Union against Tuberculosis and Lung Disease (IUATLD); Global Project on Anti-Tuberculosis Drug Resistance Surveillance / Global Alliance for tuberculosis Drug Development.

Coker, R. J., Dimitrova, B., Drobniewski, F., et al. (2003). Tuberculosis control in Samara Oblast, Russia: institutional and regulatory environment, *International Journal of Tuberculosis and Lung Disease*, 7(10): 920–932.

Dehne, K. L., Khodakevich, L., Hamers, F. F. and Schwartlander, B. (1999). The HIV/AIDS epidemic in eastern Europe: recent patterns and trends and their implications for policy-making, *AIDS*, 13(7): 741–749.

Donoghoe, M. C., Lazarus, J. V. and Matic, S. (2005). HIV/AIDS in the transitional countries of eastern Europe and central Asia, *Clinical Medicine*, 5(5): 487–490.

Donoghoe, M. C., Bollerup, A. R., Lazarus, J. V., Nielsen, S. and Matic, S. (2007). Access to highly active antiretroviral therapy (HAART) for injecting drug users in the WHO European region 2002–2004, *International Journal of Drug Policy*, 18(4): 271–280.

EuroHIV (European Centre for the Epidemiological Monitoring of AIDS) (2005). *HIV/AIDS Surveillance in Europe, End-year report 2005. No. 73*. Saint-Maurice: Institut de veille sanitaire.

Garrett, L. (2000). *Betrayal of trust: the collapse of global public health*. New York: Hyperion.

Ghys, P. D., Walker, N. and Garnett, G. P. (2006). Improved methods and tools for HIV/AIDS estimates and projections, *Sexually Transmitted Infections*, 82 (3).

Government of Ireland (2004). *Dublin Declaration on Partnership to fight HIV/AIDS in Europe and central Asia*. Dublin: Government of Ireland (http://www.eu2004.ie/templates/meeting.asp?sNavlocator=5,13&list_id=25, accessed 24 August 2006).

Hamers, F. F. and Downs, A. M. (2003). HIV in central and eastern Europe, *Lancet*, 361(9362): 1035–1044.

Institut de veille sanitaire, WHO Collaborating Centre for the Surveillance of Tuberculosis in Europe and Royal Netherlands Tuberculosis Association (KNCV) (2004). *Report on tuberculosis cases notified in 2002*. Saint Maurice: Institut de veille sanitaire (http://www.eurotb.org, accessed 27 November 2007).

Lemaine, V., Holtz, T., Zarovksa, E. S., et al. (2005). Clinical outcome of individualized treatment of multidrug-resistant tuberculosis in Latvia: a retrospective cohort study, *Lancet*, 364: 3118–3126.

Nielsen, S. (2006) Estimating HIV prevalence in concentrated HIV epidemics in eastern Europe: Application of the UNAIDS/WHO Workbook method in Ukraine. Master's thesis in Public Health Sciences. University of Copenhagen, Denmark.

Nielsen, S. and Lazarus, J. V. (2006). HIV/AIDS country profiles for the WHO European Region, in S. Matic, J. V. Lazarus and M. C. Donoghoe (eds) *HIV/AIDS in Europe: moving from death sentence to chronic disease management*. Copenhagen: WHO Regional Office for Europe.

Preker, S. and Adeyi, O. (2005). Health care, in N. Barr (ed.) *Labor markets and social policy in Central and Eastern Europe: the accession and beyond*. Washington, D.C.: World Bank.

Reichman, L. B. (2002). *Time bomb: the global epidemic of multi-drug-resistant tuberculosis*. New York: McGraw-Hill.

Ruehl, C., Pokrovsky, V. and Vinogradov, V. (2002). *The Economic Consequences of HIV in Russia*. Washington, D.C.: World Bank (http://www.worldbank.org.ru/ECA/Russia.nsf/ECADocByUnid/56435B1EA108E164C3256CD1003FBE54, accessed 20 February 2005).

Tkatchenko-Schmidt, E., Renton, A., Gevorgyan, R., Davydenko, L. and Atun, R. (2007). Prevention of HIV/AIDS among injecting drug users in Russia: opportunities and barriers to scaling-up of harm-reduction programmes, *Health Policy*, doi: 10.1016/j.healthpol.2007.07.005.

Ukraine Ministry of Health, The International HIV/AIDS Alliance in Ukraine, WHO and UNAIDS (2006). *Report on the National Consensus Estimates on HIV and AIDS in Ukraine at the end of 2005 – May 2006*. Kyiv: Ukraine Ministry of Health, The International HIV/AIDS Alliance in Ukraine, World Health Organization, Joint United Nations Programme on HIV/AIDS.

UNAIDS (2005) [web site] Geneva: Joint United Nations Programme on HIV/AIDS (http://www.unaids.org/en/resources/epidemiology/epi_softwaretools.asp, accessed 2 March 2005).

UNAIDS and WHO (2006). *2006 Report on the Global AIDS Epidemic. 1006* Geneva: Joint United Nations Programme on HIV/AIDS (http://www.unaids.org/en/HIV_data/2006GlobalReport/default.asp, accessed 27 November 2007).

UNODC, WHO and UNAIDS (2006). *HIV/AIDS prevention, care, treatment and support in prison settings: a framework for an effective national response*. Vienna, United Nations Office on Drugs and Crime.

Veen, J. and Godinho, J. (2006). HIV and TB: A critical co-infection, in S. Matic, J. V. Lazarus and M. C. Donoghoe (eds) *HIV/AIDS in Europe: moving from death sentence to chronic disease management*. Copenhagen: World Health Organization.

WHO (2004). *Interim Policy on Collaborative TB/HIV Activities*. Geneva: Stop tuberculosis Department and Department of HIV/AIDS.

WHO (2006a). *Global Tuberculosis Control: surveillance, planning, financing*. Geneva: World Health Organization.

WHO Regional Office for Europe (2002). *DOTS Expansion Plan to Stop tuberculosis in the WHO European Region 2002–2006*. Copenhagen: World Health Organization Regional Office for Europe.

WHO Regional Office for Europe (2005). *Data collected by the STIs/HIV/AIDS Programme*. Copenhagen: World Health Organization Regional Office for Europe.

WHO Regional Office for Europe (2006). *Sexually transmitted infections/HIV/AIDS programme. WHO/Europe survey on HIV/AIDS and antiretroviral therapy: 31 March 2006 update of cumulative totals*. Copenhagen: WHO Regional Office for Europe.

WHO Regional Office for Europe (2006a). European Health for All database [online database]. Copenhagen: World Health Organization Regional Office for Europe (www.euro.who.int/hfadb, accessed 2 October 2006).

WHO Regional Office for Europe (2006b). *HIV/AIDS Treatment and Care Clinical Protocols for the WHO European Region*. Copenhagen, World Health Organization Regional Office for Europe (www.euro.who.int/aids, accessed 27 November 2007).

ten

Enabling health systems in tuberculosis control: challenges and opportunities for the former Soviet Union countries

Andrei Mosneaga, Elena Yurasova,
Richard Zaleskis, Wieslaw Jakubowiak

Introduction

This chapter aims to highlight the major issues related to TB control within changing health systems and to outline the necessary actions to make TB programme efforts effective and sustainable.

In the WHO European Region the main burden of TB is borne by the countries of the former Soviet Union. All of these countries are considered as having a high TB burden within the region, with the Russian Federation among the 22 highest burden countries globally. Although the health systems in these countries have developed differently in many instances since 1991, it is still possible to identify many common features in their TB control policies.

Recent forecasts of the TB epidemic made by WHO indicate that although the achievement of the TB-related Millennium Development Goals (MDGs) globally is feasible, for two WHO Regions – the African and European Regions – this remains difficult. In Africa, this is due to the spread of the TB/HIV co-epidemic, and in the European Region (more precisely, in its eastern part), it is mainly due to the very high burden of drug-resistant TB: a "man-made" phenomenon "galvanized" by poor overall performance of the health systems.

TB control programmes, often referred to as examples of "vertical" disease control programmes with centralized management systems designed to achieve clearly defined results in a relatively short period of time, rely on the "horizontal" provision of services through primary health care, guided and monitored by national TB control programmes. However, system-wide problems do not allow for effective TB control if the control programmes are not aligned with the health system reform and development process (Bosman 2000; Kritski and Ruffino-Netto 2000; Miller 2000; Tang and Squire 2005; The Nuffield Institute 2002) (see also Chapter 7). The DOTS strategy, currently implemented in more than 180 countries worldwide (fully or partially in 44 out of 53 countries in the WHO European Region), remains the main instrument for effective TB control. Emerging challenges, such as TB/HIV co-infection and MDR-TB, have stimulated WHO and other international partners to work on the expansion of the DOTS framework. The new Stop Tuberculosis Strategy, *Building on and enhancing DOTS to meet TB-related Millennium Development Goals*, recommended by the Stop TB Partnership and WHO, embraces six main components, detailed here (WHO 2006c; WHO 2006b).

- Pursue quality DOTS expansion and enhancement, through:
- political commitment with increased and sustained financing;
- case detection through bacteriology;
- standardized treatment with supervision and patient support;
- effective pharmaceutical supply system;
- monitoring system and impact evaluation.
- Address TB/HIV, MDR-TB and other special challenges.
- Contribute to health system strengthening.
- Engage all care providers.
- Empower patients and communities.
- Enable and promote research.

The Strategy emphasizes how TB control is integral to and dependent on the health system in which it is embedded and the essential DOTS elements can be sustained only by the effective functioning of health systems. It also proposes three related approaches through which TB control and overall health system reform can be mutually reinforcing: "macro" system strengthening actions that advance TB control, advancing health systems through innovations in TB control and adapting innovations from other public health fields to strengthen tuberculosis control. Well-designed financial mechanisms and appropriate division of responsibilities within the health systems are key factors for success.

Health system reforms worldwide have tended to follow two policy paradigms since the mid-1990s: a "system design" approach, concerned with the overall operation of the health sector; and a "service provision" approach, concerned with specific disease control strategies. With varying degrees of precision, individuals and groups within the health systems have coalesced around these different approaches (Collins, Green and Newell 2002).

Since the early 1990s, health system reforms in the ECA region, including those in the countries of the former Soviet Union, have focused on macro system design and aimed at reconfiguration of the health system mainly by: separation of the roles of financing and provision and the introduction of "quasi" markets; development of alternative financing mechanisms, including application of user fees in public facilities; decentralization; limiting the scope of public sector and encouraging a greater role for the private sector; and provision of the packages of essential services prioritized using cost–effectiveness techniques (Weil 2000).

However, an integrated approach to health, education and poverty alleviation is needed if the ultimate defeat of the major communicable diseases is to be achieved. This, in turn, demands a strong society-wide effort to foster economic growth and development. This is especially true in relation to TB. TB control *is* part of any health system, and hence the frequently used phrase "TB control *and* health system development" is misleading. Saying that TB control is not part of the health system development means that the system's performance in this area is weak. There is still a tendency by national governments, as well as by external donors, to see TB control separately from the mainstream health system change.

Evolution of tuberculosis control in the post-Soviet era

In the Soviet Union, active case finding was the pillar around which TB control was built. An extensive network of specialized TB institutions was developed and emphasis was placed on lengthy hospital care, rehabilitation in sanatoria, vertical control measures led by the sanitary-epidemiology service, extensive use of administrative powers (including compulsory treatment) and extensive social support. The system was totally reliant on these separate services, while general health service providers essentially did not participate in TB control at all.

After the break-up of the USSR, the situation changed rapidly. TB re-emerged, reflecting the magnitude of social turmoil, reversing what had been a steady decrease in incidence over the previous 20 years. The economic downturn led to the disappearance of "organized collectives", along with unemployment, massive migration and pauperization of the population. In such conditions, previously quite successful active case finding had become ineffective and inefficient. While the entire health sector fell down the list of priorities for public funding, TB service fell even further within the health sector's priorities. As a result, this service was hit particularly hard; it became impossible to maintain the collapsing infrastructure and the system failed to cope with the new challenges.

At the same time, the old paradigm (that a specialized TB service is solely and fully responsible for TB control) remains very strong at all levels of the health system, from senior decision-makers to front-line health care staff. This has probably been the major barrier to the introduction of DOTS in former Soviet Union countries, as those seeking to implement change have had to deal with an extensive network of facilities and well-established but ineffective ways of working. This has often led to poor quality of the programmes and failure to progress towards the TB control targets.

Challenges for tuberculosis control in relation to the main functions of the health systems in the former Soviet Union

When defining the boundaries of a health system, WHO uses the criterion of "primary purpose", that is, actions whose main purpose is to improve health. This includes the elements normally associated with the health system, such as individual health services as well as public health services; it embraces public as well as private provision of these actions. WHO's *World Health Report 2000* (WHO 2002; WHO 2000) asserts that there are three overarching *goals* of the health system: improvement of the population's health, fairness in financing and responsiveness to people's expectations. Later, many researchers suggested that efficiency should be also considered a goal.

To achieve these four goals, all health systems carry out a set of interventions that can be grouped around four main *functions*: stewardship, financing, resource development and service delivery. The debate on the health system PAF, proposed in the *World Health Report 2000*, is ongoing; however, it has proved a useful tool for description and analysis. Looking at the main functions, it is possible to analyse not only the health system overall, but also one or several of its components. Below we seek to identify and discuss, briefly, the major challenges of TB control in the former Soviet Union through the prism of these four main functions of the health system. It is important to emphasize that this is not an overview of the specialized TB *service*, but rather an attempt to look at how the whole health system performs in relation to TB, to identify major problems that are relevant to TB control but cannot be resolved by the National Tuberculosis Programmes (NTPs), as well as systemic changes that are necessary for the successful fight against the disease.

Stewardship, governance and management

Introduced in the *World Health Report 2000* (WHO 2000), the term *stewardship*, in the context of the health system, means the careful and responsible management of health and well-being of the population; another term closely related to stewardship is *oversight*. This function is most closely associated with the policy-making role of government. There are three broad stewardship tasks: (i) formulating health policy and defining a vision for future development of the health system; (ii) exerting influence; and (iii) collection and use of intelligence.

There are a number of important issues in TB control in the former Soviet Union that can be considered pertinent to this health system function, outlined below. For practical reasons, stewardship function is extended further to include governance and management ("stewardship at lower levels"), thus allowing for a more specific overview in relation to TB.

The commitment of governments to effective TB control, one of the five pillars of the DOTS strategy, remains generally weak. While TB is often declared to be a high priority, this is rarely translated in policy and investment decisions. To a significant extent this reflects a lack of capacity in ministries of health to evaluate the relative burden of health problems as well as an inability to shift from traditional input-based decision-making to that employing at least some degree of health impact assessment and economic evaluation (WHO 2003b;

Coker and Atun 2004). The social profile of TB patients means that special strategies are needed to ensure that socially marginalized and high-risk groups (such as migrants, alcoholics, ex-prisoners, people with no fixed abode, refugees and internally displaced persons) have access to appropriate care (Jakubowiak et al. 2007).

To a significant extent, TB control efforts in the former Soviet Union countries are often driven by donors. The task of coordinating external partners, which is most definitely part of the stewardship function that should be executed by governments, is often left to the partners themselves. Joint planning and coordination among international agencies remains rare; support provided to national programmes is often "skewed" towards some elements while the other components lag behind. As a result, standardized approaches that bridge the care continuum (a key DOTS requirement) are not applied.

"Departmentality", i.e. strict vertical lines of accountability in the public service, is an important feature of former Soviet Union countries, impeding implementation of a single integrated national programme. In practical terms, shortcomings often result from simple lack of communication and cooperation between NTPs and AIDS control services, between NTPs and sanitary-epidemiology services, between TB services in the civilian sector and those in the penitentiary sector, the army and other sectors (Coker and Atun 2004).

While WHO strongly advocates to the countries to strengthen national programme management (it is a priority action recommended by the *DOTS Expansion Plan to Stop Tuberculosis in the WHO European Region 2002–2006*) (WHO Regional Office for Europe 2002), no tangible improvement has yet been seen in this regard in most of the countries concerned. The organizational identity of NTPs, or more precisely NTP Central Units or Offices, is vague; in fact these are usually a few people, in most cases TB specialists working full time in the central TB hospitals/research institutes and their functions and responsibilities are not well defined. In most instances NTPs receive no or very limited support for essential activities and are therefore very much reliant on donors. NTPs do not have sufficient authority to mobilize and coordinate with other players, such as the primary health sector, health services in prisons and AIDS control services. Even in smaller countries, it is impossible for Central Units alone to oversee the local implementation of the programme; yet the establishment of capable regional NTP structures is at a very early stage in most countries. The problems of programme management must be seen as an extremely serious obstacle to the future development of TB control in the former Soviet Union and thus to the achievement of TB control targets. This also indicates how difficult it will be to introduce and scale up the complex and demanding DOTS-Plus activities in these conditions.

One very important problem is TB surveillance and the TB recording and reporting system. The system inherited from the Soviet Union was based on meticulous collection of a large variety of data, summarized in numerous reporting forms. It uses classifications of cases and treatment outcomes that are different from those recommended by WHO; maintenance of dispensaries that require lengthy follow-up is a typical feature. Adopting the international recommendations has been difficult as it has faced much resistance. Still, in many settings, despite declarations of 100% coverage by DOTS and extensive training activities carried out with external support, a dual recording and reporting system is used. Cohort analysis of treatment outcomes remains weak, precluding adequate monitoring and evaluation of national programmes. DOTS reporting by the NTPs is "informal", as in most instances it is not incorporated in official statistics, with national health statistics departments often using different indicators and classifications. This results in discrepancies in data reported by different sources. To summarize, the current state of TB recording and reporting systems in former Soviet Union countries does not allow for either full comprehension of the magnitude of the epidemic or adequate monitoring and evaluation of programme interventions.

A systemic weakness in the region is insufficient managerial capacity at all levels. As in other settings in the health sector, managers ("head physicians") of TB facilities are medical doctors by background, with little or no management training. TB hospitals and services in general are often cited as being among the most inefficient and slow-moving parts of the health systems, and the lack of managerial competence is obviously an important contributing factor. As most TB service managers combine managerial and clinical duties, an individual (clinical) approach often prevails over a public health one (McKee, Nolte and DuBois 2006).

There are many examples in the former Soviet Union of how, instead of political commitment, "politicization" of TB issues takes place. The presence of TB is seen as an indicator of social distress and, in response to pressures from politicians (i.e. not to report much on TB lest it detract from the achievements of those in power), ministries of health are susceptible to policy reversals, and sometimes intentional "levelling down" of TB statistics takes place.

The stigma attached to TB is very significant and represents an important barrier to seeking care. Despite this, governments (and external partners) undervalue advocacy, communication and social mobilization activities; often these are just limited around the World Tuberculosis Days. Ministries and NTPs often have to respond to individual cases appearing in the mass media, which increasingly are related to drug-resistant TB and unavailability of treatment. The officials' positions in such cases are almost always defensive; in general, work with mass media and civil society to involve them in advocacy and knowledge dissemination about TB is insufficient.

Box 10.1 discusses TB control coordination in the Russian Federation.

Financing and allocation

Financing has three distinct sub-functions: (i) collection of revenues, (ii) pooling, and (iii) purchasing of services.

It is important to note that in the former Soviet Union the term *financing* is often applied to the first two sub-functions only and noticeably less importance is given to purchasing. This reflects the general pattern of health reforms in the region: often reform efforts are concentrated on changing the collection and pooling of funds and rather less on improving allocation mechanisms, whereas the latter are one of the weakest elements of the health system in the countries of concern and to a substantial extent impede the achievement of efficiency (one of a health system's fundamental goals).

Box 10.1 High-level tuberculosis coordinating body in the Russian Federation

In the **Russian Federation**, a High-Level Working Group (HLWG) on TB was established in 1999 to ensure effective cooperation and coordination among national and international partners fighting the disease. The HLWG oversees the implementation of the National Tuberculosis Control Programme and provides key advice to the Ministry of Health and Social Development on policy and strategy for TB control in the country, as well as coordinating activities of various externally funded projects. Several Thematic Working Groups have been established by the HLWG with the function of addressing specific technical issues of TB control, preparing recommendations for the HLWG. The HLWG is seen as an important mechanism for streamlining TB control efforts in the Russian Federation, which is one of 22 high-burden TB countries globally. The HLWG and the Interagency Coordinating Committee on Tuberculosis also ensure coordination and mobilization of internal and external resource for effective TB control in the country.

Different ways of reforming health financing have been employed in the region; this has resulted in a variety of arrangements. According to the main system of financing and coverage, the former Soviet Union countries may be grouped in the following way: in four countries (Estonia, Latvia, Lithuania, the Republic of Moldova) health insurance (although organized differently) is the single main source of funding; two countries (Georgia and Kyrgyzstan) have also implemented insurance but there are other sizeable complementary sources; one country (Armenia) has a centralized tax-based financing scheme; six countries (Azerbaijan, Belarus, Kazakhstan, Tajikistan, Turkmenistan and Uzbekistan) maintain a decentralized tax-based system, with a similar system in place in Ukraine, although a health insurance system is being piloted. Finally, there is a complex system in the Russian Federation, representing a mix of insurance and tax-based, central and decentralized budgetary mechanisms. In addition, direct out-of-pocket spending (including official co-payments, or user fees, at the site of service delivery) is common practically everywhere.

Despite these differences, a number of common issues may be identified. A brief analysis of key problems facing TB control in the former Soviet Union is presented below.

First, it is often very difficult to determine how much money countries spend on TB control. Budgetary classifications usually allow for aggregating expenditure across different settings of care (i.e. hospital and outpatient care) and/or items of expenditure (salaries, pharmaceuticals, equipment, etc.), but not so easily or at all by disease control programmes. For example, data are often aggregated at subnational (regional and even district) levels; whereas spending on TB hospitals is included with other inpatient institutions, TB departments are included in the general polyclinics where they are located, so distinguishing

TB spending at national level becomes impossible. Another option is aggregation by line items, whereby TB drugs are aggregated with other pharmaceuticals, salaries of TB staff, with staff of other specialties, etc. Often it is possible to see the size of the vertical "national programme", but these figures cover only centrally purchased items such as pharmaceuticals and vaccines, while other expenditure is not included. It is important to note that in some countries funds for expensive active case finding by mass miniature radiography are budgeted under the general health service and therefore are not considered as TB control. An important implication following from these policies is that assessment of the (financial) government commitment over time is difficult.

There are a few studies in which a more profound analysis was conducted (e.g. the World Bank's *Stopping Tuberculosis in Central Asia: Priorities for Action* (Godinho et al. 2005)), demonstrating that the real level of TB control financing is low as a result of several factors, detailed here.

(i)   While there is GDP growth in all countries concerned and the absolute amount of funds for health is increasing, the health financing share of GDP has not increased and has even dropped in several countries. Therefore, taking into account the rising cost of service and inflation, no or only a marginal improvement in the size of real health funding is seen.

(ii)   The public share of health funding is not increasing or is even decreasing; this does not favour TB control, which is reliant on public funding.

(iii)   Within the health system, funding of TB control is not increasing at the same pace as funding of other programmes.

TB control funding suffers from a general problem of lack of resources. The poorer the country, the lower the GDP share spent on health, and there is also a tendency for public financing to take a smaller share of overall health financing. Moreover, in countries where the health care financing is decentralized, budget equilibration mechanisms are often ineffective, leading to marked geographical inequalities in health funding (and by extension TB control funding). Consequently, the problem of inadequate TB control funding is further amplified by the unfair distribution of resources (WHO 2005c).

With few exceptions, there are no medium and longer-term plans for financial sustainability of TB control. Such plans are needed at a time when the former Soviet Union countries face the growing problem of drug resistance, requiring enhanced domestic funding for costly, but necessary, MDR-TB management programmes. The magnitude of this problem is so great in this region that it will be impossible to tackle it with external funding only. The resolution of the 58th World Health Assembly in May 2005, entitled *Sustainable financing for tuberculosis prevention and control* (WHO 2005d), expresses concern that the ". . . lack of commitment to sustained financing for tuberculosis will impede the sound long-term planning necessary to achieve the internationally agreed development goals relevant to tuberculosis contained in the United Nations Millennium Declaration" and urges the Member States ". . . to estimate the total resources required for prevention and control of tuberculosis, including HIV-related tuberculosis and multidrug-resistant tuberculosis, in the medium term, and the resources available from domestic and international sources in order to identify the funding gap".

Whether in the context of insurance-based or tax-based financing, purchasing (allocation) mechanisms in the former Soviet Union countries are in most cases rigidly oriented towards the inputs. Annual funding increases provide only for small "incremental" increases in the sums for salaries, food, and maintenance; at the same time it is difficult for the ministries of health to channel funding to important DOTS interventions such as supervision, training, improvement of TB recording and reporting systems, etc. As a result, NTPs remain highly reliant on external funding. To recapitulate, the present purchasing systems at both central and regional levels of care do not allow for the rapid scale-up of TB control interventions.

Although many countries are attempting to optimize payment systems in provider institutions, little has changed with regard to TB facilities. In TB hospitals, payment is still frequently linked to bed days, thus failing to motivate hospital managers to strive for higher efficiency; instead, the payment schemes often favour keeping patients in bed as long as possible (Godinho et al. 2005; Marx et al. 2007; WHO Regional Office for Europe 2005).

It is important to note that although TB care is often declared to be free of charge to the patients, in fact it is not. Direct user fees are often substantial. While in most settings anti-TB drugs are provided free of charge, patients have to pay other costs (additional medicines, chest X-rays, laboratory investigations, even the cost of occupying a bed). For patients with TB, the majority of whom are from low-income groups, these costs are substantial and often unaffordable and may therefore deter people from seeking care or completing the course of treatment. Patients who are treated outside NTPs because of concerns about stigma or for other reasons, may incur much higher expenses, including having to buy pharmaceuticals in pharmacies at full cost. In addition, there are informal payments to both public and private providers. Overall, direct out-of-pocket payments (both official and unofficial) represent an important financial barrier to TB care in countries of the former Soviet Union.

Staff salaries in TB services are low and often significantly lower than those in other medical specialties. Coupled with the difficulties they face in supplementing their income with informal payments (given the nature of their patients), it is unsurprising that many staff are poorly motivated. With the exception of a few pilot projects, no performance-based financial incentives exist in the field of TB care. Yet, when incentive systems have been established with external funding, they have proven effective in improving programme results; the main challenge is, however, to sustain them after the external support has ended. One study in the Russian Federation showed that salaries constitute up to 30% of the overall cost of TB control (WHO 2002).

The GFATM represents an important source of funding for TB control. During the first six GFATM rounds, 15 grants for TB were approved in 10 countries of the former Soviet Union, amounting to US$ 220 million in total. Yet this poses two sets of problems: first, there is a risk that GFATM funds may be accompanied by a reduction in core national funding for TB and, second, it raises again the question of financial sustainability after specific projects have come to an end.

Box 10.2 discusses MDR-TB management in Latvia.

Box 10.2   Local governments' support for tackling multidrug-resistant tuberculosis in Latvia

Latvia was the first country in the region to incorporate the management of MDR-TB cases in its national programme in 1997. A very important contribution to the success of the programme is the way that municipality budgets provide financial support for patients in order to cover transportation costs to medical facilities and other expenses related to direct observation of treatment. Thereby, local financing substantially contributes to the patients' adherence to treatment, which is one of the key components of MDR-TB management.

Resource generation

This health system function is concerned with investment in the diverse inputs to the health system. These inputs include human resources, physical capital (infrastructure and equipment) and consumables (pharmaceuticals, vaccines and other supplies). Appropriate decisions on these investments are of critical importance for the long-term development of the health system because they have implications for the quality and cost of care in the future.

There are a number of important challenges faced by the former Soviet Union countries' health systems in generating resources for TB. A snapshot is presented below.

Most former Soviet Union countries are experiencing acute problems in obtaining sufficient human resources for TB control:

(i)   there are acute shortages of staff in the TB services in many countries;
(ii)   many TB doctors are over retirement age (up to 60–70% in some settings);
(iii)   there is a high turnover of staff, in particular among laboratory personnel;
(iv)   few new medical graduates choose TB as a setting because of the low salaries and uncompensated professional hazards (Chen et al. 2004; Figueras, Menabde and Busse 2005).

At the same time, there is no medium- or long-term manpower planning for TB control based on a meaningful needs assessment (Harries et al. 2005). It is obvious that the TB service cannot be seen in isolation and this weakness reflects a lack of human resource planning more generally.

Few countries have created adequate postgraduate training on TB (DOTS training and retraining). What training exists is driven largely by external partners and its sustainability is uncertain.

Contemporary strategies for TB control based on DOTS are insufficiently integrated into curricula for medical students; their focus is largely on the clinical aspects of TB but not on public health aspects or organization of care. As a result, graduates of medical schools are not sufficiently "alert" to the disease, its burden in the population and the complexity of its management.

Although the shortages of pharmaceuticals that were common in the 1990s are no longer occurring (in most countries due to external support), they do happen from time to time at subnational levels as a result of unreliable supply chain management.

Anti-TB pharmaceuticals are manufactured in many former Soviet Union countries; this is encouraged by governments who support the use of domestically produced medicines by the NTPs. However, the quality of production is low or not known in many cases; the use of substandard pharmaceuticals leads to ineffective treatment and poor outcomes, including development of drug resistance. There is a need for more manufacturers in this region to obtain international certificates of good manufacturing practice (GMP), but so far progress is slow.

A common feature of the former Soviet Union countries is the wide availability of anti-TB drugs (both first- and second-line drugs) in the open market, including counterfeit drugs. Few national authorities have been able to deal effectively with this problem; it reflects a general weakness by ministries of health in regulating the pharmaceutical market. At the same time, second-line drugs are often procured by local administrations and even by individual medical institutions without proper controls. The situation is compounded by the widespread use of rifampicin and some second-line drugs for management of infections other than TB, adding to the problem of drug resistance. Box 10.3 discusses anti-TB drug procurement in Belarus.

Many TB facilities are in dilapidated conditions and lack basic amenities; in this regard one of the health system's goals – responsiveness to nonmedical needs and expectations – is not fulfilled. While most TB institutions are now adequately equipped with binocular microscopes and reagents thanks to external support, other medical equipment is often obsolete and does not encourage provision of high-quality care.

Service delivery

The delivery (provision) of health services can be divided into two categories:

(i)   interventions delivered to individuals (personal health care services); and
(ii) interventions delivered to groups of people or the entire population (population-based services).

Personal health care includes both curative and preventive services. It is important to note that some services with public (*population*) health benefits, such

---

Box 10.3   Ensuring supply of anti-tuberculosis drugs in Belarus

The Ministry of Health of **Belarus** has established a system of centralized procurement of anti-TB drugs. Timely allocation of financial resources and provision of buffer stocks avoid pharmaceutical shortages at all levels of care. The NTP ensures that the pharmaceuticals are provided free of charge to all patients with TB. In addition, a regulation to ban sales of anti-TB drugs in pharmacies has been adopted and its enforcement is being monitored closely.

as immunizations and TB treatment, are in fact *personal* care services. The distinguishing characteristic, in this case, is how the service is delivered, not the extent to which the benefits extend beyond the individual receiving the intervention.

In relation to TB, the following service delivery stages can be identified:

- case detection, diagnosis and treatment;
- in turn, the latter may be divided into the intensive phase and the continuation (follow-up) phase.

The following paragraphs set out the key issues in TB control that derive from consideration of this function in former Soviet Union countries.

A major problem impeding effective TB case detection is the limited involvement of primary health care providers; in general, except for a few donor-supported projects, they are neither trained nor "authorized" to accomplish this task. In some countries TB case detection is declared to be a primary health care function, while TB doctors establish the diagnosis and prescribe treatment (Ministry of Health of the Russian Federation 2004); however, unmotivated and overloaded primary health care providers are often uninterested in this task, leading to delayed diagnosis. This issue is addressed in more detail in the next section.

The DOTS strategy advocates bacteriology (smear microscopy and culture investigation) as the main method of TB diagnosis. Although there are a number of examples in former Soviet Union countries in which the TB laboratory networks were successfully strengthened, often by creating regional systems, serious problems with these facilities remain common. Adequate quality-assurance systems are rarely in place and performance is often poor. Clinicians often do not trust laboratory results and prefer X-ray diagnosis. The potential to integrate TB laboratories with the general health service laboratory network are being considered in many countries; again, this requires system-wide solutions that are beyond the authority of the NTPs. Decisions need to take account of the balance of the workload, geographical feasibility and quality. Box 10.4 discusses laboratory services in Georgia.

In terms of case management, despite the availability of DOTS-based guidelines and trained personnel in TB services, substantial variations in physicians' practices persist, resulting in suboptimal non-standardized treatment regimens. This problem may be overcome successfully if *system-wide* programmes of monitoring and improvement of the quality of care can be implemented.

Box 10.4 Optimizing tuberculosis laboratory services in Georgia

Georgia undertook a radical optimization of its TB laboratory network by transforming more than half its microscopy laboratories into sputum collection points and establishing a functional countrywide specimen transportation system. The resulting improvement in quality has led to a rapid improvement in the case-detection rate: for new smear-positive cases this grew from 57–58% in 2001–2003 to over 90% in 2005.

While at present DOTS coverage is alleged to be 100% in most former Soviet Union countries, direct observation of treatment and patient support, one of the key DOTS elements, is not yet in place during the continuation phase of treatment and even during the intensive phase in some countries, with the exception of a few externally supported pilot projects. If these elements are to be sustainable, they require effective involvement of the primary care sector, as they are beyond the capacity of TB services.

It is widely believed that the hospital infrastructure in former Soviet Union countries is excessive, with too many TB inpatient beds. A recent study has shown how in the Russian Federation there is no geographical correlation between need for care and provision of inpatient capacity (Marx et al. 2007). However, looking ahead, it is possible that many currently empty beds will be needed to cope with the challenge of MDR-TB, which may require a prolonged hospitalization. The key challenge is to develop an integrated system that reflects need; in some places hospital beds were substantially reduced before outpatient services were developed, leading to a shortage of capacity. This can lead to defaulting from treatment (Atun et al. 2005; Adams, Mosneaga and Gedik 2003). One study showed that only approximately 45% of TB beds could be justified from a clinical point of view and the rest were unoccupied or used for social support (WHO 2002).

An important but largely overlooked problem in the former Soviet Union countries is the role of "quasi-private" doctors working in TB control. Although the private health sector (official, licensed private practices) is commonly considered to be underdeveloped in this region, very often publicly employed providers operate on a "quasi-private" basis, that is, using public premises and other resources for the generation of private income. Many of these providers *are* involved in TB control as there is a demand for their services to treat patients outside the NTPs because of stigma or for other reasons. Having low salaries, the doctors seek to retain these patients as sources of extra informal income. This can cause the following problems:

(i)   they may not recognize TB and treat it as a trivial infection, delaying the referral to a specialized facility;
(ii) they may recognize TB but prescribe suboptimal treatment;
(iii) they may recognize TB and know how to treat it but prescribe suboptimal treatment anyway, taking into account the patient's ability to pay: few TB patients can afford to purchase TB pharmaceuticals at full cost for a 6–8 month treatment course, so doctors may recommend a 1–2 month course of treatment until the patient's condition is improved.

In all three cases, this "contribution" of quasi-private doctors to the TB epidemic is adverse, as it leads not only to improper case management but, importantly, to the development and spread of drug resistance (Newell 2002; Uplekar, Pathania and Raviglione 2001).

Involving primary health care in tuberculosis control: a golden opportunity for the former Soviet Union?

In the Alma-Ata declaration, primary health care is defined as ". . . essential health care based on practical, scientifically sound and socially acceptable methods and technology, made universally available to individuals and families in the community through their full participation and at a cost that the community and the country can afford to maintain at every stage of their development in the spirit of self-reliance and self-determination" (WHO 1978). Simply stated, primary health care is where people make their first contact with the health system; of course, they need to do it in different ways and settings.

The primary care sector carries out a wide variety of functions, such as: health education; promotion of healthy nutrition, safe water supply and basic sanitation; maternal and child care including family planning; immunization; prevention and control of locally endemic diseases; appropriate treatment of common diseases and injuries; and provision of essential pharmaceuticals. During recent years there has been an acceptance of the important role of primary health care in helping governments to achieve equity, efficiency, effectiveness and responsiveness within their health systems. The vast majority of reform efforts worldwide are targeted at this level of care, including in the former Soviet Union countries (Chen et al. 2004; Danishevski and McKee 2005; Figueras, Menabde and Busse 2005).

There is an intrinsically close relationship between primary health care and TB. Primary care involves both public health and individual care interventions. In TB control, an optimal public health impact is best achieved through rapid detection and high-quality treatment of individual patients. In many instances, however, this simple notion is not translated into action.

Whatever model of primary health care is in place, primary health care providers can and should contribute to TB control efforts through case finding, follow-up of patients, and health education. In 2004 the WHO Regional Office for Europe and the New Jersey Medical School National Tuberculosis Centre published the *Brief guide on tuberculosis control for primary health care providers for countries in the WHO European Region with a high and intermediate burden of tuberculosis* (Ahamed et al. 2004), which suggests that, although the roles of primary health care providers in TB control will differ according to individual national arrangements, primary health care providers should suspect TB in patients who present with symptoms suggestive of TB and perform (or refer for) primary evaluation and diagnosis (sputum examination and chest X-ray) to rule out the disease (Box 10.5).

The accomplishment of all or most of these functions by primary health care providers would allow former Soviet Union countries to make considerable and rapid progress in case detection and management and thus facilitate achievement of the TB control targets. MDR-TB burden, a major problem in the former Soviet Union countries compared to the other parts of the world, can be alleviated only with the active participation of the primary care sector. As re-emphasized by WHO (WHO 2006c; WHO 2006b), direct observation of treatment is very important for management of "routine" TB cases, but it becomes absolutely crucial for drug-resistant cases. Specialized TB services are

Box 10.5 Functions of primary health care providers in tuberculosis control

---

- **Suspect TB and react quickly** when patients present with symptoms suspicious of tuberculosis.
- **Ensure collection of high-quality sputum for microscopy** as the basic tool for detection of TB and monitoring of treatment.
- **Ensure** that every patient with a productive cough of greater than 2–3 weeks has **three sputum samples** examined for acid-fast bacilli in a designated laboratory.
- **Send the collected diagnostic material** for examination to a clinical diagnostic laboratory.
- Order or refer for X-ray examination.
- **Refer TB suspects** to the specialized TB services for diagnosis and treatment.
- **Communicate to patients** that TB is curable and emphasize the importance of regular and complete treatment in curing TB.
- **Communicate with specialized TB services** to be aware of diagnosis of patients who have been referred for diagnosis and treatment.
- **Emphasize the importance of screening household and close contacts** of smear-positive cases and ensuring that symptomatic contacts are evaluated, including tuberculin (Mantoux) skin testing in children.
- **Educate the community** about the signs and symptoms of TB and the need to seek medical care if these symptoms occur.
- **Provide directly observed therapy (DOT)** to completion during the continuation phase of treatment under the supervision of the TB services.
- **Report any default or complications** in DOT to the TB services immediately.
- **Complete all essential forms** and return to the TB services.
- **Monitor patients from risk groups** for TB according to the national regulations.
- **Perform BCG vaccination** and re-vaccination as well as tuberculin skin testing in children (according to national regulations).

Source: WHO and New Jersey Medical School National Tuberculosis Centre (2004).

rarely able to ensure daily DOT during more than one year of outpatient treatment of MDR-TB patients. This can, however, be accomplished by involving the primary care network, making its strengthening a key element of any strategy to boost the response to MDR-TB. When doing so, it is also important to take account of the contribution that appropriately trained nurses can make to this process.

The question, of course, is whether existing primary care services are ready to take on these new roles, either now or in the near future. A number of externally supported projects in the region, including GFATM grants, already include training on TB for primary health care providers, more or less closely structured around the tasks presented in Box 10.5. However, simply training staff is not enough. The involvement of the primary care sector in TB control can not succeed if initiated in a traditional "vertical" manner. It must go hand in hand with overall health system reform, something that has been uneven in the post-Soviet region so far.

There is a concern that having been trained, primary health care providers will not be able to accomplish the necessary tasks because the environment is unsupportive. Again, systemic changes are needed. In some cases this will require new legislation, which in this region is often enacted by presidential or ministerial decree. This has the advantage of speed of response but the disadvantage that the need for adequate resources and supportive changes in other sectors are often overlooked.

It is clear that performance-based incentives for staff can be beneficial but they need to be coordinated with the many other tasks primary health care providers must undertake. It is likely that additional support will be needed (for example, to cover transportation expenses of DOT nurses), but it many instances this will be difficult to achieve without enabling regulations on public administration and health financing schemes.

Some countries have implemented health sector reforms involving primary health care providers that enhance their role in the control of TB and other respiratory diseases (such as Kyrgyzstan, the Russian Federation, Estonia and the Republic of Moldova) (WHO 2006a). However, these decisions are often taken by ministries of health without consulting NTP managers and without preparing a "roadmap" for changing the responsibilities and functions of TB specialists and primary health care providers; this can put at risk the effectiveness and sustainability of TB control efforts in general (Baris 2000).

Box 10.6 discusses DOTS implementation in the Republic of Moldova and Georgia.

Box 10.6 Primary health care involvement in TB control in the Republic of Moldova and Georgia

Although DOTS implementation in the **Republic of Moldova** started quite late (in 2001), the programme has been successful to a large degree due to the fact that it was supported by a reformed primary health care system based on the Family Medicine Institute so that full involvement of primary health care providers was ensured from the very beginning. As an illustration, case detection has improved dramatically: the annual number of new smear-positive cases and relapses notified had increased 2-fold between 2000 and 2005.

In the Shida Kartli region of **Georgia**, engagement of primary health care nurses in patient follow-up and dispensing of TB pharmaceuticals in rural areas enabled a decrease in the default rate from 35% to 2% in just two years.

In conclusion, it is evident that active participation by the primary health care sector is essential for strengthening TB control and achieving disease control targets in the former Soviet Union countries. This is beyond the capacity of NTPs alone; the health system overall must be prepared to make it happen. The key issue is that, on the one hand, systemic changes take time but on the other hand, the TB situation demands rigorous and rapid action.

Tuberculosis control as part of the basic benefits package

Essential care packages are an important component of health system reforms worldwide; they are equally relevant to the former Soviet Union. The basic package or basic benefits package (BBP) is a set of health services (dealing with both public health and clinical interventions) covered fully or almost fully by the purchaser in the form of pre-payment from pooled funds. This definition implies that services not in the package are to be paid directly by patients out of pocket (again, fully or almost fully) at the time the service is delivered to them. Implementation of BBPs is possible with both tax-based and insurance-based financing systems.

The basic underlying economic concept is resource scarcity: in any context, available resources in society cannot cover all needs of the population as a whole (Wong and Bitrán 1999). To ensure that the available resources are spent in the best way possible way demands a system of *prioritization*. One approach to prioritization is to define an explicit package of health services that address the leading threats for the population.

A basic package of health services has three main distinguishing features:

- it typically contains a limited subset of all health care interventions made possible by today's medical technology;
- interventions are not randomly assigned to the package; rather, they result from a prioritization process to achieve specific technical and/or social objectives;
- interventions are not independent from each other within the package; many are chosen specifically to complement or reinforce each other so that there is synergism among them.

After gaining independence, many countries of the former Soviet Union have been reluctant to accept the notion of prioritization in the health sector. Instead, they have attempted to offer all services, ranging from the simplest to the most complex. However, given resource constraints, this approach has resulted in *de facto* rationing, through queues, shortages of inputs, and inefficient and inequitable use of resources. Such a "try to do everything" approach often leads to "everything being done badly". The profound disintegration of TB control services (which has not been overcome in many countries, even now) and their inability to deal with re-emergent disease are a clear illustration of the problem.

There are several reasons why explicit and comprehensive coverage of TB control interventions within the BBP is required. First, TB is a major public health threat, with serious externalities and a negative economic impact. Second, its effective control is only possible if adequate *public* funding is secured. Third, cost–effectiveness (one of the key prerequisites for an intervention to become part of the BBP) of the DOTS-based strategy is well proven.

In resource-limited settings, it is essential to ensure that financial and other resources are channelled to the needs of vulnerable population groups. However, to ration services to beneficiaries according to their level of income is very difficult in the former Soviet Union countries as many people are employed informally and a substantial part of earnings is undeclared, so official information may be misleading. This is another reason why the inclusion of TB control in the BBP is beneficial: patients with TB and those at risk of getting it are concentrated among the poor. Thus the inclusion of TB interventions for *all* will mean that, indirectly, the needs of the poor will be met.

Importantly, appropriate formulation and implementation of the BBP helps the shift away from input-based planning (and funding) towards a patient-oriented approach: first, one defines *what* needs to be done and then who will provide the service, where will it be, and how much it will cost. In the former Soviet Union countries the process is still often the other way around, strengthening existing barriers between levels of care.

Drug-resistant TB is a very important factor to be considered in defining basic benefits. If TB is to be included in the BBP, then *all* interventions should be covered if they become necessary along the patient's pathway. Thus, if a new patient is diagnosed with MDR-TB after s/he starts treatment, a second-line regimen must be provided too. The system cannot exclude that patient from the list of beneficiaries due to the lack of funds as the individual should not be blamed for having a resistant strain; rather, as already mentioned, such a turn of events is much more a result of health system failures. WHO recommends rapid scaling-up of MDR-TB management programmes in the region, but they will be sufficient without systemic changes such as ensuring sustainable funding for BBPs.

To summarize, comprehensive coverage of TB control interventions in the BBP can contribute effectively to success in fighting the epidemic of TB. Formulation of the BBP helps to reconcile the two reform paradigms: both "system design" and "service provision" to control diseases are built in. Practical implementation is, however, demanding. It is evident that a serious, integrated systemic effort is needed, and all four key health system functions need to be addressed.

Conclusions

It is evident that many of the reasons why some former Soviet Union countries are failing to achieve TB control targets lie far beyond the authority of the NTPs. They can be addressed successfully only through an integrated system-wide approach and may require changes that involve the "macro" design of the health systems (Atun et al. 2005; Coker et al. 2005). TB control provides a case for filling the macro system framework with the "contents", thus reconciling the two health reform paradigms – system design and service provision.

As for the "vertical–horizontal debate", effective TB control is impossible using either approach on its own. A number of functions need to be carried out by vertically organized NTPs (for example, programme monitoring and evaluation), while much service provision should be implemented by general health services at community level, i.e. in a horizontal manner. It is therefore more reasonable to speak about an integrated model; this integration of vertical and horizontal functions is to take place in the primary health care. To ensure sustainable and effective delivery of care, TB control programmes should plan activities complementary to and simultaneously with overall health system developments, in particular primary health care reforms (WHO 2003a).

Active involvement of primary health care in TB control seems to be an essential prerequisite for sustainable TB control in the former Soviet Union countries. Whatever the organizational model is, primary health care providers can and should contribute decisively to TB case detection, case management and follow-up, prevention and health education. A willingness to "think outside the box" will be necessary to make this happen, including a change in the persisting paradigm that envisages the specialized TB services as having sole responsibility for fighting the disease.

Work on involving primary health care in TB control has begun in a number of countries. However, it is clear that it is not enough just to train doctors and nurses in primary care. Training must be accompanied by "system design" changes that address each of the four main health system functions, all of which are equally important in TB control.

Comprehensive coverage of TB control interventions in BBPs would be an important step forward. It is necessary to note, however, that the former Soviet Union countries must undertake sometimes painful priority-setting efforts and ministries of health will need to enhance their capacities for impact assessment and evidence-based health planning. The first steps in this direction are already taking place (WHO 2005b; WHO 2005a).

Anti-TB drug resistance is a great challenge for the former Soviet Union countries. It is not a technical but rather a systemic problem, so it must be tackled by systemic measures, too. The spread of MDR-TB was, to a considerable extent, created by frailties in the health systems' overall performance.

The way forward

WHO and other international agencies provide assistance to countries in the area of health systems development as well as in TB control. Listed below are a number of areas where these two elements can contribute mutually to each other.

- *Country health system performance assessments in regard to TB control.* By adapting the *World Health Report 2000* framework, organized around the four main functions of the health system, a tool should be developed that would help the countries to identify what needs to be done with health systems to improve their ability to respond to the challenge of TB, as well as in terms of their overall performance.
- *TB financing and expenditure assessment.* Given the importance of assessing the

current levels of and gaps in TB funding, emphasized in the 2005 World Health Assembly Resolution, another tool would assist countries to develop medium- and long-term national plans for financial sustainability of TB control, as well as putting in place mechanisms for rational allocation and use of funds. Such "TB national health accounts" may be useful for other diseases such as HIV/AIDS and malaria.

- *Human resources for TB control.* Technical assistance should be provided to countries to strengthen their capacity to respond to TB.
- *Improvement of graduate medical education on TB.* A review of the existing practices should be conducted, followed by the development of a "model" manual incorporating DOTS principles and taking into account features of the health systems within the region; further adaptation by the individual countries can then be undertaken as necessary.
- *Development of a "model" for involvement of primary health care providers in TB control.* This will require a review of the existing experiences in the region, their benefits and barriers to implementation, as well as development of a set of training materials and their evaluation. This could usefully link with those GFATM projects in the former Soviet Union countries that include components of primary health care.
- *TB hospital assessment.* This should include technical assistance in determining the need for TB beds, assessment of institutional performance, recommendations and guidance for change.

References

Adams, O., Mosneaga, A. and Gedik, G. (2003). Improving institutional performance by better internal hospital management: a framework for assessing management training needs, *World Hospitals and Health Services*, 39(2): 3–10, 41, 43.

Ahamed, N., Yurasova, Y., Zaleskis, R., et al. (2004). *Brief Guide on Tuberculosis control for primary health care providers*. Geneva: World Health Organization Regional Office for Europe.

Atun, R. A., Samyshkin, Y. A., Drobniewski, F., et al. (2005). Barriers to sustainable tuberculosis control in the Russian Federation health system, *Bulletin of the World Health Organization*, 83(3): 217–223.

Baris, E. (2000). Tuberculosis in times of health sector reform, *International Journal of Tuberculosis and Lung Disease*, 4(7): 595–596.

Bosman, M. C. (2000). Health sector reform and tuberculosis control: the case of Zambia, *International Journal of Tuberculosis and Lung Disease*, 4(7): 606–614.

Chen, L., Evans, T., Anand, S., et al. (2004). Human resources for health: overcoming the crisis, *Lancet*, 364(9449): 1984–1990.

Coker, R. J. and Atun, R. (2004). Health care system frailties and public health control of communicable diseases on the European Union's new eastern border, *Lancet*, 363: 1389–1392.

Coker, R. J., Dimitrova, B., Drobniewski, F., et al. (2005). Health system frailties in tuberculosis service provision in Russia: an analysis through the lens of formal nutritional support, *Public Health*, 119(9): 837–843.

Collins, C. D., Green, A. T. and Newell, J. N. (2002). The relationship between disease control strategies and health system development: the case of TB, *Health Policy*, 62(2): 141–160.

Danishevski, K. and McKee, M. (2005). Reforming the Russian health-care system, *Lancet*, 365(9464): 1012–1014.

Figueras, J., Menabde, N. and Busse, R. (2005). The road to reform, *British Medical Journal*, 331: 169–170.

Godinho, J., Veen, J., Dara, M., Cercone, J. and Pacheco, J. (2005). *Stopping tuberculosis in Central Asia: priorities for action*. Washington, D.C.: World Bank.

Harries, A. D., Zachariah, R., Bergstrom, K., et al. (2005). Human resources for control of tuberculosis and HIV-associated tuberculosis, *International Journal of Tuberculosis and Lung Disease*, 9(2): 128–137.

Jakubowiak, W. M., Bogorodskaya, E. M., Borisov, S. E., Danilova, I. D. and Kourbatova, E. V. (2007). Risk factors associated with default among new pulmonary TB patients and social support in six Russian regions, *International Journal of Tuberculosis and Lung Disease*, 11(1): 46–53.

Kritski, A. L. and Ruffino-Netto, A. (2000). Health sector reform in Brazil: impact on tuberculosis control, *International Journal of Tuberculosis and Lung Disease*, 4(7): 622–626.

Marx, F. M., Atun, R. A., Jakubowiak, W., McKee, M. and Coker, R. J. (2007). Reform of tuberculosis control and DOTS within Russian public health systems: an ecological study, *European Journal of Public Health*, 17(1): 98–103.

McKee, M., Nolte, E. and DuBois, C.-A. (2006). *Human resources for health in Europe*. Maidenhead: Open University Press.

Miller, B. (2000). Health sector reform: scourge or salvation for TB control in developing countries? *International Journal of Tuberculosis and Lung Disease*, 4(7): 593–594.

Ministry of Health of the Russian Federation (2004). *Order 109 on tuberculosis control*. Moscow: Ministry of Health of the Russian Federation.

Newell, J. (2002). The implications for tuberculosis control of the growth in numbers of private practitioners in developing countries, *Bulletin of the World Health Organization*, 80(10): 836–837.

Tang, S. and Squire, S. B. (2005). What lessons can be drawn from tuberculosis (TB) control in China in the 1990s? An analysis from a health system perspective, *Health Policy*, 72(1): 93–104.

The Nuffield Institute (2002). *Tuberculosis & Health Systems Development. Newsletter, December*. University of Leeds: The Nuffield Institute.

Uplekar, M., Pathania, V. and Raviglione, M. (2001). Private practitioners and public health: weak links in tuberculosis control, *Lancet*, 358(9285): 912–916.

Weil, D. E. C. (2000). Advancing tuberculosis control within reforming health systems, *International Journal of Tuberculosis and Lung Disease*, 4(7): 597–605.

WHO (1978) Declaration of Alma Ata. International Conference on Primary Health Care, Alma Ata, 6–12 September 1978.

WHO (2000). *World Health Report 2000 – Health systems: improving performance*. Geneva: World Health Organization.

WHO (2002). *WHO project on cost-effective tuberculosis control in the Russian Federation*. Moscow: World Health Organization.

WHO (2003a). *Future directions for primary health care. Report by the Secretariat. EB113/11 Add.1*. Geneva: World Health Organization.

WHO (2003b). The 2nd ad hoc Committee on the tuberculosis epidemic. Recommendations of the Committee to the Stop tuberculosis Partnership. Committee Meeting 18–19 September, Montreaux.

WHO (2005a). *The efficiency of tuberculosis laboratory services in the Russian Federation. Policy brief No 5*. Geneva: World Health Organization.

WHO (2005b). *The efficiency of the WHO tuberculosis control strategy in the Russian Federation: the case of Orel Oblast. Policy brief No 1*. Geneva: World Health Organization.

WHO (2005c). *Addressing poverty in tuberculosis control. Options for national tuberculosis control programmes.* Geneva: World Health Organization.

WHO (2005d). *World Health Assembly, 58th (2005) Resolution 58.14. Sustainable financing for tuberculosis prevention and control.* Geneva: World Health Organization.

WHO (2006a). *Review of the National Tuberculosis Programme, Kyrgyzstan.* Copenhagen: World Health Organization.

WHO (2006b). *The Stop tuberculosis Strategy. Building on and enhancing DOTS to meet TB-related Millennium Development Goals. WHO/HTM/STB/2006.37.* Geneva: World Health Organization Stop Tuberculosis Partnership.

WHO (2006c). *Global Plan to Stop tuberculosis 2006-2015. Stop tuberculosis Partnership and World Health Organization. (WHO/HTM/STB/2006.35)* Geneva: World Health Organization.

WHO and New Jersey Medical School National Tuberculosis Centre (2004) *Brief guide on tuberculosis control for primary health care providers for countries in the WHO European Region with a high and intermediate burden of tuberculosis.* Copenhagen: World Health Organization and New Jersey Medical School National Tuberculosis Centre.

WHO Regional Office for Europe (2002). *DOTS Expansion Plan to Stop tuberculosis in the WHO European Region 2002–2006.* Copenhagen: World Health Organization Regional Office for Europe.

WHO Regional Office for Europe (2005). *Tuberculosis Assessment Mission to Armenia.* Copenhagen: World Health Organization Regional Office for Europe.

Wong, H. and Bitrán, R. (1999). *Designing a benefits package.* Washington, D.C.: World Bank Institute.

chapter eleven

Health systems and communicable disease control: emerging evidence and lessons from central and eastern Europe

Rifat Atun, Richard Coker

Introduction

Europe is now experiencing the fastest rate of growth of HIV in any region of the world, with rapidly increasing incidence of infection in eastern Europe and persistent endemicity in central Europe (UNAIDS and WHO 2006). Along with HIV, the countries of eastern Europe also face the public health challenge of TB and MDR-TB epidemics.

Since 1990, TB incidence has increased in eastern Europe (mostly in the countries of the former Soviet Union), with the peak incidence reached around 2001, since stabilized (Dye et al. 2005). In contrast, the incidence of TB in central Europe has continued to decline from 50 per 100 000 to reach a level of approximately 25 per 100 000. However, the incidence of TB appears still to be increasing in the central Asian republics of Kazakhstan, Kyrgyzstan, Tajikistan, and Uzbekistan (WHO 2005).

Of the 17 283 MDR-TB cases reported globally in 2004, over 60% (10 595) were from the European region and the vast majority of these from eastern Europe, including the Baltic states of Estonia, Latvia and Lithuania. Of particular concern is the fact that, as with Africa, treatment success with DOTS in Europe (particularly in eastern Europe) is substantially below what is seen in other regions of the world. The DOTS coverage and smear-positive case-detection rate remain the lowest in the world (WHO 2005). Eastern Europe now has the highest MDR-TB rate in the world (WHO Regional Office for Europe 2007). Collectively, these remain the principal obstacles to meeting the Millennium Development Goal targets for TB (Dye et al. 2005; WHO 2005).

The TB and HIV epidemics in central and eastern Europe are complex, influenced by a transition characterized by rapid political, economic, sociocultural and behavioural changes. In addition to HIV, TB and MDR-TB, eastern Europe, and to a lesser extent central Europe, face the challenge of worsening sexually transmitted illness and injecting drug use epidemics. Although many factors impact upon HIV spread in eastern Europe, especially in the countries of the former Soviet Union the epidemic has been driven principally by injecting drug use (Hamers and Downs 2003) and to a lesser extent by STIs (Grassly et al. 2003). There is a close interrelationship between HIV, drug-sensitive TB and MDR-TB.

The confluence of the HIV, TB, MDR-TB, injecting drug use and STI epidemics has significant public health implications (Drobniewski et al. 2004; Hamers and Downs 2003; Kelly and Amirkhanian 2003; Rhodes et al. 1999). Where there is an immature HIV epidemic, failure to control MDR-TB may lead to approximately a third more deaths than where there is effective treatment (Atun et al. 2005b). Further, in settings of high MDR-TB prevalence, with immature yet explosive HIV epidemics among injecting drug users, effective HIV harm-reduction and drug-sensitive TB/MDR-TB control programmes must be established concurrently if substantial numbers of deaths are to be averted. Early in an HIV epidemic centred on the injecting drug user population, inadequate attention to effective harm reduction, even in settings of good TB control, will result in substantial excess deaths (Atun et al. 2007).

This complex epidemiological picture is also of concern for the expanded EU, which now has a new eastern border that includes the Russian Federation, Ukraine and Belarus (all of which have substantial TB, MDR-TB, HIV, STI and injecting drug use epidemics). Concern also arises because of the potential for large-scale population movements and the challenges of ensuring coherent and robust public health control measures within borders. However, the countries of eastern Europe, with their frail health systems, have failed to meet these complex emerging challenges (Atun 2006; Coker and Atun 2004; Mounier et al. 2007).

The countries of eastern Europe, with health systems based on the Soviet Semashko model, were successful in curbing communicable diseases in the first half of the 20th century. However, by the late 1980s these systems were struggling to respond to the health needs of their populations. After 1991, following the break-up of the Soviet Union, the health systems in many eastern European countries collapsed in the face of serious financial shortages, which triggered reduced health sector financing, a decline in the coverage of the population and huge increases in out-of-pocket payments (Balabanova et al. 2004a). Since then, public health systems rooted in the traditional Soviet Semashko model have been unable to cope with re-emerging or emerging communicable diseases, most notably illustrated by the failure to respond effectively to the challenge of the emerging HIV and TB epidemics.

This chapter draws on a rigorous review of the empirical evidence on health system factors (namely, stewardship; financing resource allocation and provider payment systems; organization and service delivery; resource generation; and monitoring and evaluation) which have enabled or hindered an effective health system response to TB and HIV epidemics in central and eastern Europe.

The chapter is divided into five sections. Following the introduction, we present evidence on health systems responses to HIV. The third section focuses on health system responses to control TB. This is followed in the fourth section by a discussion comparing and contrasting the evidence concerning HIV and TB, while the final section identifies policy implications arising from the findings.

Health systems responses to HIV

Stewardship

In central Europe, the response of health system leadership to the HIV epidemic has been mixed. In Hungary, early in the epidemic, the response by political leaders was decisive, with mass education campaigns, peer-education programmes for commercial sex workers, compulsory testing for specific risk groups and voluntary testing for the general population (Danziger 1996a; Danziger 1996b). In Poland, sociocultural and religious barriers, combined with frequent elections and ministerial reshuffles that created policy discontinuity, initially prevented development of a rapid and comprehensive response (Danziger 1994). However, appropriate policies were soon introduced to halt the epidemic. In Romania, during the Ceausescu era, which ended in 1989, HIV was labelled as a "capitalist disease" and officially did not exist within Romanian borders. Instead, policies aimed at boosting population growth – such as banning of contraception, abortion and sex education – gave the HIV epidemic a free rein (Danziger 1996b). In 2002, following the revolution, a new law guaranteed prevention and care for people with HIV, including free, publicly funded treatment and dietary supplements for those who needed them, but the response still remains fragmented, with shortages of resources (Cocu et al. 2005; Hersh et al. 1991; Kline et al. 2004). In contrast, in the Czech Republic, following the Velvet Revolution of 1989 the response was rapid and comprehensive, underpinned by mass education campaigns and voluntary testing, as well as new laws which decriminalized same-sex relations and commercial sex work, and encouraged the implementation of HIV control programmes (Danziger 1996b).

Engagement by civil society with government began in the early 1990s in central Europe and has steadily matured. In contrast, in eastern Europe, except for the Baltic states, civil society engagement with governments, whose stewardship capacity continues to be weak, remains constrained. This is especially true in those countries with authoritarian regimes that have discouraged the development of an independent civil society (Atlani et al. 2000).

In eastern Europe, weak capacity and poor funding of civil society organizations have further hindered a multisectoral response, especially with regard to efforts to reach out to vulnerable and marginalized groups (Mounier et al. 2007). Lack of data on the numbers of civil society organizations active in the area of HIV/AIDS and the amount of financing allocated to them makes it difficult to assess objectively the extent of engagement. Consequently, in eastern Europe, and especially in the Russian Federation, health system responses to HIV remain fragmented and incoherent. Separation of civil and criminal justice systems and varying interpretations of health and criminal laws hinder HIV prevention and control activities (Atun et al. 2005d; Platt and McKee 2000). In Ukraine, where governmental leadership in the area of HIV has been limited, the bodies coordinating HIV/AIDS activities remain largely ineffective, despite support from international agencies and funding from the GFATM, in instituting a wide-ranging response that emphasizes the engagement of civil society and NGOs.

In the central Asian republics, which are on major drug smuggling routes, the response has been slow – compromised by limited abilities within governments to coordinate a response (Godinho et al. 2005). Nevertheless, in spite of a slow start and subdued leadership, there are encouraging signs of increased governmental commitment to tackling HIV. A regional AIDS strategy has been developed to provide the framework for country-specific multisectoral strategies to combat HIV. Since 2002, Kazakhstan, Kyrgyzstan, Tajikistan and Uzbekistan have developed strategic plans for multisectoral responses, which helped them to secure funding from the GFATM. The countries have also signed the Dublin and Vilnius Declarations (EC 2004; Government of Ireland 2004), which aim to galvanize commitment to fight HIV/AIDS in the area. However, these commitments have not yet been accompanied by the removal of legal obstacles to harm-reduction programmes, which is necessary if meaningful responses are to be mounted. In Turkmenistan, the Government has denied the existence of an HIV problem, having notified only two cases of infection to WHO – despite reports which suggest widespread and increasing drug use and commercial sex work (Rechel and McKee 2005).

Health system financing and resource allocation

Low levels of financing for HIV programmes, generally amounting to less than 1% of government health expenditure, and disproportionate allocation of resources to diagnostics and hospital-based services, with correspondingly low levels of funding for harm reduction create major barriers to progress in central and eastern Europe (Atun 2006).

In eastern Europe, in the period 2001–2004, international assistance for tackling HIV/AIDS (through GFATM, the World Bank and major bilateral donors) rose from US$ 52 million to more than US$ 600 million (Marquez 2005). However, significant funding gaps still exist, reflecting low domestic public health expenditure (Adeyi et al. 2003). Scaling up essential programmes for HIV/AIDS prevention, care and treatment will necessitate a 5-fold increase in funding from all sources (Futures Group and Instituto Nacional de Salud Publica 2005), to reach 2–3% of total health expenditure (far higher than the current spending levels on HIV, which amounts to approximately 0.6% of government health expenditure (Atun et al. 2005d)), with redirection of resources from equipment and HIV testing to prevention. An absence of systematic tracking of expenditure for different HIV/AIDS services and for risk groups makes it difficult to assess objectively the extent of funding gaps, inefficiencies in resource allocation and the extent of inequities.

Health system organization and service delivery

In many central and eastern European countries, health systems have been centralized, with vertical subsystems for HIV, TB, STIs and substance abuse. Services are delivered by individuals with narrow specialisms and continuity of care is fragmented. The public health function, dedicated to surveillance and enforcement of hygiene and environmental standards which manifest as the Sanitary Epidemiological Network, is also organized vertically and poorly integrated with service delivery. These organizational rigidities have hindered rapid and integrated responses to the HIV epidemic (Coker and Atun 2004), leading to a loss of confidence in public services and growth of private provision and self-care (Barr and Field 1996; Tulchinsky and Varavikova 1996).

In central and eastern Europe, despite some successful harm-reduction projects (Des Jarlais et al. 2002; Rhodes et al. 2002; Vickerman and Watts 2002), scaling-up of prevention and control activities remains a challenge. This is particularly so in the former Soviet Union countries where coverage of high-risk populations by prevention and harm-reduction programmes – in particular injecting drug users, commercial sex workers, MSM and prison inmates – remain very low (Amirkhanian et al. 2005; Barcal et al. 2005). In 2002–2003, coverage of harm-reduction programmes in the Russian Federation, most of which were implemented by externally funded NGOs, primarily the Open Society Institute, was estimated to be 1–4% of the target population (Sarang, Stuikyte and Bykov 2004). In central Asia, coverage of highly vulnerable groups by preventive services is below 15%, and is not expected to rise above 25% given existing resources (Atun, Wall and Timoshkin 2004). In contrast, in central European countries, where harm-reduction programmes are now substantially government funded, coverage levels are estimated to be higher. Poor coverage in eastern Europe means that although risk awareness has been increasing among injecting drug users and commercial sex workers, risk-reducing behaviours are far from pervasive (Amirkhanian, Kelly and Issayev 2001; Csepe et al. 2002; Grigoryan, Busel and Papoyan 2002; Kelly et al. 2001; Rhodes et al. 2004; Somlai et al. 2002).

In most of central and eastern Europe, however, education, prevention and harm-reduction programmes in prisons are few. There are exceptions, such as the Republic of Moldova, where peer educators lead needle exchange programmes (Rotily et al. 2001).

Throughout Europe there are inequities in access to ARV therapy but the situation is especially problematic in the low-income countries of central, eastern and southern Europe, where access to HAART is very limited (Colebunders et al. 2001; Kirk et al. 1998).

Surveillance, monitoring and evaluation

Although all European countries report to EuroHIV (the European Centre for the Epidemiological Monitoring of AIDS), data quality is variable. There is underreporting, especially from some countries of central and eastern Europe (Hickman et al. 1993). In eastern Europe, surveillance is bureaucratic and fails to inform policy. In most countries (except for the Baltic states) infrastructure has not been upgraded and medical staff are poorly paid. Not surprisingly, there is weak surveillance (especially for high-risk groups), with insufficient capacity of HIV programmes to engage in monitoring and evaluation.

There is a near absence of sentinel surveillance systems in central Asian countries, which instead rely on case reporting and screening to track the epidemics (Atun, Wall and Timoshkin 2004; Atun 2005a). Hence, the reported incidence and prevalence levels greatly differ from actual levels. This makes targeted responses difficult.

Health systems responses to tuberculosis

As in other regions in the world, empirical evidence on the relationship between health systems and TB control in central and eastern Europe is limited and, where available, much of the evidence relates to research from the Russian Federation. These findings are, however, relevant to all post-Soviet Union countries.

In 1994, at the First Meeting of the NTP Managers of Central and Eastern Europe and the former USSR, representatives of 25 countries agreed to adopt the WHO DOTS strategy (WHO 1997). By 2005, Croatia remained the only country which had not incorporated the five core components of DOTS into its TB control policies, while Bulgaria and Slovenia stand out as countries which have yet to produce a national TB control manual.

According to the WHO 2005 report *Global tuberculosis control: surveillance, planning, financing* (which does not include data from Ukraine), all countries in central and eastern Europe have implemented policies to use smear microscopy for diagnosis of TB (with the exception of Armenia where this policy has yet to be implemented in all TB-control units). Similarly, short-course chemotherapy is reported as being widely implemented. With the exception of Croatia, Serbia and Montenegro (then a unified country) and The former Yugoslav Republic of Macedonia, all countries reported that they had implemented outcome monitoring by cohort analysis. Implementation of DOT remains incomplete in Armenia, Georgia, and Serbia and Montenegro (WHO 2005).

In central Europe, Bosnia and Herzegovina, The former Yugoslav Republic of Macedonia, Romania, Serbia, Montenegro, Slovakia and Slovenia have all implemented guidelines for private practitioners designed to ensure well-managed public–private mix in TB control, but in eastern Europe – with the exception of the three Baltic states of Estonia, Latvia and Lithuania, and reportedly Turkmenistan – no such guidelines have been developed or implemented (WHO 2005).

However, the problem with DOTS implementation lies less with the adoption of policies to implement core components of DOTS, but more with their execution, which remain inadequate, especially in eastern Europe. This is reflected in the low treatment success of new smear-positive cases, which remain below the target of 85% in several central European countries (including the Czech Republic, Hungary, The former Yugoslav Republic of Macedonia, Poland, the Republic of Moldova and Romania) and in all of the eastern European countries except Tajikistan. The shortcomings in the implementation of the core components of DOTS are discussed in the section on service delivery (WHO 2005).

Health system responses to TB control in eastern Europe are hindered by a number of factors, but especially by (Atun et al. 2005d; Coker and Atun 2004; Coker et al. 2003; Fry et al. 2005; Zalesky et al. 1999):

- weak leadership;
- limited financing;
- vertical approaches to management of health problems – with poor horizontal linkages within the health sector and with other sectors;
- laws and regulations (and varying interpretation of these) which further reinforce these vertical approaches and prevent intersectoral and multisectoral coordination of TB control efforts; and
- ineffective coalition building with civil society.

In eastern Europe, inadequate technical capacity in ministries of health is a major barrier to the implementation of complex health reforms. In particular, there is limited capacity to analyse public health imperatives or connect public health evidence effectively to policy (Coker and Atun 2004).

Health system organization and service delivery for tuberculosis

In central Europe, case-detection rates of 70% or higher have been achieved in Bosnia and Herzegovina, Bulgaria, The former Yugoslav Republic of Macedonia, Romania, Serbia and Montenegro, but this target rate has yet to be reached in Albania, the Czech Republic, Hungary, Poland, the Republic of Moldova, Slovakia and Slovenia. The situation in eastern Europe is worse – while Estonia, Georgia, Kazakhstan, Latvia, Lithuania and Turkmenistan report case-detection rates of 70% or above, this has not been achieved in the rest of eastern Europe (including Armenia, Azerbaijan, Belarus, Kyrgyzstan, the Russian Federation, Tajikistan, Ukraine and Uzbekistan). However, given the poor state of TB services and outdated monitoring and evaluation systems in eastern Europe, these statistics should be treated cautiously.

DOTS coverage is suboptimal in the central European countries of Albania, Croatia, Romania and Serbia, Montenegro and in the eastern European countries of Azerbaijan, Lithuania, the Russian Federation, Tajikistan, Turkmenistan, Ukraine and Uzbekistan. However, as with case detection, given the poor surveillance systems, these findings (which are based on country reports rather than primary research) must be treated with caution.

In health systems based on the Soviet Semashko model, TB control is typically comprised of four vertical systems:

(i)   screening services based on X-ray fluorography
(ii) the penitentiary TB system, including prisons and pre-detention centres
(iii) hospital-based services, and
(iv) primary/community health care-based services.

Financing and management of these subsystems are separate and once funds are allocated to a subsystem, there is no opportunity for transfer of resources between them.

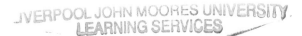

In these systems, case finding and diagnosis for TB have relied on mass population screening with fluorography and to a lesser extent bacteriology. Treatment is based on individualized regimens that include a mixture of first-line and second-line anti-TB and immune-modulating drugs, as well as surgical and physical interventions. TB patients experienced frequent and lengthy hospitalizations and were monitored for long periods after successful clinical treatment, along with patients with inactive TB, who, according to international TB control approaches, would be not classified as TB patients at all and would no longer require follow-up.

Studies from eastern Europe have shown that pilot projects can succeed in implementing TB control programmes based on WHO-approved methods (Fry et al. 2005) with treatment outcomes similar to or better than in the traditional Russian approach (Balabanova et al. 2006; Kherosheva et al. 2003; Mawer et al. 2001; Ruohonen et al. 2002). However, evaluations have identified shortcomings in the quality of the screening, treatment and services provided (Balabanova et al. 2005; Balabanova et al. 2004b).

Studies in the Russian Federation have found that the costs of treating TB using the traditional Soviet TB control system are very high compared with what is spent in other high-burden countries, reflecting intensive hospitalization policies and lengthy case management, with inpatient care accounting for more than 50% of total TB control costs (Atun et al. 2006). Further studies in the Russian Federation indicate that implementation of the DOTS strategy could lower treatment costs substantially for new smear-positive patients (Jacobs et al. 2002; Migliori et al. 1998), and that many hospital admissions for TB are not necessary. However, other factors also play a role and patients are often admitted to hospital for long periods during winter because of the lack of adequate social support systems for TB patients (Atun et al. 2005c). Indeed, in the Russian Federation, if purely clinical admission criteria were applied then less than 50% of admissions would be justified and thus less than 50% of the current number of beds would be required. Up to 85% of admissions and beds were deemed to be necessary when social need and poor access to outpatient care were included within the clinical criteria (Floyd et al. 2006).

This tendency in the Russian Federation to hospitalize patients for lengthy periods contrasts with other countries that have a high burden of TB but where treatment is generally provided on an outpatient basis. In those countries, it is unusual for patients to be hospitalized for long periods and large networks of TB hospitals do not exist. However, in spite of the emerging evidence, in many countries of eastern Europe, transition to WHO-approved methods of TB control has been difficult (Atun et al. 2005a).

Organizational barriers prevent effective multisectoral approaches to TB control (Atun et al. 2005d; Atun et al. 2005e; Fry et al. 2005; Hickman et al. 1993). In particular, close collaboration between the civil and penitentiary systems has been very challenging, with the consequence that rates of TB and MDR-TB remain very high in the prison system and prisoners released into the community without adequate follow-up continue to act as the source of a large number of new cases of TB and MDR-TB (Atun et al. 2005e; Bobrik et al. 2005; Fry et al. 2005; Kimerling 2000; Slavuckij et al. 2000; Slavuckij et al. 2002).

This inability to implement fully scaled-up TB control programmes based on WHO-approved methods of control is of profound public health concern. In eastern Europe, the institutionalization of TB care, with lengthy hospitalizations often in out-of-town facilities, create a favourable environment for nosocomial spread of TB (Coker et al. 2003) – a situation mirrored in other institutionalized settings, such as prisons and pre-detention trial centres where TB rates and, in particular, rates of MDR-TB, remain particularly high (Drobniewski et al. 2002; Drobniewski et al. 1996; Drobniewski et al. 2004; Faustini, Hall and Perucci 2006; Stern 1999).

There are, however, encouraging developments in the area of service delivery. As in other eastern European countries, in the Russian Federation there is a countrywide effort to strengthen the capacity of outpatient and laboratory services and to introduce information systems to facilitate better management of pharmaceuticals supply (WHO 2005).

Health system financing and resource allocation for tuberculosis

Evaluations in the Russian Federation have demonstrated that health system financing and provider payment systems create perverse incentives that encourage lengthy and repeated hospitalizations (beyond those stipulated in the regulations) (Fry et al. 2005). This has meant that ensuring high bed occupancy through repeat admissions or lengthy hospitalizations (because of institutional financial remuneration mechanisms) is a more profound driver of the health care system response than is clinical need. Hence, while inpatient capacity to manage patients with TB in Russian regions correlates closely with the number of new cases, the high level of utilization of that capacity has not been reduced to any noticeable extent by the introduction of DOTS (Marx et al. 2007).

In the Russian Federation and other countries of eastern Europe that have yet to reform their TB financing systems (all those except for the Baltic states), hospitals are funded according to line-item budgeting, with funds allocated according to inputs such as the number of hospital beds, the average length of stay, bed occupancy and the number of doctors. This provides a strong incentive for providers to maintain existing capacity and to hospitalize patients with TB. These funding mechanisms reward the proliferation of infrastructure and inputs rather than improving efficiency and outcomes; the quality of the care provided is neglected (Coker et al. 2005).

Surveillance, monitoring and evaluation for tuberculosis

Very few studies have examined the surveillance, monitoring and evaluation systems for TB in central and eastern Europe. Although there are efforts by WHO to strengthen the surveillance, monitoring and evaluation systems for TB in eastern Europe, weak systems have prevented appropriate and targeted responses to the emerging problems (Coker and Atun 2004; Wuhib et al. 2002).

Discussion

Emerging empirical evidence demonstrates that health system responses to HIV/AIDS and TB in central and eastern Europe are highly heterogeneous and often inadequate.

TB and HIV control programmes in most post-Soviet countries remain highly vertical, with separate sources of financing and reporting. Interaction and coordination between these programmes remains very poor. In contrast with many countries in central Europe which have made good progress to implement HIV and TB control programmes, the countries of eastern Europe, with health systems rooted in the traditional Soviet Semashko model – highly hierarchical, with vertical service delivery, inadequate multisectoral collaboration and limited civil involvement – are failing to respond effectively to the challenges of managing the TB, MDR-TB and HIV epidemics. In both central and eastern Europe, inequities in access to services persist, including HAART and TB control. Immigrants, injecting drug users, the poor and those with low levels of education suffer most.

In central Europe, health system responses to HIV have been strong, but not fully scaled up. Substantial gaps in coverage exist, and much remains to be done to control the emerging epidemics among injecting drug users and commercial sex workers, particularly in the Republic of Moldova and Romania. However, eastern European countries still face a formidable challenge, as an effective response to the epidemic must contend with the rapidly changing macro and micro environments, as well as the confluence of the HIV epidemic with those of injecting drug use, STIs and TB.

Particularly in eastern Europe, a number of health system weaknesses have hindered effective multisectoral responses to address the HIV and TB epidemics. These include:

(i)   inadequate stewardship by health ministries and an inability to build meaningful coalitions with civil society, who remain disengaged with policy and operational decisions;
(ii) low levels of financing in the health system, especially for HIV and TB, with inappropriate resource allocation mechanisms that have failed to take into account the emerging HIV epidemic;
(iii) highly vertical service delivery systems for HIV, TB, injecting drug use and STIs, with poor horizontal linkages preventing delivery of integrated responses to these colliding epidemics;
(iv) inadequate technical capacity among health professionals who remain poorly paid, and;
(v)   weak surveillance, monitoring and evaluation systems to inform decisions.

Collectively, these factors create substantial barriers to scaling up interventions. In these countries, mounting multisectoral responses is difficult, especially as there are varying interpretations of the law and as sociocultural factors influence programme design and implementation (Coker and Atun 2004).

Policy implications

Dealing with the HIV and TB epidemics requires multifaceted and multisectoral interventions. However, interactions between micro and macro contexts and health systems affect the way that policies can be translated into action. The design and implementation of these interventions should thus be shaped by the local context as their consequences may otherwise be counter-intuitive (Atun et al. 2005d). Hence, there is a need for a broader and more detailed understanding of the political, economic, social and legal contexts. But unfortunately, this rarely occurs in practice. Instead, there is a push to introduce technical solutions without understanding the broad context and the health system. It is not surprising to find that these approaches have yet to have any discernable impact on these epidemics and in many countries donor-funded programmes have failed to be scaled up beyond local projects. The key message for policy-makers, funders (such as the GFATM, bilateral and multilateral organizations) and implementing agencies is that, especially in eastern Europe, programmatic interventions are unlikely to succeed or be sustained without a good understanding of these factors and the incorporation of appropriate responses to address them.

In the Russian Federation and other countries of the former Soviet Union, where similar public health systems exist, TB hospitals still continue to shoulder not only the costs of extensive periods of clinical care but also a substantial burden of non-clinical social support, while HIV programmes remain highly medicalized and fail to inadequately embrace civil society. Joined-up interventions aimed at scaling-up of DOTS and MDR-TB treatment programmes, implementation of effective harm-reduction programmes and multisectoral public health responses, are strategies that are needed to simultaneously address these epidemics. However, this will require changes in health system norms related to planning, financing and delivery of clinical care and social services. These changes require a reform process that goes beyond TB or HIV control programmes and embraces the entire health system.

Health system frailties in eastern Europe and failure to control these epidemics pose substantial public health risks for the neighbouring countries, including those inside the EU. Given the relatively immature nature of the HIV epidemics in eastern Europe, there is still a window of opportunity for effective control of TB, MDR-TB and HIV. However, this window is unlikely to remain open for long and opportunities are unlikely to be realized if health system barriers to communicable disease control are not addressed.

References

Adeyi, O., Baris, E., Chakraborty, S., Novotny, T. and Pavis, R. (2003). *Averting AIDS crises in eastern Europe and central Asia: a regional support strategy*. Washington, D.C.: World Bank.

Amirkhanian, Y. A., Kelly, J. A. and Issayev, D. D. (2001). AIDS knowledge, attitudes, and behaviour in Russia: results of a population-based, random-digit telephone survey in St Petersburg, *International Journal of STD & AIDS*, 12(1): 50–57.

Amirkhanian, Y. A., Kelly, J. A., Kabakchieva, E., et al. (2005). A randomized social network HIV prevention trial with young men who have sex with men in Russia and Bulgaria, *AIDS*, 19(16): 1897–1905.

Atlani, L., Carael, M., Brunet, J. B., Frasca, T. and Chaika, N. (2000). Social change and HIV in the former USSR: the making of a new epidemic, *Social Science and Medicine*, 50(11): 1547–1556.

Atun, R., Wall, M. and Timoshkin, A. (2004). *Evaluation of Alliance Ukraine HIV Programme in Ukraine*. London: Imperial College London Consultants.

Atun, R. A. (2006). How the health systems responded to HIV epidemic in Europe, in S. Matic, J.V. Lazarus and M.C. Donoghoe (eds) *HIV/AIDS in Europe: moving from death sentence to chronic disease management*. Copenhagen: World Health Organization Regional Office for Europe.

Atun, R. A., Baeza, J., Drobniewski, F., Levicheva, V. and Coker, R. (2005a). Implementing WHO DOTS strategy in the Russian Federation: stakeholder attitudes, *Health Policy*, 74(2): 122–132.

Atun, R. A., Lebcir, R., Drobniewski, F. and Coker, R. (2005b). Impact of an effective multi-drug-resistant tuberculosis control programmes in the setting of an immature HIV epidemic: system dynamics simulation model, *International Journal of STD and AIDS* 16(8): 560–570.

Atun, R. A., Samyshkin, Y. A., Drobniewski, F., et al. (2005c). Seasonal variation and hospital utilization for tuberculosis in Russia: hospitals as social care institutions, *European Journal of Public Health*, 15(4): 350–354.

Atun, R. A., McKee, M., Drobniewski, F. and Coker, R. (2005d). Analysis of how health system context influences HIV control: case studies from the Russian Federation, *Bulletin of the World Health Organization*, 83(10): 730–738.

Atun, R. A., Samyshkin, Y. A., Drobniewski, F., et al. (2005e). Barriers to sustainable tuberculosis control in the Russian Federation health system, *Bulletin of the World Health Organization*, 83(3): 217–223.

Atun, R. A., Samyshkin, Y., Drobniewski, F., et al. (2006). Costs and outcomes of tuberculosis services in the Russian Federation: retrospective cohort analysis, *Health Policy and Planning*, 21(5): 353–364.

Atun, R. A., Lebcir, M. R., McKee, M., Habicht, J. and Coker, R. J. (2007). Impact of joined-up HIV harm-reduction and multidrug-resistant tuberculosis control programmes in Estonia: system dynamics simulation model, *Health Policy*, 81: 207–217.

Balabanova, D., McKee, M., Pomerleau, J., Rose, R. and Haerpfer, C. (2004a). Health service utilization in the former soviet union: evidence from eight countries, *Health Services Research*, 39(6 Pt 2): 1927–1950.

Balabanova, Y., Fedorin, I., Kuznetsov, S., et al. (2004b). Antimicrobial prescribing patterns for respiratory diseases including tuberculosis in Russia: a possible role in drug resistance? *Journal of Antimicrobial Chemotherapy*, 54(3): 673–679.

Balabanova, Y., Coker, R., Fedorin, I., et al. (2005). Intra- and inter-observer agreement in chest X-ray interpretation amongst Russian physicians: implications for active screening for tuberculosis, *British Medical Journal*, 331: 379–382.

Balabanova, Y., Drobniewski, F., Fedorin, I., et al. (2006). The Directly Observed Therapy Short-Course (DOTS) strategy in Samara *Oblast*, Russian Federation, *Respiratory Research*, 7: 44.

Barcal, K., Schumacher, J. E., Dumchev, K. and Moroz, L. V. (2005). A situational picture of HIV/AIDS and injection drug use in Vinnitsya, Ukraine, *Harm Reduction Journal*, 2(1): 16.

Barr, D. A. and Field, M. G. (1996). The current state of health care in the former Soviet Union: implications for health care policy and reform, *American Journal of Public Health*, 86(3): 307–312.

Bobrik, A., Danishevski, K., Eroshina, K. and McKee, M. (2005). Prison health in Russia: the larger picture, *Journal of Public Health Policy*, 26(1): 30–59.

Cocu, M., Thorne, C., Matusa, R., et al. (2005). Mother-to-child transmission of HIV infection in Romania: results from an education and prevention programme, *AIDS Care*, 17(1): 76–84.

Coker, R. J. and Atun, R. (2004). Health care system frailties and public health control of communicable diseases on the European Union's new eastern border, *Lancet*, 363: 1389–92.

Coker, R. J., Dimitrova, B., Drobniewski, F., et al. (2003). Tuberculosis control in Samara *Oblast*, Russia: institutional and regulatory environment, *International Journal of Tuberculosis and Lung Disease*, 7(10): 920–932.

Coker, R. J., Dimitrova, B., Drobniewski, F., et al. (2005). Health system frailties in tuberculosis service provision in Russia: an analysis through the lens of formal nutritional support, *Public Health*, 119(9): 837–843.

Colebunders, R., Schroote, W., Dreezen, C., et al. (2001). Antiretroviral treatments used among adults with HIV infection in Europe, *AIDS Care*, 13: 5–14.

Csepe, P., Amirkhanian, Y. A., Kelly, J. A., McAuliffe, T. L. and Mocsonoki, L. (2002). HIV risk behaviour among gay and bisexual men in Budapest, Hungary, *International Journal of STD & AIDS*, 13: 192–200.

Danziger, R. (1994). Discrimination against people with HIV and AIDS in Poland, *British Medical Journal*, 308: 1145–1147.

Danziger, R. (1996a). Compulsory testing for HIV in Hungary, *Social Science and Medicine*, 43(8): 1199–1204.

Danziger, R. (1996b). An overview of HIV prevention in central and eastern Europe, *AIDS Care*, 8: 701–707.

Des Jarlais, D. C., Grund, J. P., Zadoretzky, C., et al. (2002). HIV risk behaviour among participants of syringe exchange programmes in central/eastern Europe and Russia, *International Journal of Drug Policy*, 13: 165–174.

Drobniewski, F., Tayler, E., Ignatenko, N., et al. (1996). Tuberculosis in Siberia: 2. Diagnosis, chemoprophylaxis and treatment, *Tubercle and Lung Disease*, 77(4): 297–301.

Drobniewski, F., Balabanova, Y., Ruddy, M., et al. (2002). Rifampin- and multiple drug-resistant tuberculosis in Russian civilians and prison inmates – Dominance of the Beijing strain family, *Emerging Infectious Diseases*, 8: 1320–1325.

Drobniewski, F. A., Atun, R., Fedorin, I., Bikov, A. and Coker, R. (2004). The 'bear trap': the colliding epidemics of tuberculosis and HIV in Russia, *International Journal of STD & AIDS*, 15(10): 641–646.

Dye, C., Watt, C. J., Bleed, D. M., Hosseini, S. M. and Raviglione, M. C. (2005). Evolution of tuberculosis control and prospects for reducing tuberculosis incidence, prevalence, and deaths globally, *Journal of the American Medical Association*, 293(22): 2767–2775.

EC (2004). *Vilnius Declaration on measures to strengthen responses to HIV/AIDS in the European Union and in neighbouring countries [international conference declaration]*. Vilnius: European Commission (http://europa.eu.int/comm/health/ph_threats/com/aids/docs/ev_20040916_rd03_en.pdf, accessed 27 November 2007).

Faustini, A., Hall, A. J. and Perucci, C. A. (2006). Risk factors for multidrug-resistant tuberculosis in Europe: a systematic review, *Thorax*, 61(2): 158–163.

Floyd, K., Hutubessy, R., Samyshkin, Y., et al. (2006). Health systems efficiency in the Russian Federation: tuberculosis control. *Bulletin of the World Health Organization*, 84(1): 43–51.

Fry, R. S., Khoshnood, K., Vdovichenko, E., et al. (2005). Barriers to completion of tuberculosis treatment among prisoners and former prisoners in St. Petersburg, Russia, *International Journal of Tuberculosis and Lung Disease*, 9: 1027–1033.

Futures Group and Instituto Nacional de Salud Publica (2005). *Funding required for the response to HIV/AIDS in eastern Europe and central Asia*. Mexico: Institut Nacional de Salud Publica; Washington, D.C.: World Bank, UNAIDS Secretariat.

Godinho, J., Renton, A., Vinogradov, V., et al. (2005). *Reversing the tide: priorities for HIV/ AIDS prevention in central Asia*. Washington, D.C.: World Bank.

Government of Ireland (2004). *Dublin Declaration on Partnership to fight HIV/AIDS in Europe and central Asia*. Dublin: Government of Ireland (http://www.eu2004.ie/templates/ meeting.asp?sNavlocator=5,13&list_id=25, accessed 24 August 2006).

Grassly, N. C., Lowndes, C. M., Rhodes, T., et al. (2003). Modelling emerging HIV epidemics: the role of injecting drug use and sexual transmission in the Russian Federation, China and India, *International Journal of Drug Policy*, 14: 25–43.

Grigoryan, S., Busel, A. and Papoyan, A. (2002). Rapid assessment of the situation on spread of injecting drug use and HIV infection in Yerevan, Armenia, *International Journal of Drug Policy*, 13: 433–436.

Hamers, F. F. and Downs, A. M. (2003). HIV in central and eastern Europe, *Lancet*, 361(9362): 1035–1044.

Hersh, B. S., Popovici, F., Apetrei, R. C., et al. (1991). Acquired immunodeficiency syndrome in Romania, *Lancet*, 338(8768): 645–649.

Hickman, M., Aldous, J., Gazzard, B. and Ellam, A. (1993). AIDS surveillance: a direct assessment of under-reporting, *AIDS*, 7(12): 1661–1665.

Jacobs, B., Clowes, C., Wares, F., et al. (2002). Cost–effectiveness analysis of the Russian treatment scheme for tuberculosis versus short course chemotherapy: results from Tomsk, Siberia, *International Journal of Tuberculosis and Lung Disease*, 6 (5): 396–405.

Kelly, J. A. and Amirkhanian, Y. A. (2003). The newest epidemic: a review of HIV/AIDS in Central and Eastern Europe, *International Journal of STD & AIDS*, 14(6): 361–371.

Kelly, J. A., Amirkhanian, Y. A., McAuliffe, T. L., et al. (2001). HIV risk behaviour and risk-related characteristics of young Russian men who exchange sex for money or valuables from other men, *AIDS Education and Prevention*, 13(2): 175–188.

Kherosheva, T., Thorpe, L. E., Kiryanova E., et al. (2003). Encouraging outcomes in the first year of a tuberculosis control demonstration programme. Orel *Oblast*, Russia, *International Journal of Tuberculosis and Lung Disease*, 7(11): 1045–1051.

Kimerling, M. E. (2000). The Russian equation: an evolving paradigm in tuberculosis control, *International Journal of Tuberculosis and Lung Disease*, 4(12 Suppl 2): 160–167.

Kirk, O., Mocroft, A., Katzenstein. T L., et al. (1998). Changes in use of antiretroviral therapy in regions of Europe over time. EuroSIDA Study Group, *AIDS*, 12: 2031–2039.

Kline, M. W., Matusa, R. F., Copaciu, L., et al. (2004). Comprehensive paediatric human immunodeficiency virus care and treatment in Constanta, Romania: implementation of a programme of highly active antiretroviral therapy in a resource-poor setting, *Pediatric Infectious Disease Journal*, 23(8): 695–700.

Marquez, P. (2005). *Combating HIV/AIDS in eastern Europe and central Asia*. Washington, D.C.: World Bank.

Marx, F. M., Atun, R. A., Jakubowiak, W., McKee, M. and Coker, R. J. (2007). Reform of tuberculosis control and DOTS within Russian public health systems: an ecological study (doi:10.1093/eurpub/ckl098), *European Journal of Public Health*, 17(1): 98–103.

Mawer, C., Ignatenko, N., Wares, D., et al. (2001). Comparison of the effectiveness of WHO short-course chemotherapy and standard Russian anti-tuberculosis regimens in Tomsk, western Siberia, *Lancet*, 358(9280): 445–449.

Migliori, G. B., Khomenko, A. G., Punga, V. V., et al. (1998). Cost–effectiveness analysis of tuberculosis control policies in Ivanovo *Oblast*, Russian Federation. (Ivanovo Tuberculosis Project Study Group), *Bulletin of the World Health Organization*, 76: 475–483.

Mounier, S., McKee, M., Atun, R. A. and Coker, R. (2007). HIV/AIDS in central Asia, in J. L. Twigg (ed.) *HIV/AIDS in Russia and Eurasia*. New York: Palgrave, 67–100.

Platt, L. and McKee, M. (2000). Observations of the management of sexually transmitted diseases in the Russian Federation: a challenge of confidentiality, *International Journal of STD & AIDS*, 11(9): 563–567.

Rechel, B. and McKee, M. (2005). *Human rights and health in Turkmenistan*. London: London School of Hygiene & Tropical Medicine.

Rhodes, T., Ball, A., Stimson, G. V., et al. (1999). HIV infection associated with drug injecting in the newly independent states, eastern Europe: the social and economic context of epidemics, *Addiction*, 94(9): 1323–1336.

Rhodes, T., Lowndes, C., Judd, A., et al. (2002). Explosive spread and high prevalence of HIV infection among injecting drug users in Togliatti City, Russia, *AIDS*, 16(13): 25–31.

Rhodes, T., Judd, A., Mikhailova, L., et al. (2004). Injecting equipment sharing among injecting drug users in Togliatti City, Russian Federation: maximizing the protective effects of syringe distribution, *Journal of Acquired Immune Deficiency Syndromes*, 35: 293–300.

Rotily, M., Weilandt, C., Bird, S. M., et al. (2001). Surveillance of HIV infection and related risk behaviour in European prisons. A multicentre pilot study, *European Journal of Public Health*, 11(3): 243–250.

Ruohonen, R. P., Goloubeva, T. M., Trnka, L., et al. (2002). Implementation of the DOTS strategy for tuberculosis in the Leningrad Region, Russian Federation (1998–1999), *International Journal of Tuberculosis and Lung Disease*, 6(3): 192–197.

Sarang, A., Stuikyte, R. and Bykov, R. (2004). *Implementation of harm-reduction measures in eastern Europe and central Asia: lessons learned.* Vilnius: Central and Eastern European Harm Reduction Network (CEEHRN) (http://www.ceehrn.org/index.php?ItemId=939, accessed 27 November 2007).

Slavuckij, A., Sizaire, V., Lobera, L. and Kimerling, M. E. (2000). Decentralization of DOTS programme within Russian penitentiary system, *International Journal of Tuberculosis and Lung Disease*, 24: 237.

Slavuckij, A., Sizaire, V., Lobera, L., Matthys, F. and Kimerling, M. E. (2002). Decentralization of the DOTS programme within a Russian penitentiary system: how to ensure the continuity of tuberculosis treatment in pre-trial detention centres? *European Journal of Public Health*, 12: 94–98.

Somlai, A. M., Kelly, J. A., Benotsch, E., et al. (2002). Characteristics and predictors of HIV risk behaviours among injection-drug-using men and women in St. Petersburg, Russia, *AIDS Education and Prevention*, 14(4): 295–305.

Stern, V. (1999). *Sentenced to die, the problem of TB in prisons in Eastern Europe and central Asia*. London: Kings College.

Tulchinsky, T. H. and Varavikova, E. A. (1996). Addressing the epidemiologic transition in the former Soviet Union: strategies for health system and public health reform in Russia, *American Journal of Public Health*, 86(3): 313–320.

UNAIDS and WHO (2006). *2006 Report on the Global AIDS Epidemic*. Geneva: Joint United Nations Programme on HIV/AIDS (UNAIDS) (http://www.unaids.org/en/HIV_data/2006GlobalReport/default.asp, accessed 27 November 2007). Report 1006.

Vickerman, P. and Watts, C. (2002). The impact of an HIV prevention intervention for injecting drug users in Svetlogorsk, Belarus: model predictions, *International Journal of Drug Policy*, 13: 149–164.

WHO (1997). *Treatment of Tuberculosis: Guidelines for National Programmes. WHO/TB/97.220*. Geneva: World Health Organization.

WHO (2005). *Global Tuberculosis Control: surveillance, planning, financing*. Geneva: World Health Organization.

WHO Regional Office for Europe (2007). *Eastern Europe has the world's highest rate of multi-drug-resistant tuberculosis (MDR-TB). News Release on 22 March 2007*. Copenhagen:

World Health Organization Regional Office for Europe (http://www.euro.who.int/home/NewsArchive, accessed 12 April 2007).

Wuhib, T., Chorba, T. L., Davidiants, V., MacKenzie, W. R. and McNabb, S. J. (2002). Assessment of the infectious diseases surveillance system of the Republic of Armenia: an example of surveillance in the Republics of the former Soviet Union, *BMC Public Health*, 2: 3.

Zalesky, R., Abdullajev, F., Khechinashvili, G., et al. (1999). Tuberculosis control in the Caucasus: successes and constraints in DOTS implementation, *International Journal of Tuberculosis and Lung Disease*, 3(5): 394–401.

twelve

Health system reforms and communicable disease in Latin America and the Caribbean

Patricio Marquez, Oscar Echeverri, Enis Baris

Introduction

In line with international policy recommendations in the 1990s, several LAC countries began to implement health sector reforms (Marquez and Engler 1990) aimed at enhancing stewardship and oversight functions of the ministries of health and reducing their direct involvement in service delivery. Simultaneously, these reforms sought to introduce new financing models to create incentives for providers to improve their performance, decentralize services to enhance responsiveness, and redefine health benefits packages to increase coverage and improve efficient allocation of resources. New legal and administrative forms of autonomy were given to public institutions. In some countries, rationalization of health service delivery networks were accompanied by privatization of some services, in an effort to foster a more balanced and effective public–private mix in the financing and delivery of health care. Among the most important changes and innovations were the gradual transformation of supply subsidies into demand subsidies for services and the creation of new private organizations for the financing and provision of health services. However, highly traditional ministries of health and the social security institutes did not change enough to respond to the scope of the reforms. The stewardship and oversight roles of these ministries and the audit mechanisms for insurance schemes and service provision remain weak, leading to market failures, corruption and inefficiencies.

Most of these health reforms in LAC have placed an emphasis on personal health services at the expense of public health programmes and community-based interventions, with the exception of some preventive clinical programmes, such as cervical cancer screening and prevention of noncommunicable diseases (e.g. hypertension, diabetes).

Financing of public health programmes, particularly tropical disease control, was substantially reduced, or simply ignored. Decentralization, a buzzword at the time, transferred administration and financing responsibilities for health to local authorities, without strengthening their limited capacity or monitoring systems to exercise these functions.

Some reforms involved switching from vertical to horizontal implementation of communicable disease control, with integration of vertical programmes into primary health services. However, preparation was often virtually ignored.

Integration of vertical programmes or decentralizing their functions involves relocating some procurement and logistics tasks, which are inefficiently carried out at local levels due to diseconomies of scale. For instance, tropical communicable diseases are usually concentrated in very poor regions with difficult access; therefore, provision of pesticides and drug procurement are achieved more efficiently by centralized mechanisms, and logistical support for national campaigns is better coordinated by central units. Frequently, public health programmes have been weak in terms of logistics, with decentralization hampering this crucial function and leading to shortages of key inputs. Weak capacity in national health systems was one of the reasons for the choice of a vertical delivery mode by donor agencies.

The following examples of various countries' experiences illustrate how health sector reforms affected communicable disease control in LAC.

Country experiences

In Argentina, health reforms accentuated pre-existing weaknesses in the health sector. Public health and health promotion activities, despite being mentioned in the reform documents, were relegated to oblivion during implementation (Lloyd-Sherlock 2005).

In Brazil, health sector reform set in motion a gradual decentralization involving three levels: Full State Management; Basic Assistance Management, where the municipality manages the provision of basic or primary health care, and the State manages more complex types of provision; and Full Municipal System Management, where the municipality manages the provision of basic as well as complex care. Full Management status is awarded on the request of the municipal government but is dependent on the decision by the federal Government as to whether it is capable of handling this enhanced administrative role. In 1999 only 8% of all counties had Full Municipal System Management status, and 80% had Basic Assistance Management status. The probability of an uninsured individual receiving medical attention is no higher in municipalities with full control over the allocation of health care resources than in municipalities with only partial control. However, the probability of receiving attention is lower if the municipality does not have a governance plan (Mobarak, Rajkumar and Cropper 2004). Decentralization had a negative impact on key public health programmes due to weak local management capacity, poor coordination, inadequate monitoring, and lack of training of health personnel. A thorny issue has been the change of status of civil servants who are now local employees. TB deaths are increasing, in part because of the AIDS epidemic, and yellow fever, which disappeared from Brazil in the 1950s, has again become a threat to parts of the country. Dengue and cholera, once thought to be under control, have resurfaced in recent years (World Bank 1999). Administrative decentralization of health services to the municipal level seems to reduce access to services by the uninsured (Mobarak, Rajkumar and Cropper 2004). Since 1999, control of vector-borne diseases in Brazil, including malaria, Chagas, yellow fever and dengue, has become the responsibility of the former federal Family Health Program. Despite Brazil's extensive experience in vector-borne disease control, the complexity of interventions (clinical, laboratory, behaviour change, environmental control) and the logistics have created inefficiencies and frustrated this "horizontal", decentralized approach.

The *World Health Report 2000*, which focused on health system performance, ranked the Colombian health system in first place amongst the LAC countries (WHO 2000). While health insurance coverage has reached close to 60% of the population, up from approximately 20% in the early 1990s, progress in public health has been less satisfactory: coverage of vaccine-preventable diseases has deteriorated, leading to outbreaks of diphtheria and measles, and weakening of public health programmes has accompanied increased incidence of TB, malaria, and outbreaks of dengue, yellow fever and leishmaniasis. TB control performance has deteriorated in terms of a decreasing number of BCG vaccinations, reduction in case finding and contact tracing, low cure rates and increased loss of follow-ups (Arbelaez et al. 2004). A recent study, which analysed the impact of Colombia's health reform on the National network of Public Health Laboratories and the National Reference Laboratories, found that the reform did not support effective operation of these laboratories, with threats to their sustainability due to decreasing public financing, and incoherence of present regulations (López 2003).

In Mexico, the recent health sector reforms aimed at rectifying financial inequities, disparities in resource allocation between insured and uninsured individuals, and underinvestment in infrastructure. These reforms explicitly commit to funding for public health services, an integrated package of services including those for catastrophic health conditions. These services will be gradually expanded based on explicit criteria of cost–effectiveness, resource availability, social acceptability and promotion of effective participation by the non-profit-making and the private sectors. On the financing side, the reform separates funding for personal and non-personal health services, assuring explicit financing for public health programmes (Frenk 2004).

Mexico's experience with the state-level Public Decentralized Organizations has been fruitful in that it has gradually transferred financial and managerial responsibilities from the Federation to the states, and from these to the provincial and local levels. This implied new political roles for secretaries of social sectors (health, education) new state-level forms of resource allocation, and new responsibilities for local health services. The gradual transfer of political, fiscal and managerial responsibility to intermediate levels of government administrations is perhaps the greatest challenge in LAC, given the weak institutional capacity and technological capacity of local health services.

The anti-poverty Education, Health and Nutrition Program (*Progresa/ Opportunidades*) and the Coverage Expansion Program are good examples of successful vertical integration of complex and diverse health interventions, with strong decision-making at state level and full operational implementation at local level. During the 1995–2001 period, these programmes contributed to the expansion of basic health services coverage for more than 10 million poor people, most of them in dispersed rural communities with fewer than 500 inhabitants (Marquez and De Geyndt 2002).

These ongoing sectoral changes in financing, gradual decentralization, vertical integration of selected health programmes, and the prominent advocacy role of political and civil servant groups promoting effective immunization programmes have played a key role in Mexico's good experience of communicable disease control in LAC.

Lessons from the reform experience

Communicable diseases are returning with a vengeance at the beginning of the 21st century. Approximately 35 new emerging and re-emerging infectious diseases have been identified as a global threat. Some are vector-borne diseases, inflicting a heavy toll on the population of LAC. They have much less effect on developed countries, usually located beyond the tropical belt, and so are not seen as major health priorities. However, climatic and other environmental changes, migration, increased air transportation and changes in vector ecology may pose a potential threat to the whole world.

Malaria, dengue fever, cholera, TB and HIV/AIDS have many things in common that would lend them to being controlled collectively and effectively. All of them are closely related to poverty, social inequities, poor living conditions, risky health behaviours and inefficient health care delivery. Consequently, efforts to reduce poverty, improve living conditions and address social and health inequity would greatly contribute to reducing the incidence and severity of such illnesses, including tropical diseases, when combined with specific vector-control measures that take account of environmental and human behavioural changes.

The way health systems have approached the control of communicable diseases has been irregular, and for the most part, inequitable, due to health care reforms that have relegated the importance of public health to a secondary position. This has occurred since the mid-1980s in many countries of LAC, with a direct negative impact on the control of communicable diseases. The most controversial features of these reforms, in addition to ignoring public health programmes, include untimely and unfair fiscal and managerial decentralization that led to the conversion of vertical programmes into horizontal ones without careful consideration of the local capacity. Vertical integration of national programmes need to be considered, in terms of logistics, supervision, information and surveillance systems, standards setting and compliance, and clear local operational activities.

Based on the experience in LAC, the lessons outlined in the following subsections may be useful for other countries in the world.

Government leadership and sustained commitment is critically important

The commitment to public health objectives and programmes needs to be firmly entrenched in the Government's development programme and supported with the necessary budgetary allocations. Clear objectives need to be set by the Government and sustained efforts over time need to be undertaken. Financing public health is a government responsibility. In LAC, public health financing, particularly for essential public health functions, is less than 1% of the total public expenditure on health (PAHO 2002). When spending on specific public health programmes is added to this figure, the percentage increases slightly but it is still very low.

Active participation by civil society is essential

Municipal government, community involvement and active participation of the population in the design and implementation of the programmes are critical ingredients that can contribute to sustained implementation of activities while ensuring local and community ownership. In addition, mobilization of resources at the local level to complement central government financial allocations in the form of municipal government contributions and in-kind community contributions and labour tend to buffer the programmes from economic shocks and political changes.

Managed decentralization can be effective

Decentralization should be a selective and gradual process according to specific stages of managerial and governance capacities at local level. An important lesson from Mexico's experience is that centralization and decentralization can coexist and the approach should not be the "either, or" dilemma, but rather to what extent centralization and decentralization measures can go hand in hand as the most effective way to deliver health care and public health interventions, such as communicable disease control. Decentralization does not mean drastic and swift responses. It requires a long and complex set of doings and un-doings in which political decisions are only the starting point. Decentralizing the management of human, physical and financial resources may hurt the weaker regions unless central-level technical assistance aggressively supports the economically less-developed regions. Equity involves a fine line between letting go and being directive.

Vertical integration of national programmes, in terms of logistics, supervision, information, and surveillance systems, standards setting and compliance, and clear local operational activities should be considered first, when administrative reforms are proposed to make them "horizontal".

Weak logistics, particularly in communicable disease control, has been a neglected issue in health system restructuring. A good logistics system ensures the right goods, in the right quantities and condition, to the right place, at the right time, for the right cost. This makes the difference between effective control of communicable diseases and worsening incidence.

Human resources development is critical

Human resources are a fundamental and essential element for public health practice. Nevertheless, in LAC the public health workforce is one of the most neglected and least valued resources within the health sector. As a result, many countries are facing difficulties in finding the right health care professionals, in the right numbers and in the right place to carry out the new organizational and delivery reforms of health care. The importance of planning health resources has been overlooked in most health reforms but now there is growing awareness of the need to give appropriate thought to this issue and to the role of education institutions in avoiding oversupply of certain types of health workers and undersupply of others, a problem that is often compounded by inadequate training. Successful public health efforts in LAC, such as the measles eradication initiative, have depended on the improvement of the technical and managerial capability of health workers at different levels of the system, particularly at the local level.

Intersectoral policies and programmes need to be strengthened

Expansion of coverage has been difficult, not only because of financing constraints but also because primary health care has been relegated to a minimal element in the service delivery programmes, as has community participation. Likewise, intersectoral coordination is practically absent, particularly for many important interventions in health promotion and prevention. Successful communicable disease programmes need not only to emphasize such control measures as individual protection, early diagnosis and immediate treatment of suspected cases, but also include information, communication campaigns, elimination of vector reservoirs with the active participation of local governments and community organizations, and strengthening of the local institutional capacity (laboratories, health facilities and community organizations in affected areas).

Sound information and surveillance systems are urgently needed

The capacity to carry out surveillance of trends in disease, behavioural factors, accidents and exposure to toxic substances or environmental agents harmful to health is an essential public health function.

There is a need to strengthen: (i) management and monitoring of key programme activities to ensure implementation is carried out as intended; (ii) systems to ensure that the target population groups are receiving the required services; (iii) mechanisms for monitoring budget allocations and expenditure to ensure adequate and timely use of resources; and (iv) evaluations of programme impact with measurable, understandable indicators that feed into the decision-making process at the various levels of the system, particularly to facilitate finding more cost-effective strategies. This can be an important tool for the sustainability of the programmes in volatile and changing political and economic environments. However, it should be clear that serious monitoring and evaluation of programmes does not happen in the absence of well-designed health information systems and tangible incentives to stimulate them. Therefore, the promotion of meaningful monitoring and evaluation may be more successful if resource allocation decisions – either at national or programme levels – hinged on the results.

It is important to stress that high priority should be sought for the improvement of management information systems, monitoring and evaluation, and regular communication on laboratory data and performance issues. Large amounts of resources have been wasted in installing electronic information systems without regard for adequate training and standardized software for data inputs, outputs and use.

Conclusion

To conclude, it is helpful to recall Sigerist's point that ". . . it is quite obvious that the means and methods used in the prevention of disease are those provided by medicine and science. And yet, whether these methods are applied or not, does not depend on medicine alone, but to a much higher extent on the philosophical and social tendencies of the time" (Sigerist 1933). Therefore, if the successes achieved in the prevention of communicable diseases in LAC are to be sustained over the long term, the appreciation of health as a good in its own right should be promoted and supported, beginning with a reformulation of health reform initiatives to incorporate public health programmes and activities as a critical element of sectoral modernization.

References

Arbelaez, M. P., Gaviria, M. B., Franco, A., et al. (2004). Tuberculosis control and managed competition in Colombia, *International Journal of Health Planning and Management*, 19(Suppl 1): 25–43.

Frenk, J. (2004). *Fair financing and universal social protection: the structural reform of the Mexican health system*. Mexico: Ministry of Health.

Lloyd-Sherlock, P. (2005). Health sector reform in Argentina: a cautionary tale, *Social Science and Medicine*, 60(8): 1893–1903.

López, Y. L. (2003). Los laboratorios de salud pública en el Sistema de Seguridad Social en Salud, Colombia, 2000. Estudio de caso [The public health laboratories under the

Social Health Insurance, Colombia, 2000], *Revista de la Facultad Nacional de Sulud Publica*, 21(1): 9–25.

Marquez, P. V. and Engler, T. (1990). Crisis y Salud: Retos Para la Decada de los 90 [Crisis and health: challenges for the 1990s], *Educacion Medica y Salud*, 24(1).

Marquez, P. and De Geyndt, W. (2002) Mexico: reaching the poor with basic health services. Washington, D.C.: World Bank (En Breve series, March).

Mobarak, A. M., Rajkumar, A. S. and Cropper, M. (2004). *The political economy of health service provision and access in Brazil. World Bank Publication, 2004.* Boulder, Colorado: Institute of Behavioural Science.

PAHO (2002). *Public health in the Americas. Conceptual renewal performance assessment, and bases for action.* Washington, D.C: Pan American Health Organization.

Sigerist, H. E. (1933). The philosophy of hygiene, *Bulletin of the History of Medicine*, I: 365–388.

WHO (2000). *World Health Report 2000 – Health systems: improving performance.* Geneva: World Health Organization.

World Bank (1999). Health care in Brazil: addressing complexity. Operations evaluation Department *Precis*, Spring (189): 1–5.

chapter thirteen

Brazil's response to AIDS and tuberculosis: lessons from a transitional economy

Eduardo Gómez

Introduction

For quite some time now Brazil has been successful in its response to AIDS. A strong, highly centralized AIDS bureaucracy, the incorporation of a well-organized civic movement and strong relations with the world health and financial community has led to an impressive decline in AIDS deaths since the early 1990s. Yet policy analysts may not be aware of the fact that there has been no similar response to other lingering diseases, such as TB. Indeed, TB has not received nearly as much attention, notwithstanding the fact that it has emerged alongside – and in part as a consequence of – HIV/AIDS. This chapter explains why Brazil was initially much more responsive to AIDS than TB, and what this means for transitioning states and the overall quality of democracy.

However, it is important to note that Brazil's response to AIDS was not always that impressive. This chapter also shows that Brazil's new democratic federal Government (which emerged after two decades of military rule in 1985) did not immediately respond to AIDS. Rather, it initially relied on local governments as first responders. The successful response to AIDS that most people are aware of was therefore not the product of democratic deepening but instead the product of a combination of new global pressures and domestic incentives for bureaucratic and policy change. More specifically, it was the influence of new global pressures and the global reputation and domestic incentives that these pressures created that eventually led to an aggressive response to AIDS, and, though much later, TB. This chapter therefore underscores the fact that transitioning states may not be immediately responsive to local health needs, even when cognizant of the fact that new epidemics have emerged.

With regards to AIDS policy, it is argued that government apathy towards responding to the outbreak as well local governments' inability to respond was attributed to the transitioning Government's belief on what it perceived to be the most democratic and efficient means of providing health services: decentralization. However, the newly decentralized health system introduced in 1982 (*Sistema Unificado e Descentralizado de Saúde* (SUDS) or Unified Decentralized Health System) quickly decentralized policy to the states and eventually to the municipalities (through *Sestima Único de Saúde* (SUS), or Unified Health System in 1988), which were insolvent and unprepared to respond to AIDS (Table 13.1). The transitioning military's new health system, emblematic of what Smoke, Peterson and Gómez (2006) has referred to as *precocious decentralization*,[1] hampered the Government's immediate response to AIDS. Paradoxically, the military's perceived "democratic means" of rendering health services through

Table 13.1 The process of decentralization of health structures in Brazil

	1982	*1987*	*1988*
AIS	Government decentralizes health policy to the states; goal is to create Brazil's first university health care system, managed entirely by state health departments.		
SUDS		Increases authority of the states and gives them the discretion to decentralize managerial tasks to the municipalities.	
SUS			Completely decentralizes all policy and managerial functions to the municipalities, with states serving a more limited role of technical and financial assistance.

Source: Eduardo Gómez, own calculations, 2007.

Notes: AIS: Acoes Integradas de Saúde (Integrated Health System); SUDS: Sistema Unico de Sáude (Unified Decentralized Health System); SUS: Sestima Único de Saúde (Unified Health System).

[1] Precocious decentralization refers to the fast-paced timing of decentralization and the federal Government's unwillingness to ensure that state and municipal governments are adequately prepared to handle new policy responsibilities. For more on this issue, see Smoke, Peterson and Gómez (2006).

decentralization and increased local accountability in the end generated the most inefficient "policy means" for responding to AIDS.

Furthermore, decentralization allowed – and indeed encouraged – the federal Government to remain apathetic to the AIDS situation. In a sense, decentralization provided a legitimate excuse for the Government not to intervene.

Notwithstanding the transition to democracy, it would eventually take new global pressures and domestic political incentives finally to convince the Government that it should respond. By the early 1990s, pressures from the global health community and the prospect of obtaining a new loan from the World Bank generated new incentives for then President Itamar Franco (1992–1994) and Fernando Cardoso (1994–2002) to expand and strengthen the *Programa Nacional de Doencas Sexualmente Transmissíveis/AIDS* (National Program on Sexually Transmitted Infections/AIDS, PNDST/AIDS); it also provided new incentives for introducing a host of new prevention and treatment policies. Since then, the Government has been arguably the world's leader when it comes to responding to AIDS.

Did the Government learn from its earlier response to AIDS and respond just as well to other epidemics? Not at all. Regardless of the AIDS experience and again (and this cannot be emphasized enough) the transition to a so-called representative democracy, the Government *once again* failed to immediately respond to other epidemics and the needs of civil society. For example, despite its near eradication by the 1960s, TB re-emerged by the early 1980s, due in part to the spread of HIV and increased poverty in congested urban centres, such as Rio and São Paulo. Yet not even the absence of a social stigma and the needs of co-infected HIV/AIDS patients, especially the poor (who in theory stood to gain the most from decentralization), could convince the Government to respond.

The Government's lacklustre response to TB was motivated by the following structural factors. First, and in sharp contrast to AIDS, the absence of a burgeoning global health movement and attention to TB: like leprosy and malaria, TB did not receive nearly as much attention as the "mystical," globally popularized AIDS epidemic. Consequently, the Government was not racing to obtain global recognition for its response to TB, something which it eventually did for AIDS. Second, TB did not benefit from a well-organized civil society pressing for human rights, gay rights and health equality, as we saw with AIDS. Even now, there is not one TB NGO, but rather a consortium of civic organizations focusing on AIDS and other TB-related issues. Finally, the Government did not respond because of its perception that TB had been eradicated by the 1960s. These perceptions were influenced not by morals or discrimination against the poor, but rather from structural factors such as a decline in TB cases during the 1960s and 1970s and the weakened allure of treating TB.

Nevertheless, the rise of new global pressures, including direct policy criticisms from international organizations, such as WHO and the World Bank, and the recent financial incentives for responding to TB, which stem mainly from the GFATM, provide hope that the Government will finally respond. Similar to what we saw with AIDS, the Government may once again respond due to increased global pressures and incentives for change. As this chapter concludes, transitioning states may only respond to global pressures and the incentives for institutional and policy reform, rather than responding to the immediate needs of civil society whenever new epidemics emerge.

The government response to AIDS

The first confirmed case of HIV/AIDS occurred in Brazil in 1981. Initially, as in the United States, the virus spread quickly. By 1985 the total number of confirmed cases had increased to 554, with a death toll of 154. As Figure 13.1 illustrates, AIDS levels increased dramatically through 1996. After that, the increase has been less rapid, and according to UNAIDS, the HIV/AIDS epidemic has stabilized in Brazil. By 2001, an estimated 610 000 Brazilians – approximately 0.7% of the population – were living with full-blown AIDS, and in subsequent years the number of new AIDS cases has dropped significantly, from 32 526 in 2003 to only 13 933 in 2004.

The distribution of AIDS among the Brazilian population is strikingly uneven. In 1996, 32.7% of AIDS cases were among homosexual males, 21.4% were attributed to intravenous drug use and within the heterosexual population this was 18.2%. By 1998, however, the trend had changed considerably, with most of the confirmed cases found in the heterosexual population, accounting for 47.8%, while cases among homosexuals dropped to 22.4% and among intravenous drug users to 13.3%. By 2001, heterosexuals accounted for 59.4% of AIDS cases, while cases attributed to homosexuals and intravenous drug users were 18.5% and 8.0%, respectively (Bacon 2004).

The decentralization of health policy went hand in hand with the transition to democracy. In 1982, just three years before the transition to democracy in 1985, the outgoing military decided to decentralize the provision of all health

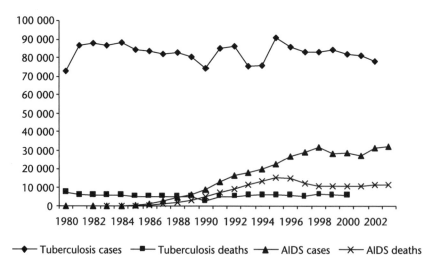

Figure 13.1   Brazil: number of cases and deaths from tuberculosis and AIDS, 1980–2003
Source: Ministry of Health 2006.

care services, management and policy regulation to the governors.[2] For the out-going military Government, health policy decentralization was perceived as an innovation that could essentially kill two birds with one stone: on the one hand, it could substantially reduce the cost to the federal Government of pro-viding health services, while on the other hand it demonstrated the Govern-ment's commitment to democratic deepening by increasing the participation of civil society in the policy reform process, in turn enhancing the quality of policy provisions. Decentralization thus reflected the interests and motivation of the Brazilian Government, not international pressures.

The first set of decentralization measures introduced was called the AIS (*Acoes Integradas de Saúde*, or Integrated Health System). In response to hyperinflation and in an effort to cut back on expenditure, the federal Government sought to offload these responsibilities rapidly to the states. The primary mission was to create, for the first time, a unified (universal) health care system, managed and controlled by the states, with an emphasis on primary care provision, an increased reliance on underutilized public facilities, rather than private ones, a greater control over high-cost medical procedures and contracted service costs (Harmeling 1999). Until that point, these responsibilities were controlled by the Ministry of Health, through INAMPS.

Even more discretion was then decentralized. In 1987, two years after the democratic transition, the Jose Sarney administration implemented the SUDS. This carried over the principles of the AIS, while giving the state health secre-tariats more control over administration and management. Furthermore, and this is key, for the first time it gave the state health secretariats complete discretion over how much financial and administrative autonomy should be decentralized to municipal health agencies (Lobato 1998; Nascimento 1999). This hinted at the federal Government's interest in devolving more authority to the municipalities.

This set the stage for a complete devolution of health financial and adminis-trative authority to the municipalities in 1988. That year, the Congress imple-mented the SUS. This was Brazil's first ever completely decentralized universal health care system. In contrast to AIS and SUDS, moreover, it was completely decentralized to the municipal health agencies. Once again, the goal was to increase efficiency in health care provision, to increase the access and avail-ability of health services (and this is important, given Brazil's 5043 municipal-ities) and to reduce costs by giving mayors more control over how much they could spend.

The problem with all of this, however, was that it was done much too quickly. That is, the SUS immediately landed into the laps of municipal health agencies that were:

[2] Note, however, that military had been debating the decentralization process for some time. The Ministry of Health was torn between those that favoured the central Govern-ment's control over policy, mainly through the Instituto Nacional de Assistência Médica da Previdência Social (National Institute for Medical Assistance and Social Security, INAMPS) and the Ministry of Health, versus those that favoured a more decentralized approach, mainly for increased economic efficiency. After several years of debating, the Government finally decided to devolve in 1982. For more on the reasons why, see Arretche and Marques (2002).

- insolvent due to their repeated inability to secure funding from state health secretariats;
- technically incompetent, such that they lacked an adequate number of doctors and nurses; and
- lacking in basic health infrastructure, such as beds.

This created a public health system that was anything but prepared for an epidemic. To make matters worse, with the exception perhaps of São Paulo, which historically has had more autonomy in health policy, from 1982 to 1988 most of the governors opposed decentralizing resources to the municipalities. Full control over health policy meant access to resources, justification for money, loans, notoriety, etc. This threatened to take away the governors' access to resources, their political popularity and thus their influence. There were therefore ample disincentives for the governors to support municipal health secretariats at the height of the AIDS epidemic.

The critical question to be asked here is where was the federal Government during the first few years of the AIDS epidemic? What happened to the Government's tradition of intervening rapidly in order to ensure that local governments had the resources needed to respond to epidemics? What happened to the rich tradition of building and/or modernizing a centralized bureaucratic agency that would immediately assist municipal health departments whenever new epidemics emerged? It should be kept in mind that this was a tradition going back to the 1920s and was maintained and even expanded under several military and democratic regimes until the re-emergence of the military Government in 1964 (Gómez [forthcoming]; Hochman 1998). Why didn't the Government do the same thing for AIDS?

The answer is simple. Authoritarian commitment to decentralization, reinforced by its perceived association with democratization, generated perceptions among the political elite that the AIDS epidemic could be more effectively handled by subnational governments. Because it was widely assumed by the President and successive health ministers that decentralization was already the most efficient policy means for responding to epidemics and other health ailments, based mainly on the expected benefits of increasing electoral accountability and transparency, there was no interest in immediately responding to the needs of local governments. There was thus no sense of urgency. It is important to note that this occurred despite the Government's full awareness that municipal health departments were in need of financial assistance and that they were both technically and administratively incapable of responding adequately on their own.

As the epidemiological data about the spread of AIDS became impossible to ignore, the Government finally responded. Impressively, in 1985 it created a new federal agency programme, the PNDST/AIDS, within the Ministry of Health. However, it was feeble and worse still, distant from the homosexual and intravenous drug user community. In essence it was a *cosmetic institution*: that is, it was built to give the impression that the Government was doing something constructive, while in reality it was not (Daniel 1991; Gómez [forthcoming]). Officials in the PNDST/AIDS rarely, if ever, met with the homosexual or the intravenous drug user community. It provided little advice to municipal health secretariats, and even at the apogee of the epidemic in 1991, one of its former directors not only decided to skip the yearly carnival festivities in Rio, but he also refrained from ordering his staff to go and distribute condoms. Meanwhile, access to AZT (an anti-AIDS drug) was at a minimum, while the Government had very little money – and thus interest – in helping local governments finance prevention and treatment programmes.

To the Government's credit, it did do a fairly good job of discussing the new disease in public and it did implement a fairly aggressive AIDS awareness campaign. Nevertheless, by the late 1990s, it became very clear to many that (a) PNDST/AIDS was very ineffective and (b) most of the municipalities were lacking the resources needed to respond to AIDS. During this period a host of municipal governments had implemented their own anti-AIDS programmes (Teixeira 1997). However, most local governments were lacking basic health infrastructure, such as beds, clean needles, surgical tables and the medical staff needed to mount an aggressive response (Teixeira 1997; Visao: Revista semanal de informacao 1985). Under these conditions, the AIDS virus continued to spread. In the end, the proud, nascent democracy, grounded in the tenants of human rights, equality and universal access to health care, had done barely anything to help municipal health agencies respond to AIDS. Yes, democratic decentralization was achieved, but to what end?

Global health movements and domestic response

Brazil's new democracy eventually responded to AIDS. Unlike what democratization theorists suggest (Gerring 2005; Haggard and Kaufman [forthcoming]), the Government did not respond to growing civic discontent, need, political accountability, elections, or in other words, the "bottom up" democratic pressures for reform. Instead, it was responding to new global pressures from the global health community (e.g., the United Nations, WHO, World Bank and PAHO) and the political incentives for responding to these pressures through new institutional and policy innovations. It was only after these new global pressures emerged that a substantive government response to AIDS finally materialized.

Indeed, as the global health community started paying more attention to AIDS, beginning in the late 1980s, so did the Brazilian Government. By this point increased international attention and commitment to fighting AIDS, coupled with direct pressures from WHO and other institutions, led to a radical shift in perceptions among the political elite and interest in responding more effectively to AIDS (Gómez 2007). With the prospect of a major World Bank loan arriving in 1992, moreover, the Government quickly increased its commitment to strengthening the PNDST/AIDS, while working more closely with civil society (Galvào 2000). Essentially overnight, the Government transformed a poorly funded national AIDS programme into a very wealthy agency that was highly autonomous and successful at implementing policy from above (Teixeira 1997). This, in turn, led to arguably the world's best institutional and policy response to AIDS, with a host of prevention and treatment measures that have contributed to a massive decline in AIDS cases and deaths since the late 1990s.

The resurgence of tuberculosis and the government response

While the Government was finally responding to AIDS, other urban diseases were nevertheless lingering and emerging as serious health threats. One in particular was TB. However, it is important to note that TB did not re-emerge in Brazil as mysteriously as the AIDS virus. Consequently, it did not trigger immediate fear and uncertainty. The gradual spread of TB in the 1970s and 1980s was attributed mainly to urbanization, free market reforms, economic crisis and unemployment (Adeodato 1991; Barrozo 1993; Jornal do Brasil 1993; Marques 1992). Some also argued that the inefficiencies of decentralization stemming from the military's SUDS programme and its repeated inability to adequately monitor and respond to TB also contributed to its resurgence (Adeodato 1991; Santos and Ezio 2006).

TB also re-emerged because of the HIV/AIDS virus (Folha de São Paulo 1991; Jornal do Brasil 1989). Because immune systems were substantially depleted due to HIV, TB's resurgence quickly spread among HIV positive individuals. This was most common within tightly concentrated urban centres, such as Rio and São Paulo. In the city of Rio, for example, the number of TB cases essentially ran parallel with the surge in AIDS cases throughout the 1980s and 1990s. During the 1980s especially, a TB/AIDS co-infection problem emerged due in large part to the difficulty of diagnosing AIDS patients with TB. For instance, the incessant coughing, vomiting of blood, and rapid weight loss commonly seen with TB patients is usually not present with the TB/HIV co-infected.[3] As a result those that were TB/HIV-positive did not seek immediate medical attention, which, in turn, contributed to TB's further spread.

As with AIDS, during this period there was also a relatively high level of social stigma associated with having TB. As in the past, it was – and still is – a disease that is mainly seen among the poor. For one to have TB is to reveal ones low income and thus social status, which in Brazil often conjures up racism and discrimination. While AIDS attacked the homosexuals, TB attacked the poor and the homosexuals – through HIV. As is discussed, one key difference between the two was that AIDS dovetailed well with the pre-existing movement for gay and human rights throughout the re-democratization period. However, this was not the case for TB. The poor had no pre-existing "pro-poor" movement that they could draw on and use to pressure the Government. What is more, they did not benefit from a "pro-TB/HIV" co-infection movement. Instead, and as explained in more detail in this chapter, it would take an increase in global pressures and the fact that the resurgence of TB was eventually perceived by international organizations as a new health threat, in turn to provide new opportunities and incentives to create a proactive civic movement.

Similar to the first few years of the AIDS epidemic, the Government also did not immediately respond to TB. In part this had to do with the fact that the global pressures and attention to TB during the late 1980s and early 1990s were not nearly as strong as they were for AIDS. As a result, the Government's interest

---

[3] Information from: interview with Dr. Margareth Delcalmo, 18 July 2006; interview with Ezio Santos Filho, Co-Chair of the Global Fund Country Coordinating Mechanism for Tuberculosis in Brazil, 30 June 2006.

mirrored that of a somewhat apathetic global health community. Under these circumstances, the Government's response depended entirely on the newly decentralized health care system (SUS), which was poorly funded and staffed. As with AIDS, during the democratic transition TB policy was also quickly decentralized to the states. The introduction of the SUS in 1988 essentially entailed the complete dismantling of the historically powerful NTP, which was created by the military dictator Guetilio Vargas in the 1940s. Once again, and similarly to the AIDS situation described earlier, the interest in decentralizing stemmed from increasing health policy efficiency and efficacy in rendering health services to the states. By 1990, the infamous NTP was completely dismantled and *all* TB policy responsibilities were decentralized to the municipalities. However, municipal health agencies were once again unprepared to effectively provide prevention and treatment services.

Why was the Government more proactive in its response to AIDS? The main reason had to do with the fact that, as has always been the case, the Government responded to a new health epidemic that garnered a lot of global attention. By responding to AIDS, Brazil was able to demonstrate to the global health community that as a modern, newly democratized state, it was capable of controlling an epidemic successfully, paving the way for social and economic prosperity. More importantly, it provided the Government with the opportunity to once again lead the global health community in response to AIDS. In other work, I have called this the "race to global fame" in international health; it generates a new level of government commitment to institutional and policy reform (Gómez [forthcoming]). In contrast, TB did not benefit from opportunities and global incentives. Since TB was not a "globally popular" disease, it provided few benefits for Brazil to illustrate its medical and institutional prowess in response to its resurgence and therefore did not provide an opportunity for Brazil to lead the global fight against it.

Civil societal response to AIDS and tuberculosis

Civil societal involvement in effective public health policy has a rich tradition in Brazil, spanning back to the First Republic. As in the past, the AIDS epidemic triggered a very aggressive response. In contrast to the past, however, this response emerged in a context of re-democratization, strongly grounded in the tenants of human rights and equality in social policy (with health being a major component of this). In addition, the movement for AIDS benefited from a burgeoning, well-organized gay rights movement that started to benefit from the outgoing military regime's somewhat progressive stance towards gay rights (Mott 2003). By the time AIDS emerged in the 1980s, there was thus a well-organized, vibrant civic network fully committed to creating a host of AIDS NGOs that would flourish throughout the 1980s and 1990s. By the mid-1990s, over 100 AIDS NGOs existed.

Unfortunately, such a movement did not occur for TB. Prior to and throughout the re-democratization period, there was not a single NGO focused on the TB problem. Despite empirical data illustrating a parallel growth in TB and HIV/AIDS, most notably in Rio and São Paulo, in sharp contrast to the past (especially when compared to the well-organized *Liga de Tuberculose* of the early 20th century), medical elites, intellectuals and local politicians were not interested in immediately creating a new civic movement for TB. In contrast to the well-organized AIDS NGO community, moreover, the urban poor (even those with HIV) had no organizational resources and support to depend on, no one to help them fight for a more effective, decentralized TB programme.[4] The whole movement for "human rights" and "human equality" in health care treatment seemed to overlook the needs of the urban poor suffering from a clandestine – yet rapidly burgeoning – TB epidemic.

Why did this occur? In large part, it was the absence of TB's "sex appeal," when combined with a decline in civic elite perceptions that TB was still a problem, which generated few incentives for a new civic movement to emerge. In contrast to AIDS, there was simply no mysticism associated with TB; it had no global allure and more importantly, there was no opportunity for medical elites to distinguish themselves by finding a cure. Successful treatment for TB had existed for decades. Moreover, the fact that TB cases had decreased tremendously since the 1960s and 1970s contributed to the misperception, both within the Government and civil society, that it was no longer a problem. Lastly, the simple fact of the matter was that TB was always, and continues to be, perceived as a poor man's disease. Its association with the poor, in marked contrast to AIDS' initial association with the homosexual white, upper-middle class community, created few incentives for civic elites to mobilize for the poor.[5]

The end result is that there was no NGO movement for TB throughout the 1980s and 1990s. AIDS NGOs and their ability to directly pressure the State flourished, while the poor and the TB co-infected became increasingly marginalized. The problem became so apparent that by the late 1990s, WHO and even the World Bank started to criticize Brazil for its biased response to AIDS at the very costly, border-line discriminatory expense of overlooking those suffering from TB and other diseases.

Global health movements – once again?

However, there is hope. For as was the case with AIDS, new global pressures started to emerge which positively influenced the Government's response to TB. In 1993, the global health community finally started to realize that TB had resurfaced as a global pandemic. That year, WHO officially declared the resurgence of TB as a global health threat. As always, the Brazilian Government was eager to respond. The NTP, which had been completely dismantled and decentralized three years earlier, was quickly *re-centralized* and given a larger staff and more resources – though, of course, still paling in comparison to the more affluent PNDST/AIDS programme. As with AIDS, shortly after these new global pressures emerged the federal Government realized that unguided decentralization

---

[4] Information from: interview with Carlos Basilia, Director of the Brazil Stop Tuberculosis Alliance, 26 July 2006.

[5] Information from: interview with Carlos Basilia, 26 July 2006.

processes were not yielding effective TB prevention and treatment policies. The NTP was thus strengthened through renewed commitment by the Lula administration (which also aligned with his emphasis on increasing social welfare distribution to the poor).

In addition to increased global recognition of the TB problem, the ability to obtain new financial resources from international donors has once again created new incentives for the Government to increase its commitment to not only the NTP but also to municipal health agencies. In 2006, the Government was the recipient of a US$ 11 million grant from the GFATM. Similar to what occurred with the first World Bank loan in 1993, the acquisition of this grant, in addition to the fact that continued funding will be contingent on grant performance, has created new incentives to strengthen the NTP and more importantly to engage in a continuous dialogue with municipal health agencies for more effective policy implementation.[6]

Once again, as with AIDS, the arrival of this foreign lending, combined with more global attention to TB, has led to the emergence of new civic movements responding to TB. In 2003 a new civic forum for TB was created in Rio by several AIDS activists, doctors, community and church leaders; a similar movement was created in São Paulo in 2005. Referred to as the "Tuberculosis Forum," this movement is dedicated to increasing awareness of TB's resurgence and to working with the federal and local governments to implement more effective policy measures (Basilia 2006). Since its existence, it has created a host of public prevention campaigns and has organized conferences with the National Tuberculosis and AIDS Program (Basilia 2006).

It is no surprise that this movement has grown in tandem with the increased attention and financial support of the global health community. The GFATM actually stipulates that a necessary condition for grant approval and renewal is the creation of a CCM, which guarantees the representation of civil society on the official committee drafting grant applications. It should be recalled that the GFATM declined Brazil's initial application for funding in 2005, based on the fact that the CCM could not prove adequate civil societal representation. Months later, it was finally approved by demonstrating to the GFATM that it had finally achieved this.[7] Elsewhere, I argue that this has created a new type of conditionality, what I call a new *institutional conditionality* for donor assistance, which requires proof of civil societal representation before grants are disbursed (Gómez [forthcoming]).

In sum, as was seen with AIDS at the beginning of the 1990s, the beginning of the 2000s has created similar incentives for the federal Government to respond to TB through the strengthening of institutions (e.g., re-centralizing the NTP) and interest in working closer with civil society and municipal health agencies. In response to the Government's efforts, new civic movements continue to emerge in order to help those suffering from TB. While no official TB NGO yet exists, several related civic associations and the church are now working together to create new TB forums throughout the nation in order to monitor

---

[6] Information from: interview with Ezio Santos Fihlo, Co-Chair of the Global Fund Country Coordinating Mechanism for Tuberculosis in Brazil, 30 June 2006.
[7] Information from: interview with Ezio Santos Fihlo, 30 June 2006.

consistently and apply pressure on the federal Government for a more timely and effective policy intervention.

Conclusion

In conclusion, this chapter has argued that transitions to democracy may not guarantee an immediate government response to epidemics. Ironically, the reforms that outgoing military elites believed would help to advance and consolidate democracy and social welfare in general, such as the devolution of health policy, was at the same time the most inefficient way of responding to an epidemic. Precocious decentralization may hamper municipal health agencies' ability to respond to new epidemics, such as AIDS, while increasing the federal Government's reliance on local governments as first responders. This generates initial political apathy towards local health needs, in turn leading to a delay in federal intervention. More importantly, it gives the impression that a nascent democracy is not completely committed to safeguarding the needs of civil society.

Indeed, when new democracies do eventually intervene, both through bureaucratic strengthening and policy intervention, it may not be in response to bottom-up pressures for reform. In a new democratic context one would expect that nascent democracies grounded in the tenants of human rights and social equality, such as Brazil's, would be more responsive to human needs. But this is not always the case. More often than not it takes global pressures and the incentives that they generate for elites to respond through institutional and policy reform. As in the Brazilian experience with AIDS, when these pressures do emerge, successful bureaucratic and policy reforms can occur.

At the same time, however, the Government's emphasis on responding to a particular type of epidemic, such as AIDS, can lead to an inequitable, biased response to other diseases. As discussed above, TB did not receive nearly as much attention as AIDS in Brazil. In large part this was due to the absence of new global pressures for reform, the absence of a well-organized, proactive civic movement for TB, and the disincentives that medical elites had in collectivizing for the poor. Nevertheless, the emergence of a new global consensus that TB has resurfaced as a world pandemic, increased international pressures and the availability of funding from the GFATM may lead to new institutional and policy innovations. Given Brazil's track record with combating epidemics in the past and more recently with AIDS, the Government may once again strive to become the world leader in the fight against TB and other epidemics, especially as international organizations and other governments start paying more attention to TB and other diseases.

Finally, a word on the nature of transitioning states. What this chapter has shown is that transitions to democracy may not guarantee an effective and equitable response to epidemics. The great irony of new democracies, especially those having transitioned from authoritarian and socialist rule, is how the downsizing of the State (in line with neo-liberal theory) and government efforts to enhance social welfare efficiency through decentralization and privatization leads not only to a decrease in policy responsiveness but also to a selectively biased, inequitable response to human needs whenever a new epidemic emerges.

Of course, this is not to deny that democracy is the preferred system of governance, or to imply that it cannot succeed in responding to epidemics. What it does say, however, is that transitioning states need to examine to what extent their federal agencies are prepared to respond immediately to epidemics through bureaucratic build-up, policy reform and, more importantly, by ensuring that municipalities have the resources needed to adequately respond. This is especially important for highly decentralized democratic federations, where local governments are often insolvent and distant from the capital (e.g., China, the Russian Federation, India, South Africa and even the United States). In other words, when it comes to public health, *expanding* the State, rather than downsizing it, may be the only way to safeguard citizens from disease and to ensure their continued prosperity within new democratic settings.

References

Adeodato, S. (1991). Rio está se transformando na capital da tuberculose [Rio is established as the capital of tuberculosis], *Jornal do Brasil*.

Arretche, M. and Marques, C. (2002). Municipalizacão da saúde no Brasil: diferencas regionais, poder do voto e estratégias de governo [The municipalization of health care policies in Brazil: regional differences, the voting power and government strategies]. Ciênc. saúde coletiva, 7(3):455–479.

Bacon, O. (2004). *HIV/AIDS in Brazil*. San Francisco: AIDS Policy Research Center, University of California.

Barrozo, J. (1993). Miséria mantém o perigo da tuberculose no Brasil (11/8/93) [Misery kills the danger of tuberculosis in Brazil], *Diario Popular (São Paulo)*.

Basilia, C. (2006). *Construando uma resposta a controle no tuberculose [Constructing a response to control tuberculosis]*. Unpublished manuscript.

Daniel, H. (1991). A doenca burocracia (6/10/91) [The disease bureaucracy], *Jornal do Brasil*.

Folha de São Paulo (1991). Tuberculose afeta mais os aidéticos e mendigos (11/29/91) [TB affects more AIDS patients and beggars].

Galvào, J. (2000). *AIDS no Brasil: A agenda de construcão de uma epidemia [AIDS in Brazil: the agenda of responding to an epidemic]*. São Paulo, Brazil: ABIA Publishers.

Gerring, J. (2005). Democracy and Economic Growth: A Historial Perspective, *World Politics*, 57(3): 323–364.

Gómez, E. J. (2007). Bureaucratizing Epidemics: The Challenge of Institutional Bias in the United States and Brazil, *Journal of Global Health Governance*, 1(1): 1–24.

Gómez, E. J. (forthcoming). Responding to Contested Epidemics: State Building and Global Politics in the United States and Brazil (1900–present) (Ph.D. dissertation, Department of Political Science, Brown University).

Haggard, S. and Kaufman, R. (forthcoming). *Re-crafting Social Contracts: Welfare Reform in Latin America, East Asia, and Central Europe*. Cambridge: Cambridge University Press.

Harmeling, S. (1999). *Health Reform in Brazil, Case Study for Module 3: Reproductive Health and Health Sector Reform*. Paper presented at the World Bank conference titled Population, Reproductive Health and Health Sector Reform, Washington, DC (October 8, 1999).

Hochman, G. (1998). *A Era do Saneamento: As bases da política de Saúde Pública no Brasil*

[The era of sanitation: the political bases of support for public health]. São Paulo, Brazil: Editora Hucitec-Anpocs.

Jornal do Brasil (1989). Falta de examen em tuberculosos pode agravar expansão da Aids [The absence of TB exams could contribute to the spread of AIDS]. 6/27/89. Sao Paolo: Jornal do Brasil.

Jornal do Brasil (1993). Lutra contra tuerculose é destaque [The fight against tuberculosis and stigma]. 9/7/93. Sao Paolo: Jornal do Brasil.

Lobato, L. (1998) *Stress and Contradictions in the Brazilian Health-Care Reform*. Paper presented at the 1998 meeting of the Latin American Studies Association, Chicago, IL (24–26 September).

Marques, C. (1992) Guilherme Álvaro registra aumento do número de casos de tuberculose (24 March). A Tribuna [Guilherme Álvaro registers an increase in the number of TB cases]. Santos, São Paulo.

Mott, L. (2003). *Homossexualidade: Mitos e Verdades [Homosexuality: myths and truths]*. Salvador, Brazil: Editora Grupo Gay de Bahia.

Nascimento, E. (1999). *Decentralización de Salud no Brasil* [Decentralization of health in Brazil]. Brasilia, Brazil: Nucleo de Investagacão em Servicos e Sistemas de Saude.

Santos, F. and Ezio, T. (2006). *Politítica de TB no Brasil: Uma Perspectiva da Sociedade Civil: Tempos de Mudancas Para O Controle Da Tuberculose No Brasil [The politics of TB in Brazil: a civil societal perspective: times of change in order to control TB in Brazil]*. Public Health Watch, the George Soros Foundation/Open Society Institute.

Smoke, P. J., Peterson, G. E. and Gómez, E. J. (2006). *Decentralization in Asia and Latin America: towards a comparative interdisciplinary perspective*. Cheltenham: Edward Elgar.

Teixeira, P. (1997). Políticas públicas em Aids, in Parker (ed.) *Políticas, instituicões e Aids: enfrentando a epidemia no Brasil [The public politics of AIDS]*. Rio de Janeiro: ABIA Publications.

Visao: Revista semanal de informacao (1985). *A verdade onde estara? [Where's the truth?]* 16 October. No. 41.

chapter fourteen

Health financing and communicable disease control: conceptual issues and implications

Rifat Atun, Claudio Politti,
Ipek Gurol-Urganci, Joseph Kutzin

Introduction

Health financing and communicable disease control is a broad and complex area. In this chapter, we explore three interrelated issues as regards financing communicable disease programmes. The first issue relates to the normative argument on priorities, i.e. whether a programme "deserves" to be funded – taking into account societal choices, the methods by which these priorities are identified, selection mechanisms, and affordability – or whether a programme can be funded, taking into account resource scarcity and fiscal space constraints. The second issue is concerned with financial design and the mechanisms of collecting, pooling and applying available funds for communicable disease programmes. The third issue pertains to provider payment systems used in the health sector and how these impact on the functioning of communicable disease programmes.

The first issue is explored from the perspective of welfare economics, in particular the nature of these interventions: i.e. whether they are considered as an "economic good" or a "good with externalities" (Serrano and Feldman 2006) and their affordability, examined in relation to health system (fiscal) sustainability and fiscal space. The second issue of financing and financial design is explored using a health financing policy analysis framework (Kutzin 2001), applied in relation in Estonia to examine collection, pooling, purchasing and provision mechanisms and to map the flow of funds to communicable disease control programmes and interventions in order to diagnose the nature of any problems in the financing system that create obstacles to the efficient delivery of these interventions. Finally, we use a proprietary toolkit, SYSRA (Atun et al. 2004), designed for simultaneous analysis of health systems and communicable disease programmes to demonstrate the importance of analysing in detail resource allocation and provider payment systems to explain provider behaviour.

This chapter is organized in five sections. The introduction section is followed by three subsequent sections, each of which deal with one of the three issues identified above and, by drawing on case studies, illustrate how these analyses can inform the design of communicable disease programmes. The chapter then concludes by summarizing policy implications arising from the findings.

Communicable disease programmes: public and private goods, affordability and fiscal space

Health services are broadly divided into either "personal" (also referred to as a "private good") or "population based" (also referred to as a "public good"). Personal services are those where an individual gains private or personal benefit from the service and the public ones are those where the benefits accrue not just to the individual but also other members of the public. This division, although rather crude, is often used to define the economic nature of the health service (the "good") and to determine whether it should be publicly funded or whether there should be individual contributions towards the cost of the service. In socialized health systems the majority of services, whether they are a "public" or a "private good" are financed through tax or social insurance. In countries which lack social insurance or mechanisms for solidarity, often the State assumes the responsibility for financing public health services or "public goods" while the "private goods" are paid for in full or in part by the individual, either directly or through a voluntary insurance mechanism.

There are different schools of thought and varied views on the nature of public and private goods and how these should be funded. The issue of whether a good is public or private is well explored in public and welfare economics and will not be discussed here in detail. Instead we briefly explore the rationale for financing public goods through public funds. More specifically, the debate centres on the issue of *externalities*. By their nature, communicable disease control interventions are not purely private goods, because their consumption benefits more than the individual receiving the intervention. Therefore, unregulated private market interactions will lead to a suboptimal level of consumption of these interventions from a social welfare perspective, because the preferences of persons 2, 3, 4, . . . N who do not receive the intervention but who derive external benefits from the intervention received by person 1 are not accounted for by the market. This is the rationale for public intervention to subsidize the provision of the intervention to the point where the sum of private optimal levels of consumption equals the socially optimal level of consumption. This is the basic economic argument for public subsidization of any good or service with positive externalities, such as communicable disease control interventions.

Conceptually, this does not imply that these services should be free of charge, but rather that they should be priced at a sufficiently low level as to encourage the socially optimal level of consumption. This "socially optimal" level of consumption can also be considered in terms of "epidemiologically optimal" level (for example) of consumption: e.g., with immunization the level to achieve herd immunity or with HIV the desirable level of population coverage for interventions to achieve control or epidemiological impact.

From the perspective of health financing policy, whether a programme/intervention with externalities is financed and the extent to which it is financed (from 0% to 100%) depends on three considerations: first, the magnitude of these externalities (i.e., it is not enough to say an intervention "has externalities", it is necessary to know how broad these external benefits are); second, the "depth" of the benefits package, i.e., the extent of co-insurance or co-payment for interventions in the essential package of services; and third, the fiscal space available to the Government (which is influenced by the second factor).

In relation to the second consideration, there are also practical concerns, namely the type of pricing regime that can be implemented. In many countries where administrative infrastructure is inadequate, it is less costly to provide certain services for free rather than at a reduced price.

Communicable disease control interventions are often considered as "public health services". This term is not strictly correct from the perspective of welfare economics or when compared with the classification of services derived from the WHO Health Systems PAF described in the *World Health Report 2000* (WHO 2000). From a welfare economics perspective, "public health services" correspond to "public goods": i.e., goods whose consumption by one person does not diminish the consumption by another and where it is impossible to exclude non-paying consumers from benefiting. While there is a link between public goods and goods with externalities, they are not identical. This is relevant for the classification of interventions as was carried out in the *World Health Report 2000*. Personal health services consist of interventions delivered to individual clients, whereas population-based services are interventions delivered to groups or the whole population. Thus, for example, when a health professional tells a client to quit smoking, that is a personal preventive service, but a billboard warning passers-by of the dangers of smoking is a population-based health service.

This error is common, as communicable disease control programmes, such as those for TB and HIV, and even immunization, are considered as "public health programmes", while the associated preventive and treatment interventions are thought of as "public health services". However, most of the interventions supported by these programmes are delivered to individual clients. This distinction is very important from an organizational perspective. Organizational arrangements should reflect how the population interacts with the services, and the financing system for these interventions should incorporate incentives for their efficient delivery.

There is, hence, a key distinction between the economic nature of the good, and the way in which the intervention is delivered. In other words, the issue of "who benefits" from an intervention is separate from the issue of "how is the intervention organized and delivered". The fact that communicable disease interventions have externalities provides the basis for their inclusion in the benefits package either free of charge or at a subsidized rate to encourage their consumption. But the existence of external benefits provides no conceptual basis for the creation of separate funding, delivery or institutional arrangements. Most communicable disease interventions consist of services delivered to individual clients, and the organizational arrangements for financing should support the mechanisms by which the interventions are to be delivered.

However, as resources in most countries are limited, the governments have to prioritize amongst competing interventions, decide on the extent to which these are funded, and the extent to which individuals contribute to the cost of a service (influenced by the government position on whether the interventions for communicable disease programmes are considered to be public or private goods, and also determined by the depth of the benefits package). What gets prioritized, how it is paid and the extent of cost sharing by the service users depend, amongst other things (such as societal choices, cultural factors, political expediency, pressure groups, etc. – factors which are beyond the scope of this chapter), on the resources available to a government and the "fiscal space". Fiscal space refers to the ability of a government to make budgetary resources available for desired purposes (for example a programme) without any prejudice to the sustainability of that government's financial position (Heller 2005).

In transition countries, and especially in those that receive external financing for health system and communicable disease control programmes, financial sustainability is of critical importance. As many of the transition countries are also subject to tight monetary and fiscal discipline imposed by international monetary organizations, the fiscal space may be rather narrow. Hence, robust planning for medium-term financial commitments and expenditure is necessary to create an environment where the existing and new funds can be appropriately utilized for communicable disease programmes that have been prioritized. In short, for any sustainable fiscal programme, resources and plans for allocation must balance. However, this is not the case in many settings and this restricts the ability of the country to attract new funds or use resources to finance communicable disease programmes. For example, the High-Level Forum has identified a lack of robust sector strategies, plans and budgets, as a barrier to the mobilization of larger aid flows for heath. This adversely affects predictable long-term financing for communicable disease programmes.

A lack of excess fiscal space means that new investments, which increase aggregate spending, lead to growing fiscal deficits that need to be funded. In turn, this leads to higher debt and accelerated inflation, which has a negative impact on the economy and government funding. Briefly, fiscal space can be created or expanded by increasing tax income, more efficient reallocation of available resources or by downsizing inefficient interventions or programmes. Alternatively, debt or international assistance can be used to plug fiscal deficits or expand fiscal space.

In many European countries, private sector funding, through public–private partnerships, have been used to expand fiscal space and to fund health investments. However, these new sources of funding must be used in a prudent manner so as to ensure allocative and technical efficiency but also to ensure new programmatic funding is not used to create inefficient vertical structures which operate in parallel to the existing health system and hinder effective horizontal linkages and coordination: so critically necessary for communicable disease programmes. Unfortunately, this is not the case in practice, and the donor funds which create fiscal space are used to develop vertical programmes which operate as separate parallel structures to the health system and which are not well-integrated into the general health system budgeting process: fragmenting the planning process, duplicating efforts, creating unnecessary transaction costs and thereby reducing chances of sustainability. These approaches also prevent any meaningful prioritization within the country to allocate scarce resources to areas of greatest need and to programmes that are most cost-effective or can be afforded.

These issues are of concern to countries in Latin America and eastern Europe, and especially relevant to countries that receive external funding to finance communicable disease programmes. Sustainable financing of these programmes and efficient allocation of resources will require effective integration of donor-financed investments for communicable diseases (and assistance) into the over-all budgeting process, aligning donor funding with the country priorities, and harmonization of donor and country processes, so that funding can be channelled through the recipient country's financing institutions (High-Level Forum 2005).

Financial design for communicable disease programmes

We apply the health financing policy analysis framework to analyse "financing systems" for communicable disease control interventions. The approach is used to identify inefficiencies arising from the financing arrangements for disease control programmes. The analytical approach and the inefficiencies are illustrated using the example of Estonia, by exploring in turn issues related to funds pooling and programme financing, budgeting and planning and parallel financing.

Estonia is a Baltic state that regained independence from the USSR in 1991 and, in 2004, joined the EU. The country is witnessing an explosion in new cases of HIV, with a rate of increase that exceeds that of all other states in the former Soviet Union. By the end of 2004 there were almost 4500 registered HIV-positive individuals. Concurrent with this increase in the number of HIV infections, TB notifications have also increased, from 26 per 100 000 in 1992 to 52 per 100 000 in 1999, although since 2000, when the WHO-recommended DOTS strategy was introduced, notifications of TB have stabilized. In 1998, Estonia had one of the highest MDR-TB rates in the world, with 14% of newly diagnosed pulmonary TB cases being MDR-TB (Atun et al. 2007b). The TB global surveillance programme identified Estonia as one of the "hot spots" for high MDR-TB prevalence (Espinal et al. 2001). Although there is an ongoing programme to manage and control MDR-TB, cure rates were initially estimated to be 20% but unpublished results indicate the cure rates may be increasing to approximately 50–60%. Weaknesses in MDR-TB control are of particular concern where HIV prevalence is also high or rising. Given the current immaturity of the HIV epidemic in Estonia, the epidemiological impact of the linkage between HIV and TB is not yet evident, but is likely to become so as populations at risk of HIV acquisition and progression mix with those who have active TB.

Although many factors impact upon HIV spread in the former Soviet Union, epidemics have been principally driven by injecting drug use. In Estonia, injecting drug use remains the main driver of the epidemic with approximately 90% of new HIV infections associated with drug use. Therefore, development of joined-up HIV, TB and substance abuse programmes is critically important to effectively address these three colliding epidemics. However, an analysis of the Estonian communicable disease control programmes and their funding, as illustrated in Figure 14.1 and explained below, shows this not to be the case.

The figure shows organizational arrangements for health services aimed at controlling HIV, TB and drug abuse interventions in Estonia, and maps the flow of funds between institutions.

The Ministry of Social Affairs is responsible for managing "public health national programmes", including those for HIV/AIDS, drug abuse and TB. These programmes, which are funded through general taxation and general budget transfers, are implemented by the National Institute of Health Development (NIHD), which is subordinate to the Ministry of Social Affairs. These national programmes are not integrated. Each programme is run as a separate "vertical" programme, with a separate line budget within the NIHD budget. The NIHD manages the ring-fenced pool of funds for each programme, which are used to

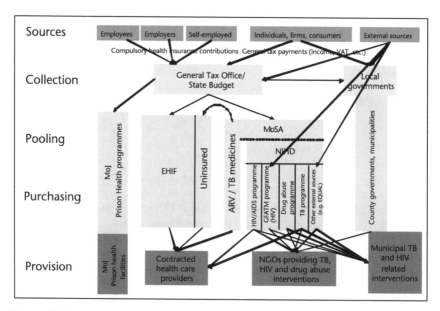

Figure 14.1 Financing of HIV, tuberculosis and drug abuse services in Estonia

Source: Alban and Kutzin 2006.

Notes: VAT: value-added tax; MoJ: Ministry of Justice; MoSA: Ministry of Social Affairs; EHIF: Estonian Health Insurance Fund; NIHD: National Institute of Health Development; ARV: anti-retroviral; GFATM: Global Fund to Fight AIDS, Tuberculosis and Malaria; TB: tuberculosis; NGO: nongovernmental organization.

contract with NGOs and municipalities to provide the necessary interventions. Municipalities also use their own funds to provide services. The prison health system (financed and managed by the Ministry of Justice), uses its separate budget to fund and deliver services to the prison population as a separate vertical programme. Budget transfer from the Ministry of Social Affairs to the Estonian Health Insurance Fund are used to fund ARV medicines for HIV and anti-TB drugs for TB for the insured (and some uninsured) populations.

Analysis of funds flows for HIV prevention and treatment demonstrates the inherent efficiencies in the system. The main risk group with HIV are the injecting drug users, mostly from the Russian Federation minority population concentrated in a few municipalities. The other main group is within the prison population. Hence, one problem immediately apparent is that the HIV control and the drug abuse programmes manage separate pools of money and engage in separate contracting processes with NGOs. Fragmentation of financing between these NIHD programmes creates disincentives to joint planning and especially pooling of resources to increase service effectiveness and efficiency. An alternative approach for the financing arrangements would be to support a "client-oriented" approach, i.e. starting with the objective of reaching the intravenous drug users to both reduce drug abuse and HIV transmission. Combining efforts and funds from the HIV control and drug abuse programmes would lead to a more efficient and effective approach, e.g. blending needle exchange or methadone substitution with the promotion of condom use and other safe-sex health promotion strategies. These strategies would be effective especially if they were combined with TB control programmes (Atun et al. 2005; Atun et al. 2007a).

The objective of a financing system is to create an enabling environment for the right interventions to reach the right clients in the most cost-effective manner possible. However, the existing arrangements in Estonia are designed to "fund programmes" on the assumption that, in turn, these programmes will reach the clients. However, a programmatic as opposed to a client-centric approach to funding leads to poor coordination between the several vertical programmes that have similar objectives and share many of the same clients. An alternative approach where the interventions are considered as personal services and where the focus is on systemic arrangements to best facilitate efficient delivery of services to clients, can more clearly identify options for reforming the financing arrangements to facilitate a "client-oriented" approach. This alternative approach will also help develop a more "horizontal" focus, with increased possibility of integrating these programmes into the primary health care level – if and when the system is ready for such an integration – as clearly, the high-risk population are not readily "captured" in the routine primary care network. Hence, in the early stages of programme development it may be more effective to use pooling of funds across programme lines within the NIHD to develop a joined-up approach that will lead to shared objectives, and "pooling" of the minds and the available expertise to facilitate joint strategy development and implementation for effective HIV, drug abuse, and TB interventions. This single pool of funds will also enable development of a unified contracting strategy that fosters the creation of a comprehensive package of prevention and treatment services, to enable more clients to be reached within a given level of budget.

Broadly, a client-oriented approach might be conceptualized as comprising the following series of steps:

- identify the clients – the high-risk groups that are top priority for the interventions and their health/social care needs (e.g. intravenous drug users, TB/ HIV co-infected individuals, etc.);
- determine the services/interventions they need;
- describe how these clients are currently served by mapping the client groups that are targets of multiple programmes;
- demonstrate how the current services are funded by undertaking a "flow of funds" analysis to demonstrate the extent of financial fragmentation in the system that creates obstacles to "doing the right thing" (i.e. that inhibits or creates disincentives to more efficient joint approaches).
- Consider alternative ways of organizing these services (given the particular context, and taking into account feasibility of organizing services in a particular way) to develop efficient joined-up intervention strategies, shared services and delivery mechanisms to effectively reach target population groups and at-risk individuals.
- Identify options to modify the health financing system (e.g. pooling currently fragmented programme budgets, joint contracting strategies, etc.) to facilitate development of suitable arrangements to deliver a cost-effective mix of prevention and treatment interventions to the defined clients.

The Estonia case illustrates the importance of exploring how financing mechanisms and approaches impact on the organization and delivery of communicable disease services. The financing framework has relevance as an analytical tool beyond the "general" or "typical" personal health services for which it is usually applied and for which it was initially developed. An important dimension of this analysis relates to the sub-function of *pooling*. This term is usually used to refer to *risk pooling*, but in this case, it is more literally the question of how the funds are actually accumulated rather than any notion of using the funds to protect individuals against financial risk. This illustrates that the pooling concept has relevance beyond that of risk pooling, and effective reform requires an understanding of this; reforming how funds are accumulated and flow through the system may be a very important category of actions one can take to improve the financing of communicable disease control.

Use of the financing analysis framework to inform joint planning and budgeting

In Estonia, as in all former Soviet Union countries, interventions against TB are planned and delivered through vertically organized programmes, with specialized hospitals, dispensaries and specialized health workers. These programmes do not interact efficiently with HIV and narcology (substance abuse) programmes. Thus, separation is reinforced by means of the fragmentation of the sources of funding, which encourages maintenance of the status quo. However, even in the presence of such fragmentation it should still be possible to introduce processes, which encourage joint planning and budgeting health services both at macro and micro levels.

For example, at the macro level, the Ministries of Health, Justice and Internal Affairs can work with the municipalities, public service providers and NGOs to jointly assess the existing arrangements for financing, purchasing and provision of services, identify gaps or overlaps and eventually collaboratively plan strategies and budgets to put in place structures for joined-up delivery of preventive and treatment interventions. At the micro level, case management can be used to promote continuity of care across different health and social sector settings, by identifying key health or social workers to provide continuity of care. Table 14.1 provides a summary of the purchasing and the provision of services by each pooling agent in Estonia in 2005.

From this summary it is possible to identify several areas of potential collaboration. For example, joined-up training; use of shared staff to coordinate delivery of services; a single procurement system for pharmaceuticals (first- and second-line treatment for TB and HAART for HIV/AIDS) by pooling or by coordinating different sources of financing; and a unified monitoring and evaluation system, including epidemiological surveillance, by integrating different registries. A joined-up approach could be used for the provision of services, even if these are financed by different sources. In this context, coordination aims to achieve both economies of scope and economies of scale, to improve the efficiency of the system. But, for this to happen, planning and budgeting both at macro and micro levels need to be coherent, so as to ensure that the services are organized around the needs of the patients, with user-centric analysis before planning to identify service gaps and any need for additional resources. Achieving such coherence is one of the main challenges for the health systems.

A key problem, yet to be addressed in Estonia and most post-Soviet states, relates to prisons: congregate settings with high prevalence of TB and HIV. This is a critical stewardship challenge, as in most of these countries the Ministry of Justice is responsible for financing and providing health care within the penitentiary institutions, as a parallel system to the civilian health system. This reinforces fragmentation and hinders development of commonly agreed and shared approaches to case finding, prevention, diagnosis, treatment, monitoring and surveillance. Further, the health professionals employed within the penitentiary systems do not have the same opportunities for continuous training as those working in the civilian system, often earn lower salaries than their civilian counterparts and do not get any opportunity to benefit from economic incentives related to performance. This leads to different levels and quality of care provided to citizens in prisons and in the general population and creates negative externalities, as the prisoners who are released at the end of their sentence would have received suboptimal treatment when in prisons, with interruptions in treatment (leading to drug resistance) and when released they are not readily picked up or followed by the civilian system, creating a high-risk group for transmitting drug-resistant forms of the diseases to the general population. It is highly likely (although there are no studies demonstrating this) that the negative externalities created by the fragmentation and lack of coordination in delivering interventions far exceed the costs of providing additional or

Table 14.1 Purchasing and provision of HIV and tuberculosis services in Estonia, by pooling agent, 2005

Purchasing	Ministry of Justice	Health Insurance Fund	Ministry of Social Affairs			Local gov't Municipalities
			TB & HAART	Public Health Programmes	GFATM*	
Staff	++			+++	++++	+
Training	++		+	+	+++	+
TB register			+			
Drugs		+++	++++		++++	+
DOTs			++++			
Syringes				+	++	
Condoms				+	+	
Other goods and services	++++	++	+	++++	++++	+
Other running costs			+	++	+++	
Investments				+	+	+
Monitoring and Evaluation	+			+	+	+

Provision	Ministry of Justice	Health Insurance Fund	Ministry of Social Affairs			Local gov't Municipalities
			TB & HAART	Public Health Programmes	GFATM*	
VCT				++		
IDU harm reduction				++++	++++	+
Prisons	++++				++	
MSM + CSW					++	
HAART		++++	+++		++++	
TB interventions			+++			
PMTCT activities		++				
Mass media – Youth awareness				++	+++	

Source: Alban and Kutzin 2006.

Notes: The level of financial resources in 2005 reported as follows: + less than € 50 000; ++ € 50 000–100 000; +++ € 100 000–200 000; ++++ more than € 200 000; VCT: voluntary counselling and testing; IDU: injecting drug user; MSM men who have sex with men; CSW: commercial sex workers; HAART: Highly Active Anti-Retroviral Treatment; PMTCT: prevention of mother-to-child transmission; GFATM: Global Fund to Fight AIDS, Tuberculosis and Malaria; DOT: directly observed treatment; TB: tuberculosis; gov't: government; * managed by the National Institute for Health Development.

differently organized services to high-risk populations. From a societal perspective, the welfare gains from a comprehensive approach to managing communicable disease financing and delivery, driven by the Government or the Ministry of Health, would be substantial.

Hence, coordination, financing and delivery of programmes are critical stewardship issues that governments need to act upon. Indeed, to address this issue, the WHO European Regional Office for Europe and WHO are working with counterparts in the three Baltic states to develop joint planning and budgeting processes for TB, HIV/AIDS and substance abuse. Government officials and stakeholders from key institutions are meeting regularly and striving to develop common national policies to effectively tackle these epidemics through collaborative interventions. At the same time, a case management approach to design interventions is developing in Estonia, centred on patient's needs and aimed at providing seamless access to appropriate health and social care. While still in its early stages, a full range of services (including voluntary testing, counselling, methadone substitution, needle exchange, HAART and DOT) have been identified together with the key health workers (family doctors, nurses and social workers) who would coordinate the referral and follow-up process.

Resource allocation and provider payment systems in communicable disease control

We use three cases, from the Russian Federation, Turkey and the Republic of Moldova, to illustrate how resource allocation and provider payment systems impact on the efficiency and effectiveness of communicable disease programmes.

Impact of provider payment systems on tuberculosis control in the Russian Federation

The Russian Federation has one of the lowest case-detection rates for new smear-positive cases and the lowest rates for treatment success for DOTS in the 22 countries identified by WHO as having a high TB burden (WHO 2005). However, despite evidence of cost–effectiveness of the WHO-approved methods in demonstration projects, to date, expansion of these in the Russian Federation has been very limited. TB patients in the Russian Federation continue to undergo unnecessary hospital admissions with long hospital stays (Floyd et al. 2006).

The study uses a proprietary toolkit (SYSRA) developed for concurrent analysis of health systems and communicable disease programmes (Atun et al. 2004). This toolkit comprises two elements: a "horizontal assessment", for analysis of the health system within which the infectious disease programme is embedded from a variety of perspectives; and a "vertical assessment", used to assess the infectious disease-specific component. Specifically, we explore how organizational arrangements, health system financing and provider payment systems in the Russian Federation create incentives and barriers that impact on the delivery of the WHO-approved methods of TB control. Samara *oblast*, which in 2001 committed to introducing WHO-approved methods of TB control, is used as an illustrative case to examine these issues in detail (Coker et al. 2003).

The TB control system in Samara comprises four vertical systems each with its own separate financing stream: (a) the screening services based on X-ray fluorography; (b) the penitentiary TB control system in prisons and pre-trial detention centres; (c) the hospital-based services and; (d) the primary/community health care-based services.

Financing for the TB system comes from federal, *oblast* and municipal budgets, the Health Insurance Fund and user fees for services provided to private patients (Figure 14.2 and Box 14.1).

Resource allocation and budgeting are driven by historic budgets and retrospective data, rather than "true" need. For example, the funds allocated to TB control increased steadily between 1998 and 2000, but in spite of worsening TB, MDR-TB and HIV epidemics declined in 2001 due to a fall in federal contributions.

The normatives and tariffs regulated by Federal Law define Clinical Statistical Groups (CSGs) under which a number of diagnoses of similar complexity, intensity of resource use, and average length of hospital stay are pooled. These normatives are based on the Russian national TB classification system that differs from the WHO or internationally adopted classification systems. CSGs stipulate length of stay and clinical management of TB cases and define a "completed case" for episodes of care and payment levels. The CSGs are refined regionally within federal regulatory boundaries.

Hospital admissions are costed according to the average length of stay and the average daily cost of stay by clinical specialty. Rates are set not according to real costs of the provider institutions but according to set costs based on norms specified by regulations and available regional health care resources.

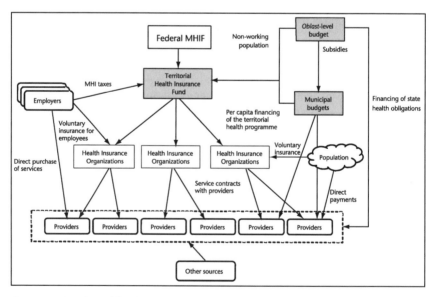

Figure 14.2 Flow of funds in the health system of the Russian Federation's Samara Region

Source: Atun et al. 2005a.

Notes: MHIF: mandatory health insurance fund; MHI: mandatory health insurance.

Box 14.1   Financing of the Tuberculosis Control System in the Samara Region of the Russian Federation

The *oblast* **budget** is composed of two elements, the *oblast*-level budget and the local budgets of the districts and city municipalities under the *oblast* jurisdiction.

Health finance comes from two main sources: a payroll tax levied on the working population under the regulations for the Mandatory Health Insurance Fund (MHIF) and the *oblast* budget. These resources are pooled at the Territorial Health Insurance Fund (THIF).

The *Oblast* **Health Department** is responsible for the organization of health services and implementation of the package of health services specified in the State Guarantees for Health (SGH), which determines the list of diseases (interventions, volume of services, conditions of provision of services) and pharmaceutical benefits financed from the THIF programme. These services are free at the point of delivery. On the basis of the SGH, regions define a free Regional Benefits Package that can be larger than the SGH.

The **Mandatory Health Insurance System** has three components: (a) the Federal Health Insurance Fund; (b) the Territorial branch of the Federal Health Insurance Fund, THIF, and; (c) private insurance companies. The THIF allocates finances to a number of health insurance companies according to a risk-adjusted per capita formula. These insurance companies provide health insurance to the working and non-working population (Figure 14.2).

There are five groups of TB services compensated by the insurance companies: (a) complex outpatient phthisiatry (TB) service provided in the community to patients registered with a TB dispensary; (b) completed cases of hospital inpatient treatment; (c) complicated cases of suspected TB requiring tests as inpatients to establish a diagnosis; (d) certain health services commissioned by the primary health care sector (consultation, examination) and; (e) sanatoria services.

Primary care TB providers receive a risk-adjusted per capita payment for each registered case under "dynamic supervision" according to the estimated resource use for each case grouping. The per capita payment system for ambulatory care providers without the performance-related element creates perverse incentives to retain patients in the system as each patient under "dynamic supervision" attracts payment. This payment system prevents execution of the "gatekeeping function" as the primary care level providers benefit from maximizing the number of patients registered, increasing hospital referrals, and minimizing the scope of services delivered. The study reveals approximately 40 100 patients under dynamic supervision in 2002. Of these, over 80% were clinically cured cases and contacts, and only 12% were new or suspected active pulmonary TB cases.

TB hospitals are paid a fee-for-service for "completed cases", classified according to CSGs which define the complexity of the case, taking into account the clinical guideline used to treat the case and the prescribed length of stay at first admission. Each CSG attracts a different payment rate. This payment-per-case system creates perverse incentives for the providers and encourages "supplier-induced demand" to increase the number of admissions and investigations to attract funding, to "upcode" diagnoses so that they will attract higher pay levels, and to encourage interventions that attract higher daily payments rates, such as surgery, at the expense of other more cost-effective options. Not surprisingly, between 1999 and 2001 approximately 40% of patients were hospitalized more than once and over 7% of all TB-related hospitalization episodes were associated with complex investigations and surgery that attracted higher pay levels: this is a very high proportion compared with international practices.

A further problem with the hospital payment rate is that it is weighted according to the category of the hospital. Provider units with a greater proportion of qualified staff, expensive equipment, larger numbers of beds and more space per bed attract a higher rate per completed case. This in turn encourages retention of staff, large numbers of beds, preservation of a sizeable space per bed, and investment in equipment, but discourages downsizing of the hospital sector to achieve efficiency improvements, as a downsized hospital attracts less payment per case and a service shift to community results in a net loss of revenue. Consequently, attempts at downsizing the number of beds have faltered, while hospital expenditures increased (Atun et al. 2006).

Clearly, the current organizational arrangements, resource allocation and provider payment and financing systems for TB services provide few incentives for improving efficiency or effectiveness of the TB control system. Instead, the system encourages prolonged supervision in dispensaries, multiple admissions and lengthy hospitalizations.

Impact of provider payment systems on human resources for tuberculosis control in Turkey

The health system in Turkey is undergoing major reforms (Atun 2006). The "Transformation in Health Programme", launched in December 2003, aims to reverse the decades of underperformance of the health system and relatively poor health outcomes, by incorporating major principles stated as "human centrism", "sustainability", "continuous quality improvement", "participation", "reconcilement", "volunteerism", "division of power", "decentralization" and "competition in service". Within the "Health Transition Project", financed through a loan from the World Bank, significant changes are planned for the financing and provider payment systems (Ministry of Health of the Republic of Turkey 2003).

As part of these reforms, the health system will be financed through a unified social insurance scheme, with the social insurance premia collected as a payroll tax by the Treasury and then allocated to the General Health Insurance Scheme, established to pool resources from the three current social insurance organizations ("SSK" for employees, "Bag-Kur" for artisans and self-employed and "Emekli

Sandigi" for pensioners). The General Health Insurance Scheme will also receive budget contributions to cover those unable to contribute.

New provider payment systems have been introduced, whereby the primary care level will be paid according to a per capita formula, augmented by performance-related, activity-based fee-for-service (FFS) pay. Hospitals, currently funded through a mix of Ministry of Health budget and activity-based FFS funding from the social insurance organization, will be paid according to diagnosis-related groups (DRGs), which are being developed. The additional activity-based FFS revenues are pooled as a "revolving fund" and used by the providers for profit sharing.

The incidence and prevalence of TB in Turkey began to increase after a 7-year period of decline. In 2003 the incidence was 28 per 100 000 and the prevalence 45 per 100 000. Approximately 2.8% of the new cases comprise MDR-TB cases. DOTS implementation in Turkey began in 2003 in four pilot areas, but in spite of strong political commitment to TB control and relatively favourable organizational arrangements, the official coverage rate, at 3%, is still very low. The treatment success rate in terms of the DOTS pilot sites was 93%.

The NTP is managed by the Department of Tuberculosis Control, which is directly accountable to the Minister of Health. The TB services in Turkey are currently financed directly from the Ministry of Health budget (through direct budgeting), social insurance organizations (through social insurance payments to hospitals providing TB services), NGO funding, and out-of-pocket payments for private services. Detailed and accurate data exist only for the Ministry of Health budget transfers, thus an aggregate figure for total expenditure for TB cannot be calculated. The TB programme budget as a proportion of the Ministry of Health budget has declined from a peak level of 3.5% in 1987 to a level of 1.2% in 2006.

The TB dispensaries and laboratories account for 86–87% of the total expenditure. Of this, approximately 80% is allocated to staff salaries, and 16% to consumables, medical devices and pharmaceuticals. In addition to the Ministry of Health budget allocations, TB dispensaries and laboratories receive a fee-for-service payment from the social insurance organizations for services delivered, used towards the "revolving fund" scheme. The remaining 13–14% of the total expenditure is by the Central Tuberculosis Control Department. Of this, 16% is allocated to staff salaries and 75% to consumables, medical devices and pharmaceuticals.

In the Turkish health system and the TB system within that, the number of health care professionals per patient is low compared to average levels for these in the WHO European Region. The scarce resources are distributed inequitably, with low numbers of staff in poor and rural areas compared with richer regions and cities. The skills within the country's TB staff are also inefficiently distributed, as the number of administrative staff is high in proportion to the number of clinical staff. Despite the willingness of the staff to engage in further training, there is no capacity to undertake these tasks. There is no line item in the Ministry of Health TB control budget for training or for effectively expanding or evaluating the DOTS programme.

The staff employed at the Central Tuberculosis Control Department and the dispensaries are salaried, with a small amount of performance-related pay linked to the fee-for-service revenue generated from the social insurance payments. This contrasts with the large amount of additional payment received by doctors and other staff working in hospitals and, to a lesser extent, in primary care units, which can add up to 10 times their salary – far greater than the amounts received by doctors and staff working in TB dispensaries, which amounts to less than 20% of their salary. There is significant dissatisfaction amongst the TB dispensary staff regarding the inequalities in income levels due to the revolving fund scheme. This has led to staff leaving the TB dispensaries to move to hospital and primary health care institutions that offer higher remuneration. Since 2003, there has been a reduction of approximately 10% in the number of staff in TB dispensaries, including general practitioners, nurses, lab technicians and radiographers. Many dispensaries are also expanding their services to include family medicine and primary health care services, to generate additional funding for their centres and staff. The introduction of the fee-for-service payment and the revolving fund scheme for the general health system has clearly created disincentives for TB organizations and their staff and "crowded out" TB services.

Recognizing that sustainable TB services in Turkey will need modification of the financing and resource allocation system to create appropriate incentives and to generate capacity for effective TB control, the Ministry of Health has recently introduced a new regulation to increase performance-related pay to health care staff working in TB services. However, the TB services remain separate from the rest of the health services and it will be interesting to see whether the attempt to redress imbalances in payment will halt the outflow of staff from the TB services.

Impact of hospital payment systems on tuberculosis services in the Republic of Moldova

The Republic of Moldova is the poorest country in Europe, with an average life expectancy at birth of 64 years for women and 71 years for men (Atun 2005).

In the early 1990s, coinciding with the transition period, the health sector almost collapsed due to very low public funding and correspondingly low provider payments. This led to increasing inequalities, emigration of health professionals, rent-seeking behaviour and informal payments, which created barriers to accessing health services and further exacerbated inequalities.

To address these inequalities the Government has introduced an ambitious health reform programme with decentralization to improve the overall efficiency and equity, launch of the Mandatory Health Insurance to improve pooling of health sector funds, and introduction of a contracting mechanism by establishing a Health Insurance Company to act as the purchaser of health services. A "minimum package" of health services is provided free of charge to the citizens.

In 2004, the Republic of Moldova had the fourth highest incidence (138 per 100 000) and the second highest prevalence (214 per 100 000) of TB amongst the 52 member countries of the WHO European Region. Approximately 15% of the new TB cases are MDR-TB. The NTP was established in 1996 as a response to the sharp increase in TB incidence in the 1990s. The implementation of the DOTS programme began in 2001. The programme has achieved 100% coverage since 2004, with 56% case-detection and 65% treatment success rate.

Health care expenditure as a share of GDP increased from 3% in 1996 to 7.5% in 2004, of which approximately 57% is government expenditure and 43% is private expenditure. There is no separate budget for TB services, but WHO estimated that approximately 14% of government spending on health care would be used for TB services in 2006. A substantial part of the NTP budget comes from external donors, especially from the GFATM.

The Health Insurance Company and directors of the *rayon* (district) hospitals negotiate annual budgets, based on FFS payments approved by the Ministry of Health and the number of inhabitants in a particular *rayon*. The *rayon* hospital director decides on the allocation of these funds to different health services. Secondary health care services are reimbursed according to the volume of services provided (i.e. "per treated case") within a maximum annual budget, while the primary health care services are financed according to a simple capitation formula. It is not possible to calculate the exact amount of TB funds allocated within primary and secondary health care, as TB financing is integrated with the general financing of the health care sector.

Public health care personnel are salaried. In 2004, the average monthly salary was US$ 125 for doctors and approximately US$ 90 for nurses. Although performance indicators and bonus payments were recently introduced in the health system, these are not substantial and the impact on provider behaviour is not yet known. Performance-based incentives were introduced for primary health care providers to implement the DOTS strategy, providing for a 5% salary increase for both the family doctor and his/her nurse for every TB notification and another 5% for proper DOT provision during the continuation phase of treatment. Although the system is encouraging, proper monitoring and feedback systems are not yet in place and the payment levels are determined solely by the assessment of performance of the family doctor and by the TB specialists.

Issues related to financing of hospital tuberculosis services

Between 1998 and 2002, the number of hospitals was reduced from 305 to 65 and the number of beds from 14.4 to 6.5 per 1000 people. Following the restructuring of the hospital system and the introduction of the DOTS programme, the bed occupancy days for TB patients in the Physiopneumonology Institute declined from 349 days in 1997 to 303 in 2003, but increased to 339 in 2004 (Nejdlova 2005).

In 2004, the Health Insurance Company introduced a "maximum length of stay" policy, whereby the Health Insurance Company only pays for the first 47 days of hospitalization for a TB patient. Following the policy change, the average period of hospitalization decreased significantly from 62.4 days in 2002 to 51.1 in 2004. However, these levels are incongruous with the recommended hospitalization levels defined in the local DOTS programme, which stipulates hospitalization of two months for a new TB case and a period of six months for a new MDR-TB case. To ensure consistency with the Health Insurance Company rules, the Physiopneumonology Institute now admits the MDR-TB patients for two months at a time, discontinuing hospital treatment for a few days in between these admissions. Further, for regular TB patients, the difference of 13 days between the 2-month hospitalization period stipulated by the DOT programme and 47 days stipulated by the Health Insurance Company has to be financed from other sources, as these days are not covered by the Health Insurance Company. Expenses for uninsured TB patients are covered from the budget for "social diseases" but those for the insured are not. This creates funding difficulties for the resource-strapped Physiopneumonology Institute. As the Health Insurance Company does not cover expenses for concomitant diseases, these are often financed by out-of-pocket payments. When the TB patient cannot afford to pay these amounts, hospital special funds are used for treatment, which leads to rationing of services, with only the most urgent cases treated.

The Moldovan case, as with the Turkish one, shows how general health system reforms of provider payment systems can have unintended consequences for TB control systems. Clearly, in the case of the Republic of Moldova, the hospital reimbursement criteria need to be re-evaluated to ensure the continuity, sustainability and success of the DOTS programme.

Conclusions

This chapter illustrates the importance of understanding health financing issues as regards communicable disease programmes, which are often run as vertical interventions with limited interaction with the general health system. This separation has inherent risks as we have demonstrated with a number of case studies. Communicable disease control programmes have to be closely integrated into the reform processes in a given country and carefully analysed as to how any financing reform may impact on the financing, design and delivery of the programme. This needs to be done not retrospectively and in a reactive fashion but engaging early on in the debate on the general health system and financing reforms.

In particular, three areas need to be carefully considered. First, the fiscal space available in the country, which determines the magnitude of investment for communicable disease programmes. In turn, this requires identifying priority areas for investment, if the fiscal space is narrow and if the investment available is not adequate to meet the needs. Alternative sources of financing may be considered to expand the fiscal space.

Second, the financial design for these services, in particular the mechanisms for funds pooling and allocation, which, as the Estonia case illustrates, can substantially influence the design, planning, delivery, monitoring and evaluation of communicable disease programmes and the extent to which these functions are executed efficiently and effectively.

Third, the provider payment system – as illustrated by the case studies from the Russian Federation, Turkey and the Republic of Moldova – which can adversely influence provider and human resource behaviour. If the changes in provider payment methods in the general health system are introduced without due consideration for the communicable disease control programmes, there are substantial risks to programme effectiveness due to unintended policy consequences.

Understanding how health systems elements, in particular financing, affect communicable disease programmes is critical to ensuring sustainability, efficiency and effectiveness of these programmes.

References

Alban, A. and Kutzin, J. (2006). *Scaling up treatment and care for HIV/AIDS and TB and accelerating prevention within the health system in the Baltic states (Estonia, Latvia, Lithuania): economic, health financing and health system implications.* Copenhagen: WHO Regional Office for Europe Health Systems Financing Programme.

Atun, R. (2005). *Review of Experience of Family Medicine in Europe and central Asia – Moldova Case Study.* Washington D.C.: World Bank Human Development Sector Unit. World Bank, Europe and central Asia Region, Report No. 32354-ECA.

Atun, R. A. (2006). *WHO Mission to Turkey: Assessment of the Turkish National TB Programme* (2006) – "Review of the National Tuberculosis Programme". Unpublished document.

Atun, R. A., Lennox-Chhugani, N., Drobniewski, F., Samyshkin, Y. and Coker, R. (2004). A framework and toolkit for capturing the communicable disease programmes within health systems: Tuberculosis control as an illustrative example, *European Journal of Public Health*, 14: 267–273.

Atun, R. A., Lebcir, R., Drobniewski, F. and Coker, R. (2005). Impact of an effective multidrug-resistant tuberculosis control programmes in the setting of an immature HIV epidemic: system dynamics simulation model, *International Journal of STD & AIDS*, 16 (8): 560–570.

Atun, R. A., Samyshkin, Y.A., Drobniewski, F., Gusarova G., Skuratova, N. M., Kuznetsov, S. I., Fedorin, I.M., Coker, R.J. (2005a). Barriers to sustainable tuberculosis control in the Russian Federation, *Bulletin of the World Health Organization*, 83 (3): 217–223.

Atun, R. A., Samyshkin, Y., Drobniewski, F., et al. (2006). Costs and outcomes of tuberculosis services in the Russian Federation: retrospective cohort analysis, *Health Policy and Planning*, 21(5): 353–364.

Atun, R. A., Lebcir, R. M., Drobniewski, F., McKee, M. and Coker, R. J. (2007a). High coverage with HAART is required to substantially reduce the number of deaths from tuberculosis: system dynamics simulation in the setting of explosive HIV epidemic and tuberculosis, *International Journal of STD & AIDS*, 18: 267–273.

Atun, R. A., Lebcir, M. R., McKee, M., Habicht, J. and Coker, R. J. (2007b). Impact of joined-up HIV harm-reduction and multidrug-resistant tuberculosis control programmes in Estonia: system dynamics simulation model, *Health Policy*, 81: 207–217.

Coker, R. J., Dimitrova, B., Drobniewski, F., et al. (2003). Tuberculosis control in Samara *Oblast*, Russia: institutional and regulatory environment, *International Journal of Tuberculosis and Lung Disease*, 7(10): 920–932.

Espinal, M. A., Laszlo, A., Simonsen, L., et al. (2001). Global trends in resistance to anti-tuberculosis drugs. World Health Organization International Union against Tuberculosis and Lung Disease Working Group on Anti-Tuberculosis Drug Resistance Surveillance, *New England Journal of Medicine*, 344(17): 1294–1303.

Floyd, K., Hutubessy, R., Samyshkin, Y., et al. (2006). Health systems efficiency in the Russian Federation: tuberculosis control, *Bulletin of the World Health Organization*, 84 (1): 43–51.

Heller, P. S. (2005). *Understanding Fiscal Space*. IMF Policy Discussion Paper. PDP/05/4. Washington D.C.: International Monetary Fund.

High-Level Forum (2005). *Paris Declaration on Aid Effectiveness: Ownership, Harmonization, Alignment, Results and Mutual Accountability*. Paris: High-Level Forum (http://www-1.worldbank.org/harmonization/Paris/FINALPARISDECLARATION.pdf, accessed 27 November 2007).

Kutzin, J. (2001). A descriptive framework for country-level analysis of health care financing arrangements, *Health Policy*, 56(3): 171–204.

Ministry of Health of the Republic of Turkey (2003). *Transformation in Health*. Ankara: Ministry of Health of the Republic of Turkey.

Nejdlova, M. (2005). *Analysis of contextual factors impacting on implementation of DOTS Programme in The Republic of Moldova*, MSc Thesis. London: Imperial College.

Serrano, R. and Feldman, A. (2006). *Welfare economics and social choice theory. 2nd ed.* New York: Springer.

WHO (2000). *World Health Report 2000 – Health systems: improving performance*. Geneva: World Health Organization.

WHO (2005). *Global Tuberculosis Control: surveillance, planning, financing*. Geneva: World Health Organization.

fifteen

Health systems and communicable diseases: predicting and responding to future challenges

Richard Coker, Ana Mensua, Rifat Atun, Martin McKee

Introduction

In December 2003, Donald Rumsfeld, then United States Defence Secretary, won an award from the British Plain English Campaign. The prize was for the most nonsensical remark made by a public figure. Rumsfeld's now famous statement, ridiculed by many others at the time it was made in February 2002, referred to uncertainties in relation to the Iraq war. He said, "As we know, there are known knowns. There are things we know we know. We also know there are known unknowns. That is to say, we know there are some things we do not know. But there are also unknown unknowns, the ones we don't know we don't know" (Rumsfeld 2002).

Yet, whilst perhaps lacking some elegance, Rumsfeld's statement is not, despite what the Plain English Campaign and others might assert, nonsensical. Indeed, scientists, public health experts, and policy-makers would perhaps do well to reflect on his suggestion a little more profoundly regarding uncertainties that permeate practice and policy-making. While science is often seen as a repository of known knowns, increasingly we are becoming aware of gaps in our knowledge, of "known unknowns" – it is these defined unknowns that enable us to develop and test hypotheses and thus scientists, if not policy-makers, should be cognizant of these known unknowns; it is these that drive their search to further knowledge, after all. Yet scientists and policy-makers alike have still to come to terms with the equally unavoidable "unknown unknowns" that necessarily dog any attempt to model reality, anticipate the future unfolding of events, and determine the most resilient, sustainable and effective courses of action influenced as they are by unpredictable forces.

This concluding chapter aims to summarize the critical "knowns" in our evolving and understanding of the complex relations between the wider contextual environment of transitional economies, man and microbial agents, and the challenges faced by health systems. We then attempt to draw out what some of the known unknowns are, what issues should be deserving of greater attention and research such that our understanding may become fuller and more sophisticated. Finally, and necessarily briefly, we speculate on some potential unknown unknowns.

Known knowns; health systems, hosts, agents and the environment

Earlier chapters have drawn attention to our understanding of the complex challenges faced by health systems in the transitional societies of Latin America and eastern European countries. Chapters 2 to 4 addressed contextual factors that influence the relationship between microbe and man, be that changes in ecosystems or the changing socioeconomic conditions witnessed in transitional societies of Latin America and the former Soviet Union. Since mankind existed, and even before, microbes have evolved to take selective advantage of changing conditions. Mankind is, however, unlike other animals, not only susceptible to microbes but also able to modify his environment in ways that are far more profound than any animals. The changes mankind makes to his environment, with the intention of providing benefit to either some or all of mankind result in sometimes unpredictable consequences. Microbes take advantage of this. Antimicrobial resistance, a scourge of the late 20th century and early 21st century is an iatrogenic phenomenon. Though mutations would have arisen in the natural course of events, conferring drug resistance before the use of antimicrobials, because no selective advantage resulted, expansion of such strains did not occur. But with the discovery and widespread use of antimicrobials since the mid-1950s, producing momentous benefits for mankind through reductions in mortality and morbidity, has also resulted in microbes that are now practically untreatable.

Antimicrobial resistance, it is argued, is an almost perfect lens through which to examine the impact of health systems on the man, microbe and environment. The prevalence of MDR-TB (or the likely prevalence of resistant strains of HIV) in many countries of the former Soviet Union bears witness to this. The public health challenges of transitional economies highlight two issues that compound one another. Such economies can play host to the emergence of sociobehavioural shifts that result themselves in increased mortality and morbidity. The explosive outbreaks of HIV amongst injecting drug users in the former Soviet Union reflect one consequence of such seismic social change. Likewise, a second example is illustrative. A criminal justice system that incarcerates its nation's poor and most vulnerable in such huge numbers and under such circumstances, as is the case in the Russian Federation and its neighbours, promotes communicable disease transmission and then discharges them into the wider community where transmission of disease continues. So transitional economies help generate the challenges that arise from communicable disease. Yet they also, afflicted as they are by health systems that are often rooted in the past, struggle to respond flexibly and effectively to new public health threats including communicable diseases (such as HIV), or changed communicable diseases (such as drug-resistant TB).

In this book, the terms "transitional societies" and "transitional economies" have been used synonymously and to encompass countries undergoing significant changes to their political, economic and social institutions. Traditionally the term has been used to describe countries of the former Soviet Union, which are moving from centrally planned to market economies. We also include countries of Latin America because many have pursued fundamental political and economic reform programmes in recent decades. In Chapter two, McKee and Falkingham outline what we understand by transitional economies and characterize them. In the former Soviet Union, "countries experienced a seismic transition in the years after 1989, as communist regimes fell like dominoes". The results varied. In some countries, democracy flourished. In others, one authoritarian regime was replaced by another. Some transitional periods were peaceful, others violent. Yet across the board, profound social and economic change resulted. For Latin America, though there was no seismic shock such as the collapse of communism to auger in a new transitional phase, transition has nevertheless happened, albeit in a more piecemeal fashion. The oil crises of the 1970s, followed by economic depression through the 1980s and further economic crises in the 1990s have resulted, as in the former Soviet Union, in a period of marked socioeconomic change. And microorganisms, not surprisingly, have taken advantage of these changing circumstances, as Chapters 5 and 6 testify.

In recent decades the pattern of communicable diseases in the European region has been characterized by contrasting patterns. For vaccine-preventable diseases such as pertussis and measles, where health systems are failing – for a variety of reasons – to provide herd immunity, outbreaks have been witnessed and incidence is climbing. These failures in health systems are not unique to transitional economies but illustrate fault lines readily because their transmission dynamics are acutely sensitive to falls in immunization rates below relatively high population coverage thresholds.

Communicable diseases that have been a particular concern in transitional economies include TB and HIV. Although some countries, notably the United Kingdom and Sweden, have reported increases in TB in recent years, the rate of rise has been slow, and reflects several factors outside the health system, such as migration. In eastern Europe and former Soviet Union countries the high prevalence of MDR-TB testifies to the profound failings of the health systems. Whilst the climbing incidence of TB has been driven by wider social ills, drug resistance has resulted from fractured health systems that mean treatment has been erratic, incompatible with international standards, and based not on evidence but on clinicians' judgements alone.

The spread of HIV through the former Soviet Union, though currently a relatively immature epidemic, portends grave consequences. As individuals currently infected grow older, their immune function will deteriorate, and the maturing HIV epidemic will, as other regions in the world have discovered, impact on other communicable diseases, most worryingly TB. The collision of these two epidemics means some countries in the former Soviet Union will be challenged profoundly. Health systems dedicated to specific diseases are already highly vertical. These systems risk becoming silos where the two complex diseases of TB and HIV are concerned. Individuals suffering from both diseases will fall in the gaps between these silos.

Patterns of communicable diseases in LAC are more mixed. Population growth, urbanization, climate change and development, and widening inequalities have influenced the epidemiology of many diseases. Tropical diseases such as dengue, yellow fever and malaria have, broadly, remained constant, and cholera has largely been controlled. Control of HIV and TB is more patchy. Only three countries' health systems, Cuba, Barbados and Brazil, can be said to be effectively managing their HIV epidemics. In other countries, the HIV pandemic continues to expand remorselessly.

Given these communicable diseases challenges, how should states, including transitional states, respond? What should they do, if anything? What, as Lee and Owen ask in Chapter 3, is the "appropriate role of government"? They argue cogently that a major challenge "facing all societies today is defining and agreeing what essential functions governments must provide to best protect and promote health." In stating that the management of shared risk resulting from communicable diseases means that government has an obligation to act, this chapter then defines what functions should be incumbent upon government – these are known knowns.

The authors develop a notion of "resilience" whereby, in an ideal world, governments have "the ability at every level of the system to detect, prevent, control and recover from disruptive challenges." Yet the functions of transitional economies have been hampered for a variety of reasons. Governments may be unable or unwilling to perform the necessary functions. This may be because of a lack of capacity, a lack of political will, insufficient financial resources or inefficient use of resources, or administrative and managerial frailties. The picture that emerges from the transitional societies examined in this book is multifaceted. Government functions have failed for a variety of often interconnected reasons. For example, the Russian Federation's failure to respond to its HIV epidemic is the result of a delayed political commitment, a reluctance to address the needs of societies marginalized and excluded, a failure of health systems to respond flexibly and draw on other countries' experience and lessons learned elsewhere in a timely manner, and a ponderous reform process that remains centrally controlled and draws on local innovative policies and practices only unwillingly.

Known unknowns: predicting future challenges

In the early chapters of this book, several contributors explored the epidemiological consequences of health system failures for communicable disease control, the causes of these failures and the wider contextual milieu within which health systems operate. If health systems are to operate effectively, efficiently, equitably and respond in a timely manner to anticipated and unanticipated challenges then lessons need to be learned that inform reform processes. These lessons should tell us not only *whether* a health system delivers results, but also *why* and through *what* mechanisms. As Atun and Menabde make clear in Chapter 7, unfortunately, with the exception of a small number of studies, our understanding of interaction between health systems and communicable disease programmes remains limited (Atun et al. 2004; Atun et al. 2005a; Atun et al. 2005b). Whilst the research community has often been able to discern whether an intervention "works", through, for example, randomized controlled studies or observational epidemiological studies, traditional approaches depend upon controlling potentially confounding variables. This requires the adoption of approaches to evaluation that capture the dynamic interplay of individual, institutional, processual and structural relations within a complex wider environment, to inform policy implementation. Understanding this complexity is a testing challenge. Part of the challenge results from the fundamental epistemological and ontological tensions that exist between researchers of different disciplines. Yet, a more nuanced framework to evaluate health systems and communicable disease control is needed, one that draws effectively and coherently on qualitative and quantitative research methods, from experimental, sociological, epidemiological, management and political science fields (Coker, Atun and McKee 2004). Through a more sophisticated approach to evaluating whether, how and why health systems impact on communicable diseases we can start to identify and define known unknowns, that is, to determine what the critical issues are that we need to understand more fully if health system reforms are to be more effective.

Atun and Menabde explore approaches and frameworks used for health system analysis and describe a novel framework developed for analysis of health systems that draws on systems thinking. Their choice of this discipline for analysis is posited on the notion that it is critical to understand the relationships between institutions, actors and events over time if patterns are to be identified and organizational dynamics to be understood in terms of their impact on programmes through health systems. Such an approach, the authors argue, should facilitate the anticipation of events (rather than just enable reactions) such that systems can prepare for emerging challenges.

If we can anticipate future challenges, we can start to determine where our knowledge gaps are in responding to those, and thus define our known unknowns.

Preparing for the future: anticipating unknown unknowns

Anthony McMichael, in Chapter 4, reminds us that mankind has always been and always will be challenged by novel and unpredictable microbial challenges. The interactions between man and his environment and the forces of development and globalization mean that not only are novel diseases likely to emerge ever more frequently but that the geographic spread of these diseases, if transmitted between humans, also occurs ever more rapidly. Whilst the 1918 pandemic of human influenza took months to become global, SARS in 2003 took advantage of the aviation industry to become an intercontinental outbreak within weeks. The next influenza pandemic may take a matter of only days to become global. The world is now more interconnected than ever. This means that not only do we all face the consequences of known communicable disease challenges (TB, measles, HIV, pertussis, etc.), we also face together anticipated but as yet non-existent challenges (pandemic influenza). Yet we will also be challenged by as yet unknown threats. Who foresaw how changes in food processing would threaten the beef industry in the United Kingdom posed by the emergence of BSE, or its consequences for human health in the form of vCJD? Who anticipated in the 1970s the emergence, a decade later, of a global STI that would leave millions suffering and dying and that would challenge the scientific, political and public health communities for decades? Who predicted the emergence of a novel coronavirus in China (SARS) that would act as a dry-run and wake-up call to the international community of the threat of far greater magnitude of pandemic influenza?

Whilst we cannot hope to anticipate unknown unknowns, by their very nature, we can hope to build health systems that respond effectively and flexibly to threats of different types, whether they are sexually transmitted viruses, airborne microbes, or novel agents that have arisen from our highly industrialized food manufacturing processes. Health systems have responded effectively to novel challenges. The response to SARS is a case in point. The future may not be entirely unpredictable (though its exact form is). To respond effectively, health systems need to have generic capacity, be flexible and above all be alert. Or, as Donald Rumsfeld stated, again rather inelegantly "I would not say that the future is necessarily less predictable than the past. I think the past was not predictable when it started."!

References

Atun, R. A., Lennox-Chhugani, N., Drobniewski, F., Samyshkin, Y. and Coker, R. (2004). A framework and toolkit for capturing the communicable disease programmes within health systems: Tuberculosis control as an illustrative example, *European Journal of Public Health*, 14: 267–273.

Atun, R. A., McKee, M., Drobniewski, F. and Coker, R. (2005a). Analysis of how health system context influences HIV control: case studies from the Russian Federation, *Bulletin of the World Health Organization*, 83(10): 730–738.

Atun, R. A., Samyshkin, Y., Drobniewski, F., et al. (2005b). Health system barriers to sustainable tuberculosis control in the Russian Federation, *Bulletin of the World Health Organization*, 83: 217–223.

Coker, R. J., Atun, R. A. and McKee, M. (2004). Untangling Gordian knots: improving tuberculosis control through the development of programme theories. *International Journal of Health Planning and Management*, 19: 217–226.

Rumsfeld, D. (2002). *Department of Defence Press Briefing, 12 Feb*, Washington DC: Department of Defence.

Index

MENTAL HEALTH POLICY AND PRACTICE ACROSS EUROPE

Martin Knapp, David McDaid, Elias Mossialos and Graham Thornicroft

We are proud to announce that this book is joint winner of the EHMA Baxter Award 2007.

> A genuinely fantastic resource; such a rare text that provides such factual information for students and lecturers. A rich review of the subject areas from across Europe. Fantastic text. *Chris Kelly, Programme Leader, Bournemouth University*

This book maps the current state of policy, service provision and funding for mental health care across Europe, taking into account the differing historical contexts that have shaped both the development and delivery of services. A holistic approach is adopted that aims to assess the influence on mental health of environmental factors such as housing, poverty, employment, social justice and displacement.

Covering a wide range of policy issues, the book:

- Examines the legal rights of people with mental health problems
- Addresses the impact of stigma, social exclusion and discrimination
- Reviews the role of users and their families in the development of mental health services and policy
- Reflects on approaches to reform and on the future development of services
- Evaluates opportunities for the rehabilitation of people with mental health problems
- Discusses the financing and organisation of mental health systems
- Reflects on approaches to reform and the future development of services

Mental Health Policy and Practice Across Europe is key reading for policy makers, professionals involved in the delivery of health and social care services, voluntary agencies, non-governmental organizations, academics and students of health policy.

Contents

Series editors' introduction – Foreword 1 – Foreword 2 – Acknowledgments – Mental health policy and practice across Europe: An overview – The historical development of mental health services in Europe – Inequalities, social exclusion and mental health – Financing and funding mental health care services – The evidence base in mental health policy and practice – A policy framework for the promotion of mental health and the prevention of mental disorders – Common mental health problems in primary care: Policy goals and the evidence-base – Reforms in community care: The balance between hospital and community-based mental health care – Developments in the treatment of mental disorders – Psycho-pharmaceuticals in Europe – Mental health policy in former eastern bloc countries – Addiction and substance abuse – Housing and employment – Developing mental health policy: A human rights perspective – The user and survivor – Movement in Europe – Carers and families of people with mental health disorders – The mental health care of asylum seekers and refugees – Global perspective on mental health policy and service development issues.

2006 488pp
978–0–335–21467–9 (Paperback)   978–0–335–21468–6 (Hardback)

PRIMARY CARE IN THE DRIVER'S SEAT
ORGANIZATIONAL REFORM IN EUROPEAN PRIMARY CARE

Richard Saltman, Ana Rico and Wienke Boerma (eds)

- What is the best way to structure primary care services?
- How can coordination between primary care and other parts of health care systems be improved?
- How should new technologies be integrated into primary care?

There is considerable agreement among national policy makers across Europe that, in principle, primary care should be the linchpin of a well-designed health care system. This agreement, however, does not carry over into the organizational mechanisms best suited to pursuing or achieving this common objective. Across western, central and eastern Europe, primary care is delivered through a wide range of institutional, financial, professional and clinical configurations. This book is a study of the reforms of primary care in Europe as well as their impacts on the broader co-ordination mechanisms within European health care systems. It also provides suggestions for effective strategies for future improvement in health care system reform.

Primary Care in the Driver's Seat is key reading for students studying health policy, health economics, public policy and management, as well as health managers and policy makers.

Contributors
Richard Baker; Sven-Eric Bergman; Wienke Boerma; Mats Brommels; Michael Calnan; Diana Delnoij; Anna Dixon; Carl-Ardy Dubois; Joan Gené Badia; Bernhard Gibis; Stefan Greß; Peter Groenewegen; Jan Heyrman; Jack Hutten; Michael Kidd; Mårten Kvist; Miranda Laurant; Margus Lember; Martin Marshall; Alison McCallum; Toomas Palu; Ana Rico; Ray Robinson; Valentin Rusovich; Richard B. Saltman; Anthony Scott; Rod Sheaff; Igor Svab; Bonnie Sibbald; Hrvoje Tiljak; Andrija Štampar; Michel Wensing.

Contents

2005 280pp
0 335 21365 0 (EAN: 9 780335 213658) Paperback
0 335 21366 9 (EAN: 9 780335 213665) Hardback

HUMAN RESOURCES FOR HEALTH IN EUROPE
Carl-Ardy Dubois, Martin McKee, and Ellen Nolte

Health service human resources are key determinants of health service performance. The human resource is the largest and most expensive input into healthcare, yet it can be the most challenging to develop. This book examines some of the major challenges facing health care professions in Europe and the potential responses to these challenges.

The book analyses how the current regulatory processes and practices related to key aspects of the management of the health professions may facilitate or inhibit the development of effective responses to future challenges facing health care systems in Europe. The authors document how health care systems in Europe are confronting existing challenges in relation to the health workforce and identify the strategies that are likely to be most effective in optimizing the management of health professionals in the future.

Human Resources for Health in Europe is key reading for health policy-makers and post-graduates taking courses in health services management, health policy and health economics. It is also of interest to human resource professionals.

Contributors
Carl Afford, Rita Baeten, James Buchan, Anna Dixon, Carl-Ardy Dubois, Sigrún Gunnarsdóttir, Yves Jorens, Elizabeth Kachur, Karl Krajic, Suszy Lessof, Ann Mahon, Alan Maynard, Martin McKee, Ellen Nolte, Anne Marie Rafferty, Charles Shaw, Bonnie Sibbald, Ruth Young.

Contents

2005 288pp
0 335 21855 5 (Paperback)   0 335 21856 3 (Hardback)

PURCHASING TO IMPROVE HEALTH SYSTEMS PERFORMANCE

Edited by Josep Figueras, Ray Robinson and Elke Jakubowski

Purchasing is championed as key to improving health systems performance. However, despite the central role the purchasing function plays in many health system reforms, there is very little evidence about its development or its real impact on societal objectives. This book addresses this gap and provides:

- A comprehensive account of the theory and practice of purchasing for health services across Europe
- An up-to-date analysis of the evidence on different approaches to purchasing
- Support for policy-makers and practitioners as they formulate purchasing strategies so that they can increase effectiveness and improve performance in their own national context
- An assessment of the intersecting roles of citizens, the government and the providers

Written by leading health policy analysts, this book is essential reading for health policy makers, planners and managers as well as researchers and students in the field of health studies.

Contributors
Toni Ashton, Philip Berman, Michael Borowitz, Helmut Brand, Reinhard Busse, Andrea Donatini, Martin Dlouhy, Antonio Duran, Tamás Evetovits, André P. van den Exter, Josep Figueras, Nick Freemantle, Julian Forder, Péter Gaál, Chris Ham, Brian Hardy, Petr Hava, David Hunter, Danguole Jankauskiene, Maris Jesse, Ninel Kadyrova, Joe Kutzin, John Langenbrunner, Donald W. Light, Hans Maarse, Nicholas Mays, Martin McKee, Eva Orosz, John Øvretveit, Dominique Polton, Alexander S. Preker, Thomas A. Rathwell, Sabine Richard, Ray Robinson, Andrei Rys, Constantino Sakellarides, Sergey Shishkin, Peter C. Smith, Markus Schneider, Francesco Taroni, Marcial Velasco-Garrido, Miriam Wiley.

Contents
*List of tables – List of boxes – List of figures – List of contributors – Series Editors' introduction – Foreword – Acknowledgements – **Part One** – Introduction – Organization of purchasing in Europe – Purchasing to improve health systems – **Part Two** – Theories of purchasing – Role of markets and competition – Purchasers as the public's agent – Purchasing to promote population health – Steering the purchaser: Stewardship and government – Purchasers, providers and contracts – Purchasing for quality of care – Purchasing and paying providers – Responding to purchasing: Provider perspectives – Index.*

2005 320pp
0 335 21367 7 (Paperback)   0 335 21368 5 (Hardback)

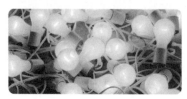
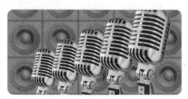
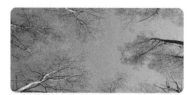
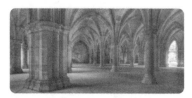
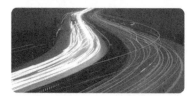
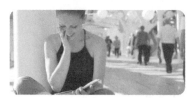
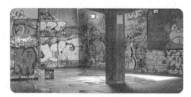